MW01674808

Case Studies in Implant Dentistry

Case Studies in Implant Dentistry

Editor: Drew James

AMERICAN
MEDICAL PUBLISHERS
www.americanmedicalpublishers.com

AMERICAN
MEDICAL PUBLISHERS
www.americanmedicalpublishers.com

Cataloging-in-Publication Data

Case studies in implant dentistry / edited by Drew James.
p. cm.
Includes bibliographical references and index.
ISBN 979-8-88740-605-3
1 Dental implants. 2 Mouth--Surgery- 3. Implants, Artificial 4. Dentures.
5. Dentistry I. James, Drew.
RK667.I45 E95 2023
617.693--dc23

© American Medical Publishers, 2023

American Medical Publishers,
41 Flatbush Avenue,
1st Floor, New York,
NY 11217, USA

ISBN 979-8-88740-605-3 (Hardback)

This book contains information obtained from authentic and highly regarded sources. Copyright for all individual chapters remain with the respective authors as indicated. All chapters are published with permission under the Creative Commons Attribution License or equivalent. A wide variety of references are listed. Permission and sources are indicated; for detailed attributions, please refer to the permissions page and list of contributors. Reasonable efforts have been made to publish reliable data and information, but the authors, editors and publisher cannot assume any responsibility for the validity of all materials or the consequences of their use.

Trademark Notice: Registered trademark of products or corporate names are used only for explanation and identification without intent to infringe.

Contents

Preface

The world is advancing at a fast pace like never before. Therefore, the need is to keep up with the latest developments. This book was an idea that came to fruition when the specialists in the area realized the need to coordinate together and document essential themes in the subject. That's when I was requested to be the editor. Editing this book has been an honour as it brings together diverse authors researching on different streams of the field. The book collates essential materials contributed by veterans in the area which can be utilized by students and researchers alike.

Implant dentistry is a branch of dentistry that uses dental implants to restore missing teeth. Dental implants refer to artificial tooth roots made of biocompatible materials that are surgically placed into the jawbone to provide a strong foundation for replacement teeth or dental prostheses. This field combines principles from various fields such as oral surgery, prosthodontics, and implantology. The process of implant dentistry involves several stages. The first stage is an evaluation to study the patient's oral health and suitability for dental implants. Following, the surgical stage takes place where the implant is placed into the jawbone through a surgical procedure. The implant then integrates with the surrounding bone through a process called osseointegration. After the osseointegration period, the restorative phase of implant dentistry begins. This involves the placement of an abutment, which connects the implant to the replacement tooth or dental prosthesis. This book unravels the recent studies on implant dentistry. It will serve as a valuable source of reference for graduate and postgraduate students.

Each chapter is a sole-standing publication that reflects each author´s interpretation. Thus, the book displays a multi-facetted picture of our current understanding of application, resources and aspects of the field. I would like to thank the contributors of this book and my family for their endless support.

Editor

1

Analysis of Digital Workflow in Implantology

Gustavo Vargas da Silva Salomão,[1] **Eliseo Pablo Chun**,[2] **Renato dos Santos Panegaci**,[2] **and Fernando Toledo Santos**[2]

[1]*Department of Oral Rehabilitation, School of Dentistry, Ibirapuera University (Unib), Av. Interlagos, 1329, Chácara Flora, São Paulo, SP 04661-100, Brazil*
[2]*Department of Prosthodontics, School of Dentistry, Ibirapuera University (Unib), Av. Interlagos, 1329, Chácara Flora, São Paulo, SP 04661-100, Brazil*

Correspondence should be addressed to Gustavo Vargas da Silva Salomão; gvs.salomao@usp.br

Academic Editor: Sukumaran Anil

Digital workflow is increasingly accessible in daily dental practice. It has several benefits in implantology, such as the possibility of precise planning, which results in faster and safer surgery and, consequently, reduced prosthetic complications. There are also disadvantages that must be taken into consideration for successful treatment, such as deviations between the planned and placed implant position and intraoral scanning inaccuracies. We report a clinical case in implantology in which digital workflow was used throughout the process, pointing out its facilities and complications in the daily practice of dental surgeons. The patient had grade II mobility and external root resorption of tooth 11. After virtual planning, a surgical guide was fabricated by a CAD/CAM system, with immediate placement of a dental implant using the guided surgery technique. At the end of the osseointegration period, intraoral scanning was performed for fabrication of the final prosthesis also by a CAD/CAM system. After placement, the patient approved the aesthetic and functional results of the implant. We observed advantages such as simplification of clinical steps and safety of the proposed planning, but there were also disadvantages such as the complexity of digital tools, deviations of the placed implant, and inaccuracy in color selection. It was concluded that digital workflow is a reality that can be integrated into daily dental practice, resulting in greater safety, predictability of results, and ease of use in all clinical stages. However, it should be noted that there are still inaccuracies in digital tools and that a steep learning curve is needed in this area, which, if neglected, may lead to unsatisfactory results.

1. Introduction

Digital workflow in dentistry has increased rapidly in recent years due to advances in technologies such as software and intraoral scanners [1, 2]. This evolution resulted in benefits such as predictability of treatment, simplification of clinical steps, and quick and easy communication between professionals [3, 4]. The possibilities of treatment involving digital workflow have also evolved with new materials and techniques. The fabrication of laboratory works by a computer-aided design (CAD) and computer-assisted manufacturing (CAM) system associated with several digital tools has allowed a range of options for the proposed work [5].

In implantology, digital workflow has several advantages, such as precise planning and simplified surgical approach, which result in a faster and more predictable surgery [6]. At the prosthesis manufacturing stage, it is possible to reproduce the implant position virtually by intraoral scanning [7], thus avoiding distortions generated by conventional impression materials, promoting greater patient comfort, and eliminating the need for plaster dental casts [8, 9].

Digital techniques also have disadvantages, such as deviations between the planned and placed implant position [10] and inaccuracies of the intraoral scanning technique [11, 12]. These factors are extremely important for clinical treatment because, if they are not taken into account during planning, undesirable results may occur, such as invasion of the space of noble areas and misfit of prosthetic components.

Although apparently easy to perform, digital workflow requires extensive experience of the operator, as it can produce unsatisfactory results if not performed accurately and appropriately [13, 14]. Digital treatment options do not obviate the need for theoretical knowledge. Therefore, the clinician needs to have both a conceptual understanding of the procedures to be performed and the ability to use digital tools to achieve the expected success [13].

The present clinical case report has the novel purpose of demonstrating all clinical stages of digital workflow in implantology, pointing out its facilities and complications in the daily practice of dental surgeons.

2. Case Presentation

This case was reported according to the Case REport (CARE) statement and checklist [15], and written informed consent was obtained from the patient to publication of this case report.

A 29-year-old female patient, nonsmoker, who reported not consuming alcoholic beverages, not taking any long-term medication, and having no clinically relevant family history information, complained of pain on touching the maxillary left central incisor (tooth 11). Her dental history included injury to the tooth in question due to a fall from standing height during childhood, and the tooth began to be dislodged over the years. In a specialized dental care clinic, she received endodontic treatment that did not achieve the expected success.

Clinical examination showed grade II mobility of tooth 11. Radiographic examination revealed the presence of external root resorption that resulted in extensive resorption of the buccal wall in the area (Figures 1 and 2).

After evaluating the case, extraction of tooth 11 was proposed to the patient, followed by immediate placement of a dental implant associated with guided bone regeneration, because her gingival biotype was classified as thick [16], and the remaining bone tissue allowed immediate implant placement [17]. The management option of choice was a fully digital treatment, from surgical planning to fabrication of the final crown, for the current analysis of digital workflow in dentistry.

A computed tomography (CT) scan of the complete maxilla was obtained in Digital Imaging and Communications in Medicine (DICOM) format, and intraoral scanning was performed using the Trios 3® pod scanner (3shape) to obtain stereolithography (STL) files.

Once these 2 files had been obtained, the coDiagnostiX® software (Dental Wings) was used for virtual planning. After DICOM and STL images were superimposed, surgical planning was performed by placing the implant in the optimal position for future prosthetic rehabilitation (Figure 3). Once the implant had been virtually planned, a software for manipulation of 3D objects (Meshmixer®) was used to remove tooth 11 from the original STL file in order to fabricate a tooth-supported surgical guide. This new STL file was imported, and the process of guide fabrication was started by using the "Add surgical guide" tool in coDiagnostiX®. The final virtually designed guide (Figure 4) was then printed with a Rapid Shape®-Straumann 3D printer.

At the time of surgery, before the sterile drapes were applied, intraoral antisepsis was performed by mouth rinses with 5 mL of 0.12% aqueous chlorhexidine, and extraoral

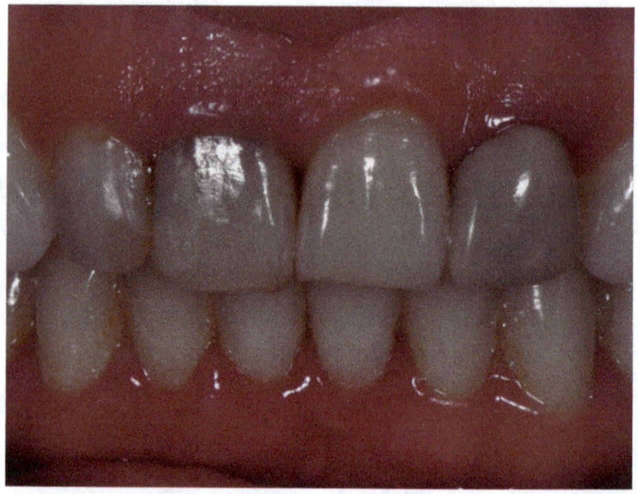

FIGURE 1: Initial clinical image of the case.

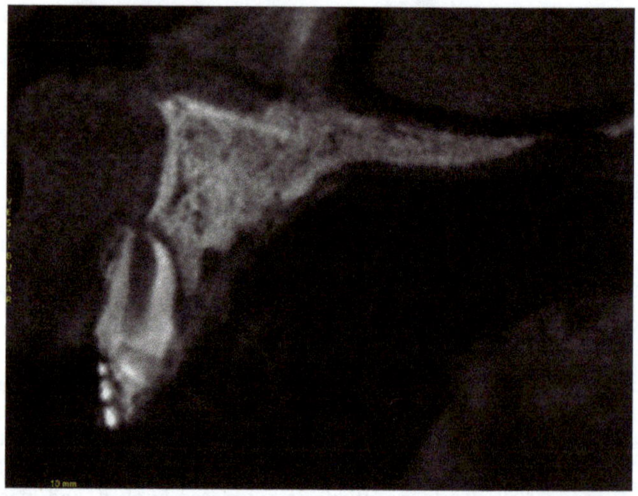

FIGURE 2: CT scan of tooth 11 area, where it is possible to note external root resorption and extensive resorption of the buccal wall.

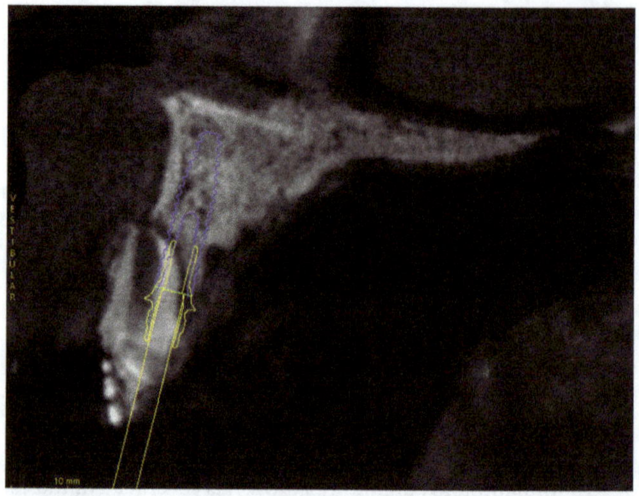

FIGURE 3: Virtual implant placement in the optimal position for future prosthetic rehabilitation.

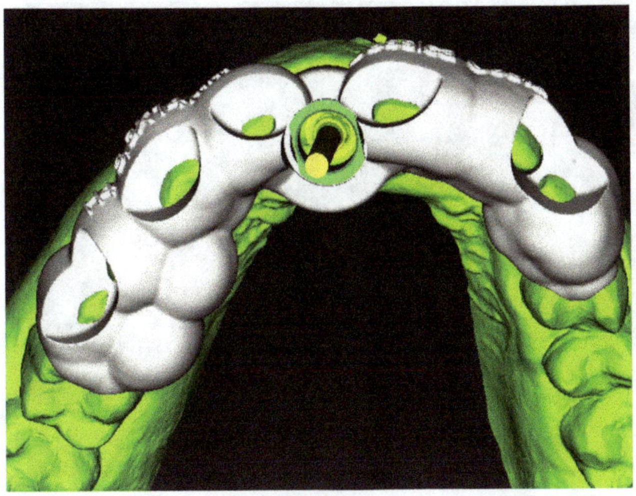

Figure 4: Image of the surgical guide virtually designed using virtual planning software.

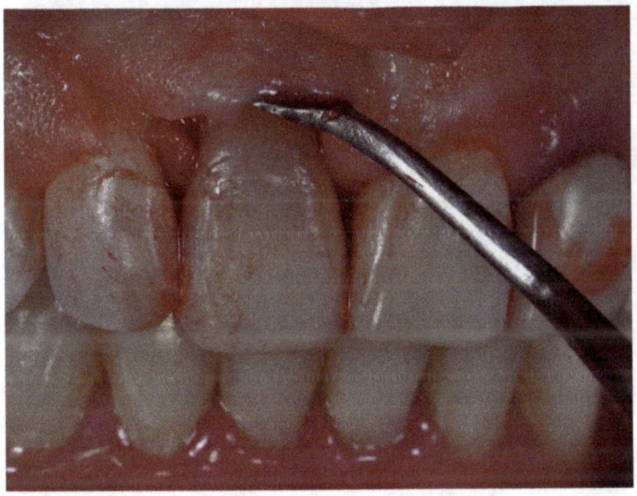

Figure 5: Incision made prior to extraction. Note that the papillae were preserved.

antisepsis was performed with 2% aqueous chlorhexidine. Anesthesia was obtained with 4% articaine with 1 : 100,000 epinephrine (4% Articaine DFL®). Initially, a buccal incision was made 2 mm above the mesial papillae (from tooth 21 to 12), in order to have them preserved, followed by a divergent relaxing incision in the mesial side of tooth 12 extending to the mucogingival line [18] (Figure 5). The flap was then elevated, and tooth 11 was extracted using a minimally invasive approach with periotomes (Quinelato). After extraction, the surgical guide was placed in position to assess proper fitting through the inspection windows. After this stage, the implant bed was prepared with drills from the Straumann ® Guided Surgery–BLT system, as described in the protocol printed by the planning software (Figure 6(a)). Subsequently, a 3.3 × 14 mm Straumann SLActive® Bone Level Tapered Roxolid implant (NC) was placed, reaching a maximum torque of 45 Ncm (Figures 6(b) and 6(c)). Its respective tap was then inserted. Particulate bone substitute (Geistlich Bio-oss®) was placed on the exposed threads, as planned virtually, for the purpose of guided bone regeneration [19, 20] (Figure 6(d)). Once bone grafting had been completed, the flap was repositioned and secured with simple interrupted sutures (4-0 silk suture, Ethicon) for healing by first intention. Postoperative care included administration of antibiotics (amoxicillin 500 mg, every 8 hours for 7 days), anti-inflammatory drugs (dexamethasone 4 mg, every 12 hours for 2 days), and analgesics (acetaminophen 750 mg, every 6 hours for 3 days in case of pain).

The crown of tooth 11 was prepared and temporarily bonded with light-cured resin (Tetric N-Ceram®-Ivoclar Vivadent) to the adjacent teeth (teeth 21 and 12) until the time of implant uncovering.

After 45 days, the implant was uncovered. The surgical guide was again positioned in the mouth, and using a 3.4 mm diameter mucosa punch (Straumann Guided Surgery®–BLT), the gingival tissue was removed, and the tap was exposed. A temporary abutment for NC–BLT implant (Straumann) was then placed, while the provisional crown was captured in the mouth (artificial teeth–Trilux–Euro-VIPI). After polishing and finishing, the temporary abutment was tightened with manual torque (Figure 7).

The patient was scheduled to return in 4 weeks for evaluation of the peri-implant tissue. At this visit, minor adjustments were also made to the crown to improve the gingival contour. The patient was then scheduled to return in 6 months for fabrication of the final prosthesis. At this return visit, the provisional crown was removed, and a scanbody (NC Straumann) was placed. After checking the scanbody for proper position, another intraoral scanning was performed (Trios 3® pod–3shape) for fabrication of the final prosthesis. During scanning, the patient's tooth shade was determined by using the scanner's shade measurement tool (Figure 8) and the VITA Classical shade guide. Subsequently, both the STL files and the visually selected shades were sent to the laboratory for fabrication of the final prosthesis.

Given the precision of the digital workflow, the final abutment (3.8 mm diameter, 5.5 mm height, 1 mm gingival height; NC–Variobase®), preselected during virtual planning, was sent to the laboratory, which was requested to send us the final crown, thus obviating the need for an appointment for metal framework try-in. A specific CAD dental software (Dental System–3shape®) was used to design the crown, which was subsequently milled with the Ceramill® Motion 2 milling machine (Amann Girrbach) (CAM system). On delivery, minor adjustments were made to the prosthesis to eliminate occlusal interference. After polishing and patient's approval of aesthetics and function, the crown was placed on the implant with a torque of 35 Ncm.

The coDiagnostiX® "treatment evaluation" tool was used to assess how much the implant deviated from the preoperatively planned position. The STL image produced by intraoral scanning through the scanbody was superimposed onto the software planned implant position, thus generating the deviations (Figure 9).

The patient returned for treatment evaluation 3 months after crown delivery, when she reported satisfaction with the aesthetic and functional results of the final crown (Figure 10), without any complications since its placement.

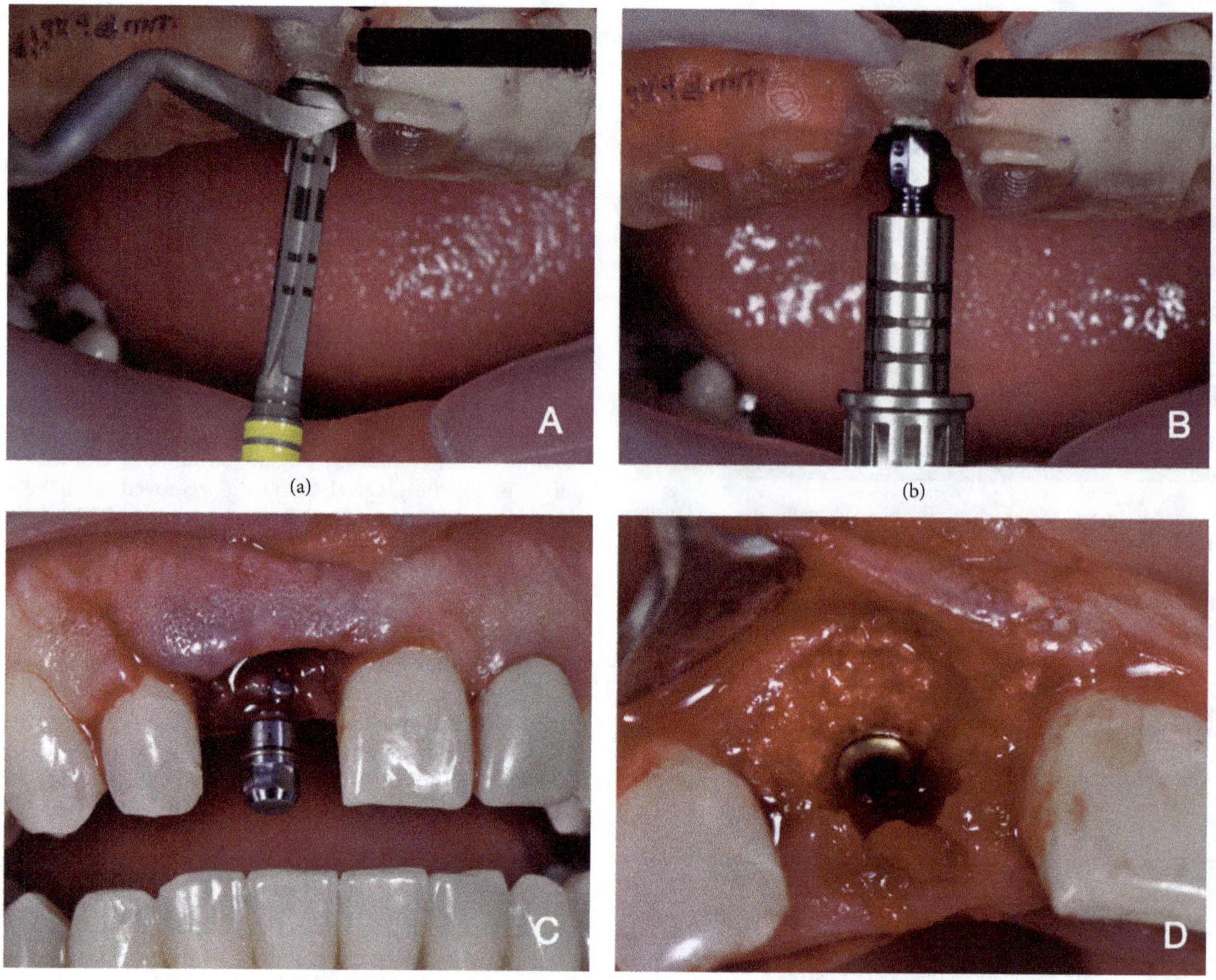

(a) (b) (c) (d)

Figure 6: Presentation of the guided implant placement surgery: (a) implant bed preparation; (b) fully guided implant placement; (c) checking the implant for proper final position in relation to the adjacent teeth; (d) guided bone regeneration after implant placement.

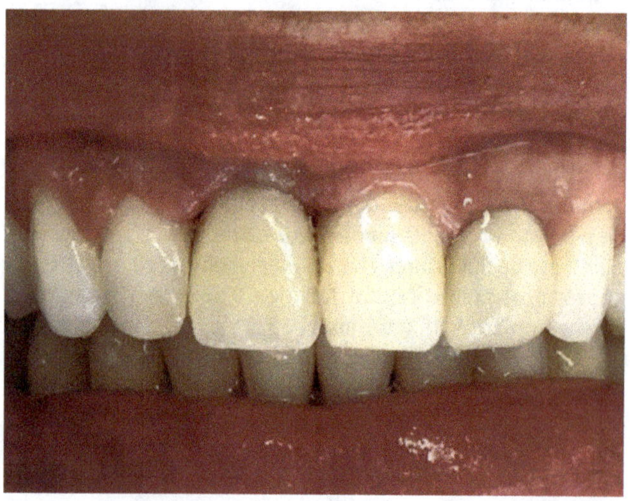

Figure 7: Placement of the temporary abutment on the implant, after implant uncovering.

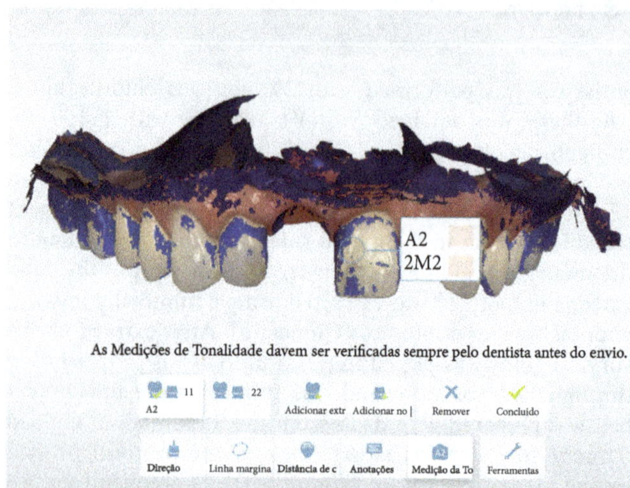

Figure 8: Selection of the final crown shade using the intraoral scanner.

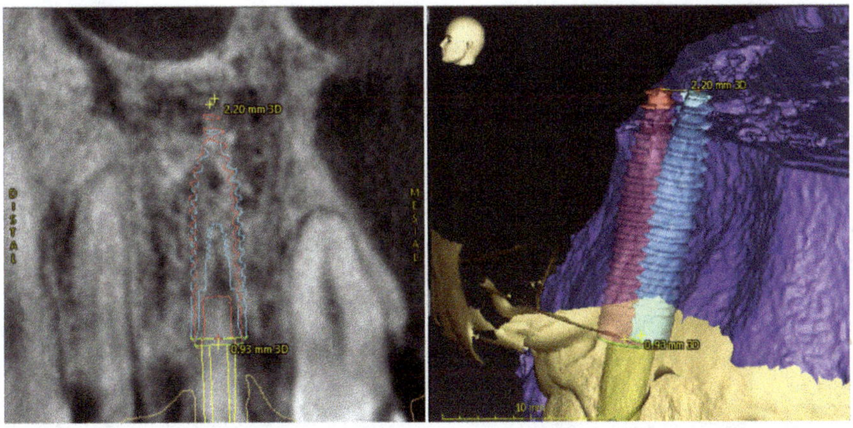

FIGURE 9: Deviations observed in superimposed images of the placed and planned implant position in the tangential and axial views, respectively.

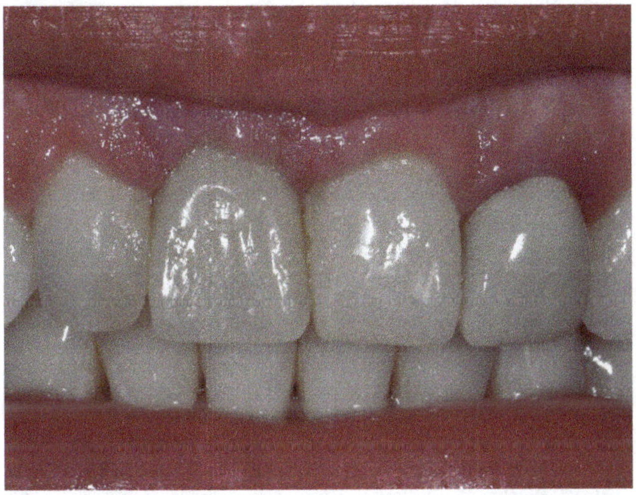

FIGURE 10: Aesthetic result 3 months after final crown placement.

3. Discussion

Digital workflow is constantly and rapidly evolving in implant dentistry, resulting in increasingly more accurate works and, consequently, reducing the number of analog steps in the clinician's daily practice [21, 22]. Despite the simplicity of the various stages of treatment, digital workflow requires a steep learning curve as well as an understanding of the complications that may occur, such as deviations in implant position and intraoral scanning inaccuracies [13, 14].

Experience in digital treatment begins with planning. Software programs used in implantology for virtual planning require some steps that are essential for clinical success, including segmentation, deletion of artifacts, superimposition of images (DICOM/STL), and virtual implant placement [13]. Another important factor is the type of printer with which the virtual surgical guide is to be printed. The accuracy of surgical guides has been shown to be strongly associated with both the printing device and printing method [23]. Therefore, it is clear that there are many subtle points at the stages of planning and manufacturing the guide, in which the sum of errors may lead to disastrous results [13, 24].

Regarding the surgical procedure, guided implant surgery is generally faster than conventional freehand surgery and results in greater comfort for the patient in the postoperative period [25, 26]. Similar findings were observed in the present case report, in which guided surgery was performed without any complications, and the patient reported no pain or discomfort in the postoperative appointment. Although a guided surgery is mostly indicated in cases of flapless surgical implant placement [27], in our case, we opted for a guided surgery technique due to the limitations of the case. In bordering regions, such as the one reported here, there is a high risk of failure both in the surgical procedure, due to the extensive bone defect, and in aesthetic terms, due to possible gingival recession. In these cases, guided implant surgery is a favorable alternative to achieve the necessary precision for implant placement [4].

The precision of the guided surgery technique has already been demonstrated in the literature [28]; however, there are deviations that must be taken into consideration when developing virtual planning [13, 29]. In the current case report, we observed a deviation of 0.93 mm at the entry point, 2.2 mm at the apex of the implant, and an angular deviation of 5.5°, results different from those reported in a systematic review by Tahmaseb et al. [29], who observed a mean of 1.3 mm at the entry point, 1.2 mm at the apex of the implant, and 3.3° of angular deviation (Table 1). Although the deviation at the entry point in this case report was less than the average reported in the literature [29], apical and angular deviations were greater. These data alert us to the care needed in virtual planning, in the preparation of the surgical guide and in its printing, since there was no surgical complication. This can be considered a confounding factor in our study because, due to the several thorough steps of digital workflow prior to the surgical procedure, we were unable to understand what might have caused the observed deviations.

Another important stage in digital workflow is prosthesis fabrication. In the present case, we opted for intraoral scanning to digitize the implant. Advantages included greater comfort for the patient and the possibility of clearly assessing

Table 1: Comparison between the deviations presented in the current case report and the mean deviations in partially edentulous patients reported in a systematic review by Tahmaseb et al. [29].

Deviations	Entry point (measured in mm)	Apex (measured in mm)	Angular deviation (measured in degrees)
Current case report	0.93 mm	2.2 mm	5.5°
Tahmaseb et al. [29]	1.3 mm	1.2 mm	3.3°

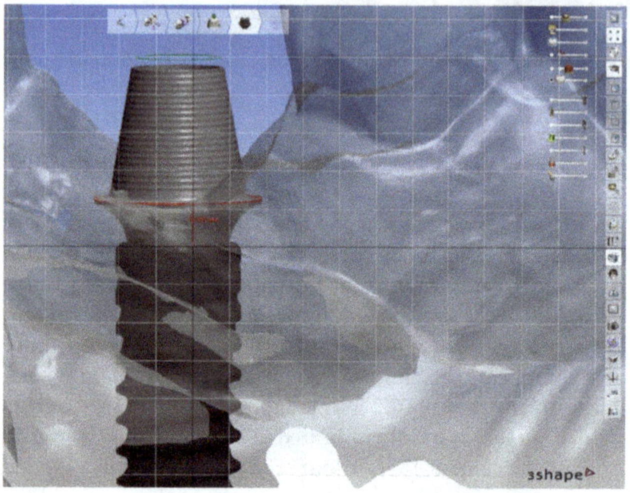

Figure 11: Evaluation of the abutment selected prior to the surgical procedure, demonstrating the accuracy of the technique.

the details of the scanned object, which allowed us to rescan any part that was not clear [14]. Obtaining a digital model also brings many benefits, such as not occupying any physical space and posing no risk of fracture. A great efficiency of the digital model, which we noticed in our case, was the ease of sending it to more experienced peers to exchange information about planning [30]. Evaluation of the final abutment in the virtual model (Figure 11) showed that our selection of abutment prior to surgical planning was accurate, leading us to believe that the observed deviations were not detrimental to the success of the final rehabilitation.

Given the precision of intraoral scanning [31], we decided to request the laboratory to send us the final crown, thus obviating the need for metal framework try-in. To this end, the final crown shade was selected using the intraoral scanner, and observed differences were compared to the VITA Classical shade guide. These results are compatible with those reported in the literature suggesting not to use intraoral scanning as the first option for color selection [32]. In our case, we sent the results of the two selections made (digitally and manually) to the laboratory for greater precision in the fabrication of the prosthesis. At the time of implant placement, only minor adjustments were needed, which indicates that digital workflow can simplify the clinical steps [21]. These data support the patient's positive assessment of treatment outcome. The patient reported that the procedures were not painful, especially the surgical procedure, for which she had great expectation of success. Also, she was comfortable in the postoperative period, and the prosthetic appointments were rapid and objective, meeting the patient's aesthetic and functional expectations.

4. Conclusion

Digital workflow is a reality in dentistry and can be integrated into daily dental practice. The clinical case reported here enabled us to demonstrate that virtual planning is safe, leading to faster clinical procedures with simplification of clinical steps as well as to a more predictable final result. It is important to note that there are still inaccuracies in digital tools, which must always be taken into consideration. We highlight that there is a learning curve for using these techniques, in which the sum of errors throughout the process may result in treatment failure.

Consent

Written informed consent was obtained from the patient to publication of the case report and images.

References

[1] R. Richert, A. Goujat, L. Venet et al., "Intraoral scanner technologies: a review to make a successful impression," *Journal of Healthcare Engineering*, vol. 2017, Article ID 8427595, 9 pages, 2017.

[2] W. Renne, M. Ludlow, J. Fryml et al., "Evaluation of the accuracy of 7 digital scanners: an in vitro analysis based on 3-dimensional comparisons," *The Journal of Prosthetic Dentistry*, vol. 118, no. 1, pp. 36–42, 2017.

[3] G. Cervino, L. Fiorillo, A. V. Arzukanyan, G. Spagnuolo, and M. Cicciù, "Dental restorative digital workflow: digital smile design from aesthetic to function," *Dentistry Journal*, vol. 7, no. 2, p. 30, 2019.

[4] P. S. Wöhrle, "Predictably replacing maxillary incisors with implants using 3-D planning and guided implant surgery," *The Compendium of Continuing Education in Dentistry*, vol. 35, no. 10, pp. 758–762, 2014.

[5] T. Miyazaki and Y. Hotta, "CAD/CAM systems available for the fabrication of crown and bridge restorations," *Australian Dental Journal*, vol. 56, pp. 97–106, 2011.

[6] A. Azari and S. Nikzad, "Flapless implant surgery: review of the literature and report of 2 cases with computer-guided surgical approach," *Journal of Oral and Maxillofacial Surgery*, vol. 66, no. 5, pp. 1015–1021, 2008.

[7] W. J. van der Meer, F. S. Andriessen, D. Wismeijer, and Y. Ren, "Application of intra-oral dental scanners in the digital workflow of implantology," *PLoS One*, vol. 7, no. 8, article e43312, 2012.

[8] E. Yuzbasioglu, H. Kurt, R. Turunc, and H. Bilir, "Comparison of digital and conventional impression techniques: evaluation of patients' perception, treatment comfort, effectiveness and clinical outcomes," *BMC Oral Health*, vol. 14, p. 10, 2014.

[9] G. J. Christensen, "Impressions are changing: deciding on conventional, digital or digital plus in-office milling," *The Journal of the American Dental Association*, vol. 140, no. 10, pp. 1301–1304, 2009.

[10] G. S. Unsal, I. Turkyilmaz, and S. Lakhia, "Advantages and limitations of implant surgery with CAD/CAM surgical guides: a literature review," *Journal of Clinical and Experimental Dentistry*, vol. 12, no. 4, pp. e409–e417, 2020.

[11] J. Winkler and N. Gkantidis, "Trueness and precision of intraoral scanners in the maxillary dental arch: an in vivo analysis," *Scientific Reports*, vol. 10, no. 1, article 1172, 2020.

[12] M. Imburgia, S. Logozzo, U. Hauschild, G. Veronesi, C. Mangano, and F. G. Mangano, "Accuracy of four intraoral scanners in oral implantology: a comparative in vitro study," *BMC Oral Health*, vol. 17, no. 1, article 92, 2017.

[13] D. N. Tatakis, H. H. Chien, and A. O. Parashis, "Guided implant surgery risks and their prevention," *Periodontology 2000*, vol. 81, no. 1, pp. 194–208, 2019.

[14] H. Kihara, W. Hatakeyama, F. Komine et al., "Accuracy and practicality of intraoral scanner in dentistry: a literature review," *Journal of Prosthodontic Research*, vol. 64, no. 2, pp. 109–113, 2020.

[15] J. J. Gagnier, G. Kienle, D. G. Altman, D. Moher, H. Sox, and D. Riley, "The CARE guidelines: consensus-based clinical case reporting guideline development," *Global Advances in Health and Medicine*, vol. 2, no. 5, pp. 38–43, 2013.

[16] T. De Rouck, R. Eghbali, K. Collys, H. De Bruyn, and J. Cosyn, "The gingival biotype revisited: transparency of the periodontal probe through the gingival margin as a method to discriminate thin from thick gingiva," *Journal of Clinical Periodontology*, vol. 36, no. 5, pp. 428–433, 2009.

[17] C. Hu, T. Gong, W. Lin, Q. Yuan, and Y. Man, "Immediate implant placement into posterior sockets with or without buccal bone dehiscence defects: a retrospective cohort study," *Journal of Dentistry*, vol. 65, pp. 95–100, 2017.

[18] S. Aslan, N. Buduneli, and P. Cortellini, "Entire papilla preservation technique: a novel surgical approach for regenerative treatment of deep and wide intrabony defects," *The International Journal of Periodontics & Restorative Dentistry*, vol. 37, no. 2, pp. 227–233, 2017.

[19] R. E. Jung, A. Ioannidis, C. H. F. Hämmerle, and D. S. Thoma, "Alveolar ridge preservation in the esthetic zone," *Periodontology 2000*, vol. 77, no. 1, pp. 165–175, 2018.

[20] S. T. Chen, I. B. Darby, and E. C. Reynolds, "A prospective clinical study of non-submerged immediate implants: clinical outcomes and esthetic results," *Clinical Oral Implants Research*, vol. 18, no. 5, pp. 552–562, 2007.

[21] D. J. Fasbinder, "Digital dentistry: innovation for restorative treatment," *Compendium of Continuing Education in Dentistry*, vol. 31, 2010Spec No 4:2-11.

[22] C. Monaco, L. Scheda, L. Ciocca, and G. Zucchelli, "The prototype concept in a full digital implant workflow," *Journal of the American Dental Association*, vol. 149, no. 10, pp. 918–923, 2018.

[23] B. Sommacal, M. Savic, A. Filippi, S. Kühl, and F. M. Thieringer, "Evaluation of two 3D printers for guided implant surgery," *The International Journal of Oral & Maxillofacial Implants*, vol. 33, no. 4, pp. 743–746, 2018.

[24] M. Vercruyssen, R. Jacobs, N. Van Assche, and D. van Steenberghe, "The use of CT scan based planning for oral rehabilitation by means of implants and its transfer to the surgical field: a critical review on accuracy," *Journal of Oral Rehabilitation*, vol. 35, no. 6, pp. 454–474, 2008.

[25] C. H. Hämmerle, P. Stone, R. E. Jung, T. Kapos, and N. Brodala, "Consensus statements and recommended clinical procedures regarding computer-assisted implant dentistry," *The International Journal of Oral & Maxillofacial Implants*, vol. 24, pp. 126–131, 2009.

[26] S. Y. Youk, J. H. Lee, J. M. Park et al., "A survey of the satisfaction of patients who have undergone implant surgery with and without employing a computer-guided implant surgical template," *The Journal of Advanced Prosthodontics*, vol. 6, no. 5, pp. 395–405, 2014.

[27] N. Van Assche, D. van Steenberghe, M. Quirynen, and R. Jacobs, "Accuracy assessment of computer-assisted flapless implant placement in partial edentulism," *Journal of Clinical Periodontology*, vol. 37, no. 4, pp. 398–403, 2010.

[28] F. Younes, J. Cosyn, T. De Bruyckere, R. Cleymaet, E. Bouckaert, and A. Eghbali, "A randomized controlled study on the accuracy of free-handed, pilot-drill guided and fully guided implant surgery in partially edentulous patients," *Journal of Clinical Periodontology*, vol. 45, no. 6, pp. 721–732, 2018.

[29] A. Tahmaseb, V. Wu, D. Wismeijer, W. Coucke, and C. Evans, "The accuracy of static computer-aided implant surgery: a systematic review and meta-analysis," *Clinical Oral Implants Research*, vol. 29, no. S16, pp. 416–435, 2018.

[30] P. S. Fleming, V. Marinho, and A. Johal, "Orthodontic measurements on digital study models compared with plaster models: a systematic review," *Orthodontics & Craniofacial Research*, vol. 14, no. 1, pp. 1–16, 2011.

[31] M. Tallarico, E. Xhanari, Y. J. Kim et al., "Accuracy of computer-assisted template-based implant placement using conventional impression and scan model or intraoral digital impression: a randomised controlled trial with 1 year of follow-up," *International Journal of Oral Implantology*, vol. 12, no. 2, pp. 197–206, 2019.

[32] H. I. Yoon, J. W. Bae, J. M. Park, Y. S. Chun, M. A. Kim, and M. Kim, "A study on possibility of clinical application for color measurements of shade guides using an intraoral digital scanner," *Journal of Prosthodontics*, vol. 27, no. 7, pp. 670–675, 2018.

2

Rehabilitation of Maxillary Defect using Zygomatic Implant Retained Obturator

Mounika Ayinala and Gautam Shetty

Department of Prosthodontics, Rajarajeswari Dental College and Hospital, Bengaluru, Karnataka, India

Correspondence should be addressed to Mounika Ayinala; mounika.a13@gmail.com

Academic Editor: Konstantinos Michalakis

Tumors involving the hard palate, maxillary sinus, or nasal cavity require maxillectomy based on the extent of the lesion. Lack of these boundaries affects the speech, esthetics, and masticatory function. Prosthetic rehabilitation of these defects can be done utilizing zygomatic implants. This present case describes the use of a zygomatic implant to retain a maxillary obturator in a 22-year-old male patient following partial maxillectomy (Brown's Class 2b) due to odontogenic myxoma. A surgical obturator was secured in position subsequent to the implant placement. Following the healing period, an interim obturator using heat cure acrylic was fabricated. Mechanical retention for the definitive obturator was obtained through the ball attachment suspended from the multiunit abutment of the zygomatic implant. The case was followed up closely for a year to evaluate the function of the prosthesis. The prosthetic rehabilitation not only promoted esthetics and function but also improved the patient's quality of life.

1. Introduction

A challenging endeavor for prosthodontists is rehabilitating patients with maxillectomy/atrophic maxilla as it is a complex area. Carcinomas involving the hard palate, maxillary sinus, and nasal cavity will require maxillectomy, causing dysfunction of the stomatognathic system and thus affecting the patients' quality of life [1]. Tumors such as odontogenic myxoma are uncommon and have the potential for destruction of the jaws. They arise from the dental papilla, dental follicle, or periodontal ligament and occur during the second/third decade of life. These tumors are painless, slow-growing, and invasive with the expansion of bony cortices, causing asymmetry of the face [2, 3]. Management of these carcinomas is through a surgical approach which ranges from enucleation with curettage, segmental resection to hemimaxillectomy depending on the size, and extent of the lesion. They cannot be managed through radiotherapy and chemotherapy as they are not radiosensitive [4, 5].

A custom-made dental prosthesis such as an obturator plays an important role to promote function and esthetics and helps in maintaining the oro-nasal separation. Obtaining retention and stability depends on the extent of the defect, the remaining number of natural teeth, the amount of residual bone, and the patients' ability to adapt to the prosthesis [6]. Usually, because of limited bone support and large defects, the function of an obturator is compromised. But, with the advent of osseointegrated implants, better retention and support can be derived for the implant-retained obturator with less discomfort, complications, and time [7]. Apart from endosseous implants, zygomatic implants have gained popularity over recent years. Branemark introduced it in 1998 for its use in the atrophic maxilla, tumor resection defects, and congenital defects. Later, in the year 2001, Branemark and his team published the first paper on the survival of zygomatic implants placed to obtain prosthetic anchorage in patients with maxillary defects [8]. The 12-year cumulative survival rate of these implants is 95.2% and can be used in rehabilitation after tumor resection/trauma/atrophic maxilla without hard and soft tissue augmentations [9].

This clinical report describes the successful management of a patient with maxillary odontogenic myxoma who underwent partial maxillary resection followed by prosthesis using a zygomatic implant.

2. Case Report

A 22-year-old male patient was referred to Rajarajeswari Dental College and Hospital with a complaint of swelling in the left maxillary posterior region. On extraoral examination, no gross facial asymmetry was noticed. Intraorally, there was no pain/mobility of the teeth. The swelling extended from 23 to 26 region as shown in Figure 1. Radiographic and histopathological examinations confirmed the diagnosis, i.e., odontogenic myxoma involving the left maxilla. A partial left-sided maxillectomy was planned, and the patient was referred to the department of prosthodontics for the fabrication of a surgical obturator. A preoperative impression was made using irreversible hydrocolloid, and the casts were poured using dental stone. The area of resection was delineated by the surgeon and accordingly, the cast was scrapped to fabricate a surgical obturator.

Through the intraoral approach, partial maxillectomy was carried out by preserving the frontal wall of the maxillary antrum, zygoma, and the floor of the orbit. The anterior cut was undertaken through the left lateral incisor and limiting the posterior cut up to the 1st molar as seen in Figure 2. The histopathological report revealed that the tissue was excised with good margins and did not require any adjunctive therapy. A 42.5 mm zygomatic implant (NobelZygoma, Nobel BioCare, United States) as seen in Figure 3 was placed in the left zygomatic bone with maximum stability, ensuring the retention of the obturator through proper positioning of the prosthetic head beneath the body of the prosthesis. The buccal and palatal flaps were saved and sutured before the placement of a surgical obturator which was screwed in with the help of a multiunit abutment and a prosthetic screw. The surgical obturator was cleaned every now and then until an interim obturator was fabricated.

After 4 weeks of the healing period, the patient was recalled for the fabrication of an interim obturator. There was no evidence of infection with good healing of the soft tissues around the abutment as seen in Figure 4. A removable interim obturator was fabricated conventionally using heat cure acrylic resin by making the preliminary impressions. Jaw relation and teeth arrangement were done by relieving the abutment area. The interim obturator was fabricated using compression molding technique, and retention was obtained by placing retainers on the central incisor, molar, and premolars of the contralateral arch.

Five months following the surgery, a fixed-removable prosthesis was planned by utilizing precision attachments. The diagnostic casts were mounted on a semiadjustable articulator following a face bow transfer, and the amount of space available for the attachment was evaluated using a putty index. As the available space was more than required

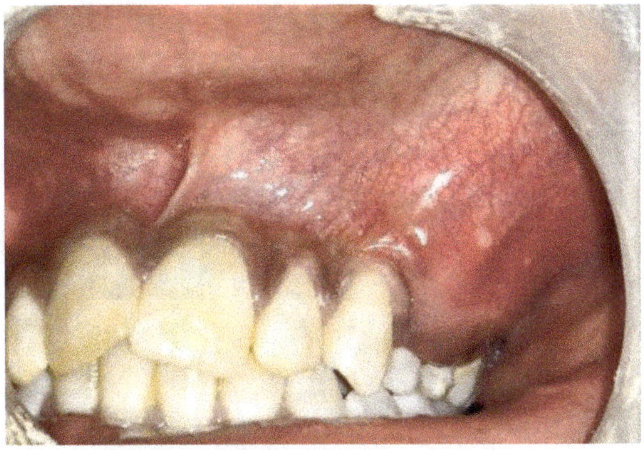

FIGURE 1: Intraoral view of the lesion.

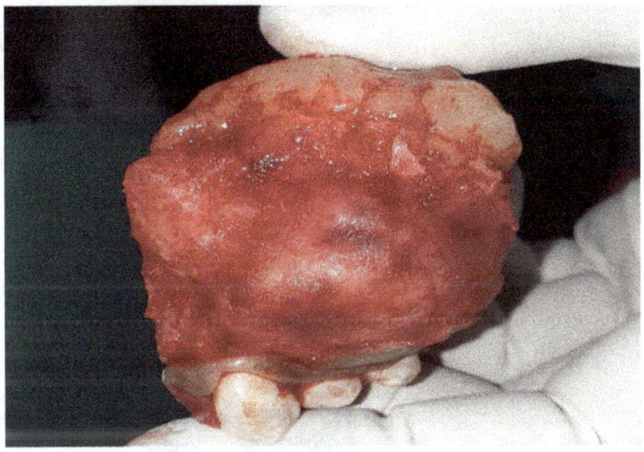

FIGURE 2: Excised tissues.

(15 mm), a ball and socket attachment system was planned with a cast partial denture. Occlusal rest seats were prepared on 15 and 16 to receive an embrasure clasp, and the guide planes were prepared on 21 and 27, respectively. Following mouth preparation, a custom tray was fabricated to make an abutment level impression using heavy and light body consistency of polyvinyl siloxane impression material as seen in Figure 5. The accuracy of the definitive cast was verified using a jig trail. Two microballs of 2.5 mm diameter (Rhein 83, NY) were casted and secured using a prosthetic screw on the multiunit abutment, and the fit was confirmed using an IOPA as seen in Figure 6. The definitive cast with ball attachment was scanned using an optical scanner, converted to .STL (Standard Tessellation Language) format for computer-aided designing of cast partial denture as seen in Figure 7. A selective laser melting of cobalt-chromium was employed for the fabrication of the denture, and the trail fit was verified. Following jaw relation, the esthetics and speech were verified with the trail denture in place. Chairside pickup of the final denture was done to incorporate the metal housings with nylon caps for retention. The patient was educated about oral hygiene and how to handle the prosthesis. The clinical outcome included improvement of esthetics; function and the sense of confidence and

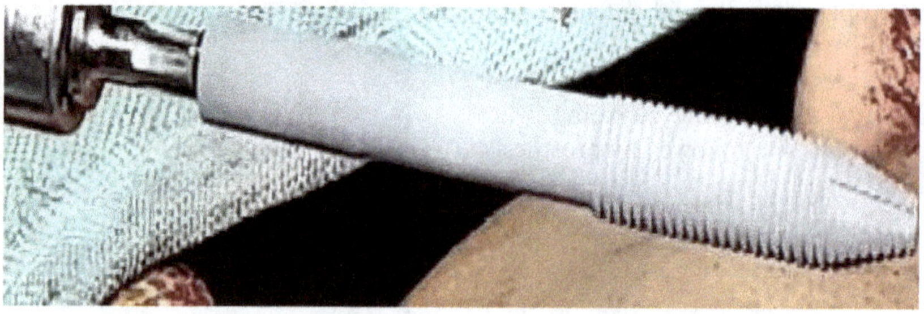

Figure 3: Zygomatic implant.

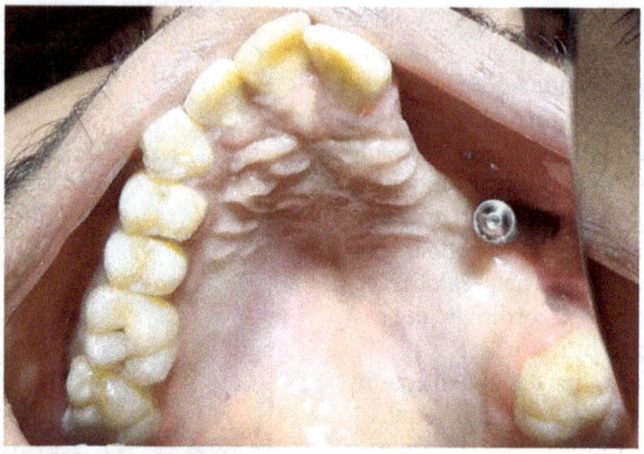

Figure 4: Intraoral view after 5 weeks of healing period.

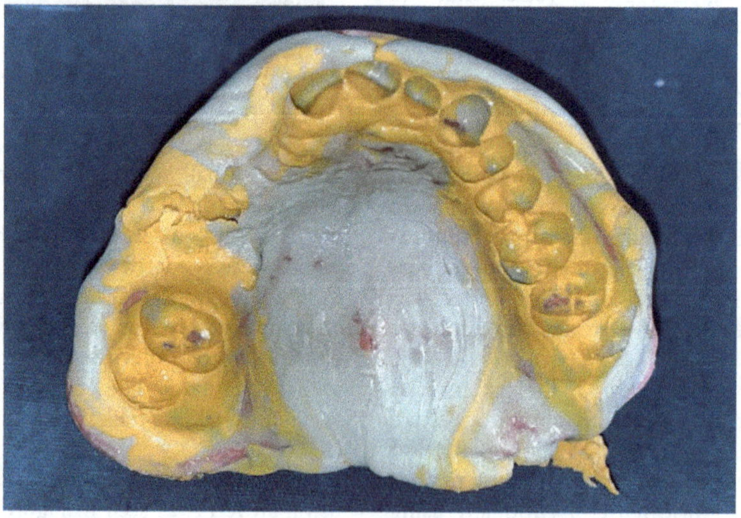

Figure 5: Definitive impression following mouth preparation.

security were restored in the patient as seen in Figure 8. A twelve-month follow-up did not show any evidence of infection, and the patient was asked to return for check-ups at 6-month interval.

3. Discussion

Various procedures such as obturators, local flaps, and microvascular flaps have been advocated to reconstruct the maxilla following the surgical resection [10–13]. Microvascular reconstruction poses certain clinical risks as there could be donor site morbidity, failure of flap or fibrous union, etc. [14]. Also, the retention and stability factors of the conventional obturators are compromised in extensive maxillary defects. The supporting bone plays an important role in the success of a prosthesis, and hence, it is easier to restore subjects with partial/hemi maxillectomy compared to total maxillectomy.

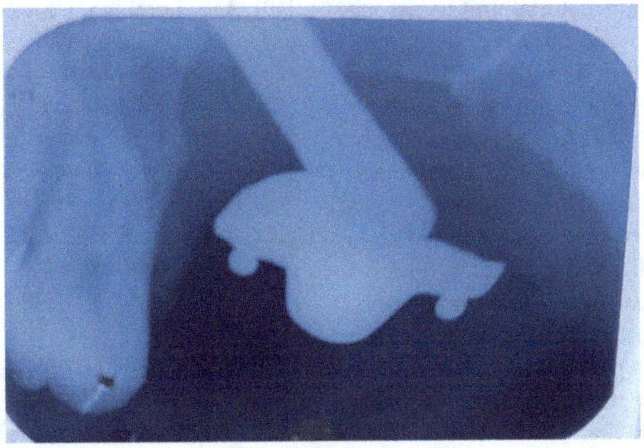

FIGURE 6: IOPA of O-ball attachment secured with prosthetic screw over multiunit abutment.

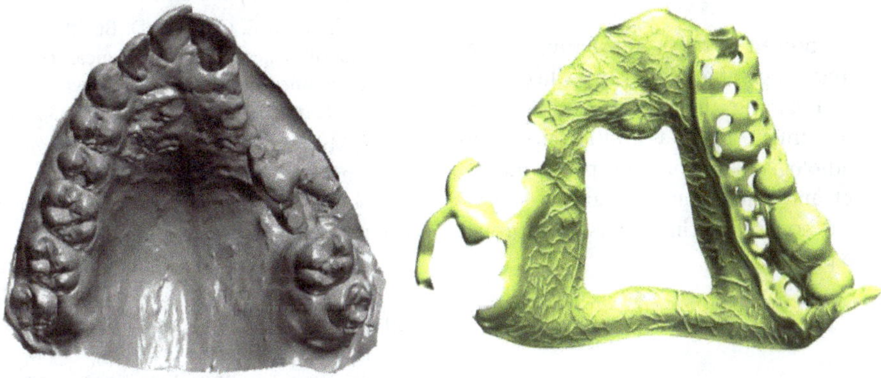

FIGURE 7: .STL file of the scanned cast and designing of cast partial denture.

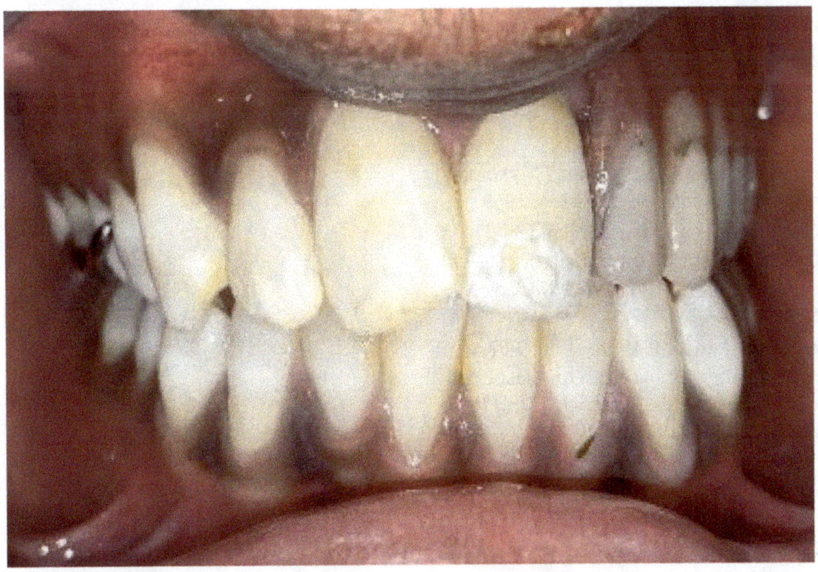

FIGURE 8: Final prosthesis.

The amount of remaining horizontal component is the deciding factor in restoring the subjects with an obturator. A significant amount of forces can be distributed on the remaining dentition through clasps to retain the prosthesis in position [15]. Due to the limited availability of the bone, the success of endosteal implants in the long term is questionable. In the present case, since the hard palate was sectioned, the prosthetic rehabilitation was planned with an obturator supported by a zygomatic implant considering the age of the patient. The major advantage of these implants is that they eliminate the use of graft material and its associated infections [16, 17].

Apart from this, there are certain complications associated with the placement of zygomatic implants, such as orbital injury/penetration, oroantral fistula formation, sensory nerve deficits temporarily, and vestibular cortical fenestration [18]. To overcome these complications, it is important to plan the placement of the implant based on a CT/CBCT imaging, and the skill of the surgeon plays a crucial role. As mentioned previously, there were no postoperative complications in the present case except for the sensitivity of soft tissue around the implant during the 12-month follow-up period, but this did not limit the functionality of the prosthesis.

4. Conclusion

Zygomatic implants have proven to be an alternative to the traditional methods in restoring subjects with maxillectomy defects as they help in retaining the obturators. With a proper diagnosis and treatment plan, a multidisciplinary approach involving a radiologist, surgeon, and prosthodontist helps to reconstruct and rehabilitate at various stages of treatment. The ultimate goal of the clinician is to improve the quality of life of the patient.

References

[1] T. D. Taylor, *Clinical Maxillofacial Prosthetics*, Quintessense Publishing Co, Inc., 1st edition, 2000.

[2] W. Shafer, M. Hine, and B. Levy, *A Textbook of Oral Pathology*, Saunders, Philadelphia:PA, 4th edition, 1983.

[3] I. Kramer, J. Pindborg, and M. Shear, *Histological Typing of Odontogenic Tumours*, Springer Verlag, Berlin, 2nd edition, 1992.

[4] R. E. Barros, F. V. Dominguez, and R. L. Cabrini, "Myxoma of the jaws," *Oral Surgery*, vol. 27, no. 2, pp. 225–236, 1969.

[5] P. B. Deron, N. Nikolovski, J. C. den Hollander, H. A. Spoelstra, and P. P. Knegt, "Myxoma of the maxilla: a case with extremely aggressive biologic behavior," *Head & Neck*, vol. 18, no. 5, pp. 459–464, 1996.

[6] S. Koyama, K. Sasaki, T. Inai, and M. Watanabe, "Effects of defect configuration, size, and remaining teeth on masticatory function in post-maxillectomy patients," *Journal of Oral Rehabilitation*, vol. 32, no. 9, pp. 635–641, 2005.

[7] E. Roumanas, R. D. Nishimura, and B. K. Davis, "Clinical evaluation of implants retaining edentulous maxillary obturator prostheses," *The Journal of Prosthetic Dentistry*, vol. 77, no. 2, pp. 184–190, 1997.

[8] S. M. Parel, P. I. Brånemark, L. O. Ohrnell, and B. Svensson, "Remote implant anchorage for the rehabilitation of maxillary defects," *The Journal of Prosthetic Dentistry*, vol. 86, no. 4, pp. 377–381, 2001.

[9] B. R. Chrcanovic, T. Albrektsson, and A. Wennerberg, "Survival and complications of zygomatic implants: an updated systematic review," *Journal of Oral and Maxillofacial Surgery* vol. 74, no. 10, pp. 1949–1964, 2016.

[10] A. B. Kornblith, I. M. Zlotolow, J. Gooen et al., "Quality of life of maxillectomy patients using an obturator prosthesis," *Head & Neck*, vol. 18, no. 4, pp. 323–334, 1996.

[11] P. G. Cordeiro and E. Santamaria, "A classification system and algorithm for reconstruction of maxillectomy and midfacial defects," *Plastic and Reconstructive Surgery*, vol. 105, no. 7, pp. 2331–2346, 2000.

[12] T. Mücke, F. Hölzle, D. J. Loeffelbein et al., "Maxillary reconstruction using microvascular free flaps," *Oral Surgery, Oral Medicine, Oral Pathology, Oral Radiology, and Endodontics*, vol. 111, no. 1, pp. 51–57, 2011.

[13] M. Sakuraba, Y. Kimata, Y. Ota et al., "Simple maxillary reconstruction using free tissue transfer and prostheses," *Plastic and Reconstructive Surgery*, vol. 111, no. 2, pp. 594–598, 2003.

[14] A. Dattani, D. Richardson, and C. J. Butterworth, "A novel report on the use of an oncology zygomatic implant-retained maxillary obturator in a paediatric patient," *International Journal of Implant Dentistry*, vol. 3, no. 1, pp. 1–6, 2017.

[15] D. J. Okay, E. Genden, D. Buchbinder, and M. Urken, "Prosthodontic guidelines for surgical reconstruction of the maxilla: a classification system of defects," *The Journal of Prosthetic Dentistry*, vol. 86, no. 4, pp. 352–363, 2001.

[16] S. Mittal and M. Agarwal, *Case Reports in Dentistry*, vol. 2018, Article ID 3437417, Rehabilitation of posterior maxilla with obturator supported by zygomatic implants, 2018.

[17] R. Agbara, E. Goetze, F. Koch, and W. Wagner, "Zygoma implants in oral rehabilitation: a review of 28 cases," *Dental Research Journal*, vol. 14, no. 6, pp. 370–375, 2017.

[18] F. Tzerbos, F. Bountaniotis, N. Theologie-Lygidakis, D. Fakitsas, and I. Fakitsas, "Complications of zygomatic implants: our clinical experience with 4 cases," *Acta Stomatologica Croatica*, vol. 50, no. 3, pp. 251–257, 2016.

3

Management of Buccal Screw Access Hole Positioning for Implant Fixed Complete Dentures: A Report of Two Patients and a Proposed Decision Tree

Fawaz Alzoubi

Department of General Dental Practice, Faculty of Dentistry, Kuwait University, Jabriya, Kuwait

Correspondence should be addressed to Fawaz Alzoubi; fawaz.alzoubi@ku.edu.kw

Academic Editor: Asja Celebic

The present report demonstrated the use of two methods to correct the positioning of buccal screw access holes in both implant- and abutment-level implant-supported fixed complete dentures in two patients. The report suggests that nonaxially tightened abutments (in this report, dynamic abutments), angled multi-unit abutments, and the use of a milled framework with individual crowns aid in masking buccal screw access holes while maintaining the benefits of a screw-retained design. A decision tree is also proposed to facilitate the workflow when faced with such clinical scenarios.

1. Introduction

Implant fixed complete dentures (IFCDs) are a well-documented, predictable, and reliable treatment method [1–4]. Nevertheless, the installation of IFCDs is a complex procedure, and issues related to its execution are common. One of the primary issues encountered involves the buccal emergence of screw access holes (SAHs).

Screw-retained implant prostheses are generally preferred because of their advantageous design, especially in relation to retrievability [5–8]. However, an esthetic problem arises in cases where the implant trajectory results in a buccally positioned SAH; hence, a cement-retained design may be used to mask the buccal SAH [9]. Although this technique might be acceptable for partially edentulous cases, it is generally not recommended to have cement-retained designs in IFCDs [9]. The reasons to avoid this technique include an extreme difficulty in retrieving the prosthesis without damaging it [10], increased likelihood of having remnant cement around the implants, potentially causing peri-implant disease [11–14], and a high chance of cement setting before the complete seating of the prosthesis, leading to possible misfit.

During the retrieval of a cement-retained IFCD, it is very likely to damage the prosthesis while accessing the prosthetic screws, a scenario that not only requires a considerable amount of time and effort but also carries a financial burden because of the likelihood of having to reexecute the entire prosthetic treatment. Removing excess cement from single or partial implant-supported fixed dental prostheses [14] is a challenging procedure because of the limited accessibility to the peri-implant environment, which would be even more complicated if it was executed for a full-arch prosthesis including four to eight implants. In case of IFCDs, a passive fitting (or minimal misfit) of the prosthesis is desired in order to minimize any biomechanical complications and possible failure [15–18]. With a cement-retained IFCD, the clinician must ensure that the cement is mixed and applied evenly throughout multiple implant abutments. This constitutes a significant challenge because the cement is likely to start setting on the first abutment before the clinician is able to apply any of it on the last abutment. This difference in application and setting time impedes the complete seating of the prosthesis because of the hard consistency of the cement that begins to set in the abutments where it was first applied, hence impeding passive seating of the framework and increasing the likelihood of misfit and biomechanical problems.

The literature currently reports a great understanding of several factors related to the proper installation of IFCDs. However, authors are inclined to report technical methods to address any potential obstacles (such as positioning of buccal SAHs) to assist colleagues in managing these scenarios and optimize implant-based treatment involving buccal SAH, which is a current challenge in the field of dentistry. Hence, the aim of this paper is to describe two methods for managing the positioning of buccal SAHs for IFCDs by reporting two clinical cases and proposing a decision tree to facilitate clinicians' workflow when faced with similar scenarios. This may have significant clinical implications, as it will aid clinicians in making informed and appropriate clinical decisions in this type of scenario.

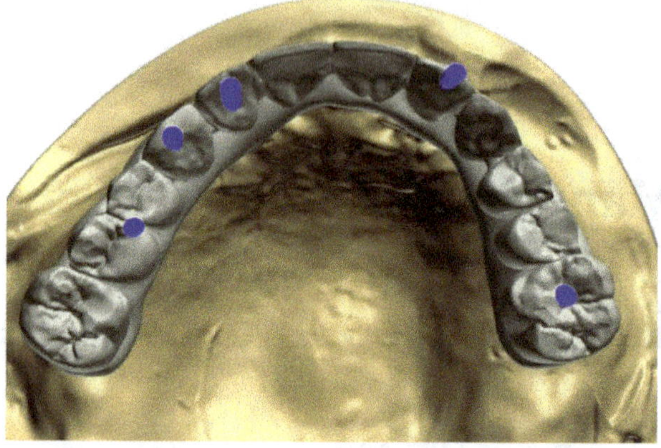

Figure 1: Digital superimpositions of the tooth setup and implant master cast scans for case one indicating buccal SAH on site 22 and insufficient thickness of buccal material in site 13.

2. Case Presentations

2.1. Case One. A 53-year-old female patient presented to the clinic requesting replacement of her missing and compromised teeth with a fixed prosthesis. Medical history was reviewed and considered noncontributory. After clinical and radiographic examinations, the proposed treatment was a maxillary IFCD supported by five implants. Five 4.5 × 11 mm implants (NobelReplace Conical Connection, Nobel Biocare, Kloten, Switzerland) were placed as planned, and an immediate removable complete denture (RCD) was relined and delivered after surgery. This approach was selected because of the sufficient availability of bone on the maxillary right side and the lack of bone on the maxillary left molar side. To avoid a sinus augmentation procedure, the left maxillary posterior implant was tilted, and the trajectory was corrected using a 30° multi-unit abutment.

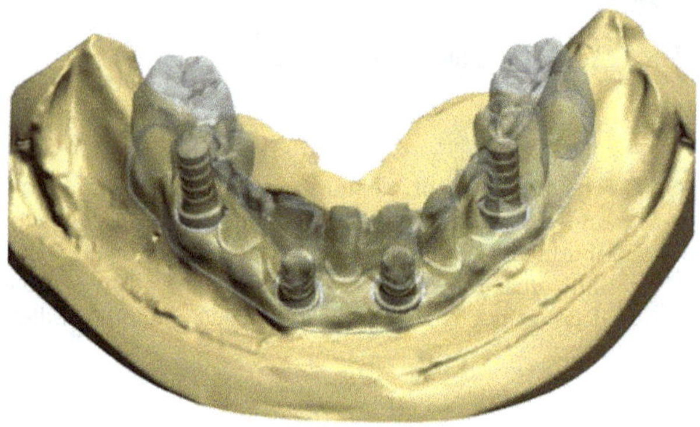

Figure 2: Digital superimpositions of the tooth setup and implant master cast scans for case two indicating buccal SAHs in the two anterior implants.

2.2. Case Two. A 70-year-old female patient presented to the clinic requesting replacement of her missing mandibular teeth with a fixed prosthesis. Medical history was significant for diabetes mellitus, hypertension, hyperlipidemia, hypothyroidism, benign positional vertigo, anemia, and nonalcoholic steatohepatitis. The patient used multiple medications to control her underlying conditions. After clinical and radiographic examinations, the proposed treatment was a mandibular IFCD supported by four implants using an All-on-4 approach. Two 5 mm × 10 mm tilted implants (NobelReplace Conical Connection, Nobel Biocare, Kloten, Switzerland) were placed in the posterior sites using 30° multi-unit abutments, and two 4.3 mm × 10 mm axial implants (NobelReplace Conical Connection, Nobel Biocare, Kloten, Switzerland) were placed in the anterior sites using straight multi-unit abutments. An immediate RCD was relined and delivered after surgery. This approach was selected because of the lack of bone in the area posterior to the mental foramina and to avoid considerable bone grafting procedures in an already medically compromised patient.

2.3. Clinical Outcomes. Fixed implant rehabilitation was selected for both patients to enhance quality of life by improving mastication, esthetics, and psychological well-being, since both patients could not tolerate removable prostheses. Furthermore, in both cases, resin-template guides were produced after duplicating the respective complete dentures and were used during surgery to guide the initial drills into the planned osteotomy sites.

Both patients were followed up after approximately 4 months of uneventful healing. Temporary milled polymethyl methacrylate- (PMMA-) provisional IFCDs were fabricated. In both patients, it was noticed during the digital design phase of the provisional IFCDs that the implant trajectories of some anterior implants led to buccally positioned SAHs. Furthermore, in case one, the implant trajectory at site 13 (maxillary right canine) did not present sufficient thickness of material buccal to a the SAH (Figures 1 and 2). Nonetheless, the lab was instructed to proceed with fabricating screw-retained, PMMA-provisional IFCDs with an understanding of the aforementioned issues. Both provisional IFCDs were delivered, and the buccal SAHs were masked with resin in an attempt to match the tooth shade as accurately as possible (Figures 3, 4, and 5). After approximately 8 weeks, patients were recalled for evaluation and did not report any significant complaints; however, it was noticed

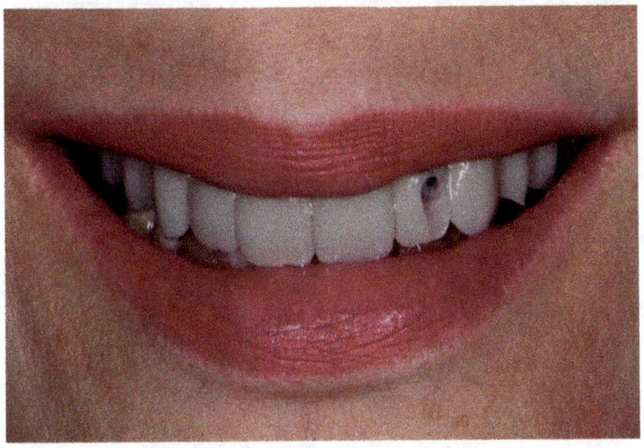

Figure 3: Case one: maximum smile with provisional implant showing visibility of the buccal SAH.

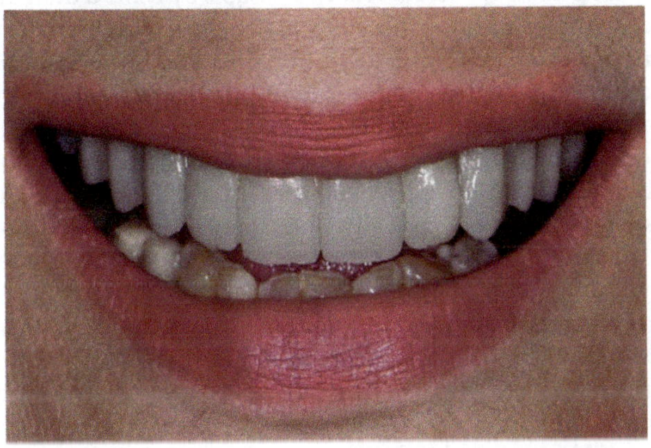

Figure 4: Case one: maximum smile after masking with resin.

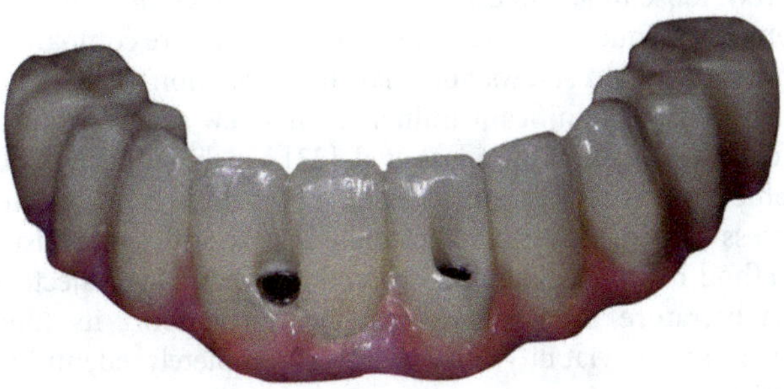

Figure 5: Provisional IFCD with buccal SAH in case two.

that the resin masking the buccal SAHs was stained, compromising the esthetic result.

For case one, nonaxially tightened dynamic abutments (DA) were used to correct the buccal SAH in implant 22 (maxillary left lateral incisor) and lingualize the SAH in implant 13 to allow for increased thickness of the prosthetic material that was buccal to the SAH. Finally, a combination of an implant- and abutment-level (only on the left maxillary posterior implant) splinted IFCD with a milled zirconia framework, which was layered with lithium disilicate on the anterior teeth, was fabricated and delivered (Figures 6 and 7).

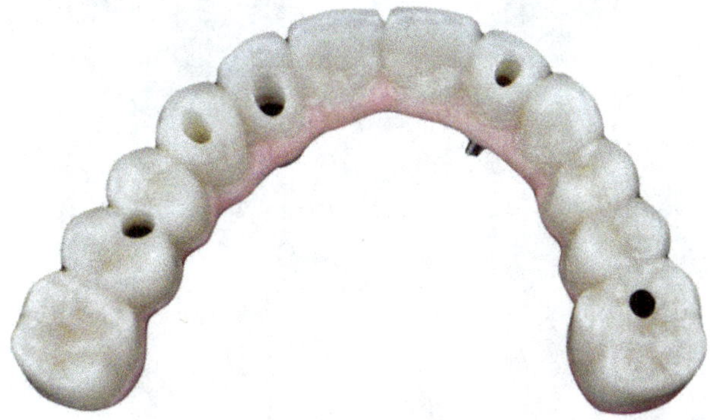

Figure 6: Case one: occlusal view of the final IFCD demonstrating lingual SAH on site 22 and improved thickness of buccal material in site 13.

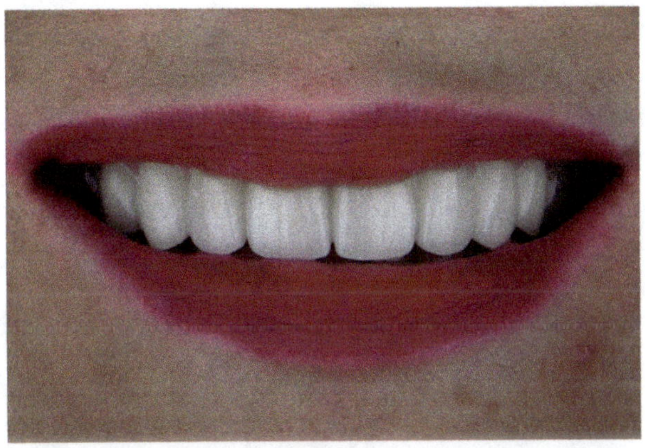

Figure 7: Case one: maximum smile after installation of the final IFCD with lingualized SAH using DA.

For case two, to correct the buccal SAHs in the anterior two implants, the lab was instructed to fabricate an abutment-level splinted milled zirconia framework with individual lithium disilicate crowns for the buccal SAH sites (Figures 8 and 9). This design lends itself to a screw-retained approach and masks buccal SAHs via the intraoral cementation of individual crowns. The prosthesis was then delivered, screws were torqued according to manufacturer's recommendations, and individual crowns were cemented with resin only on the sites presenting buccal SAHs (Figures 10 and 11).

3. Discussion

Although implant placement should be prosthetically driven and placed to accommodate a screw-retained position, bone topography and quantity might obstruct such placement, especially in the anterior region. Bone augmentation may be recommended; however, in completely edentulous cases, this procedure might be challenging and present questionable prognosis due to factors such as age (older age is often accompanied by medically compromised health) and the amount of augmentation necessary to regain lost bone.

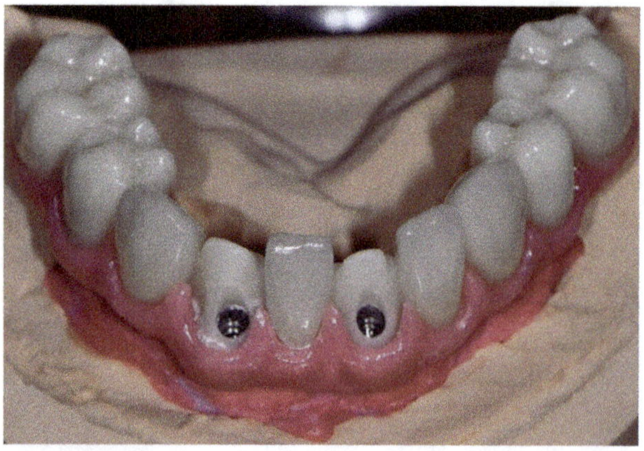

Figure 8: Final milled zirconia framework with individual crowns in case two: abutments milled for anterior teeth with buccal SAH.

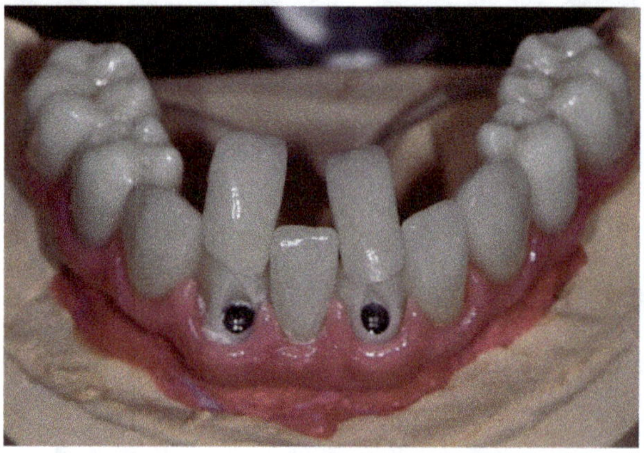

Figure 9: Final milled zirconia framework with individual crowns in case two: individual *E*max crowns fabricated to be cemented intraorally.

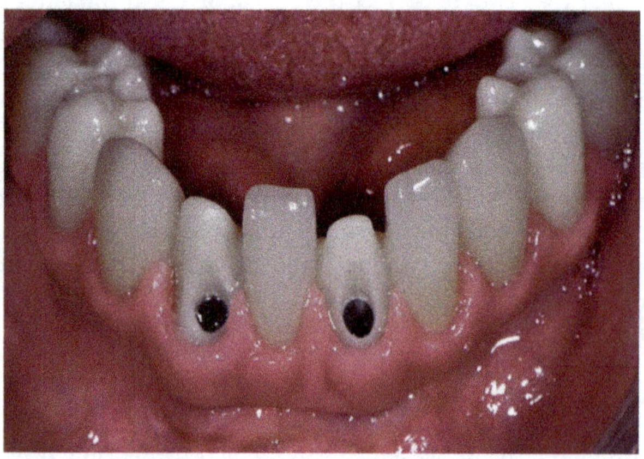

Figure 10: Final milled zirconia framework with individual crowns in case two: after securing the implants and torquing the prosthetic screws.

Hence, interest has been invested into prosthetic solutions to overcome these surgical limitations [19–23], such as DAs and angled multiunit abutments.

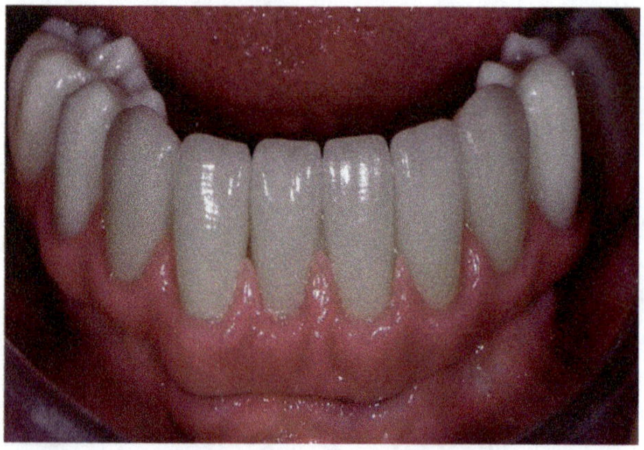

Figure 11: Final milled zirconia framework with individual crowns in case two: after intraoral *e*.max crown cementation.

DAs allow for screw-retained designs by using a titanium screw that is torqued in a nonaxial manner [22], permitting angular correction by up to 28° [24]. In addition, a significant advantage is that an implant-level prosthesis can be fabricated. Hence, there is no need for additional restorative components to correct for angulation (e.g., angled multi-unit abutments), which might compromise available space and esthetic outcomes, especially when there is not sufficient soft tissue around the implant (such as in case one). If an angled multiunit abutment was used to lingualize implant trajectories at sites 13 and 22, then not only would the metal collar show, leading to an esthetic issue, but it would also compromise the already-limited prosthetic space available. A considerable limitation of DAs is that the screw torque values required to secure the abutments to the implant are generally lower than conventional values; hence, it is plausible to hypothesize the subsequent occurrence of issues involving screw loosening. Goldberg et al. [22] concluded that the removal torque and fatigue strength of DAs were comparable to those of gold screws and that the angulation of the abutment had no significant influence on screw removal torque values. However, Swamidass et al. [23] concluded that torque values presented greater torque differences in angulated access channel crowns. Although this is still a promising method for the angulation correction of implant trajectory, the literature lacks strong evidence to support its long-term clinical viability, especially in completely edentulous patients.

In case two, an All-on-4 approach was used, with angled multi-unit abutments for the posterior implants and with straight multiunit abutments for the anterior implants. It was noticed during the digital design of the provisional IFCDs that the implant trajectories for the anterior two implants led to the buccal placement of SAHs. A solution for this could have been to retrieve the straight multi-unit abutments and replace them with angled multi-unit abutments to lingualize the SAH. Nonetheless, this procedure might have interrupted the established soft tissue seal between the abutment and gingiva, leading to potentially negative effects on soft tissue and marginal bone levels [25]. In addition, this option was not feasible as we strived

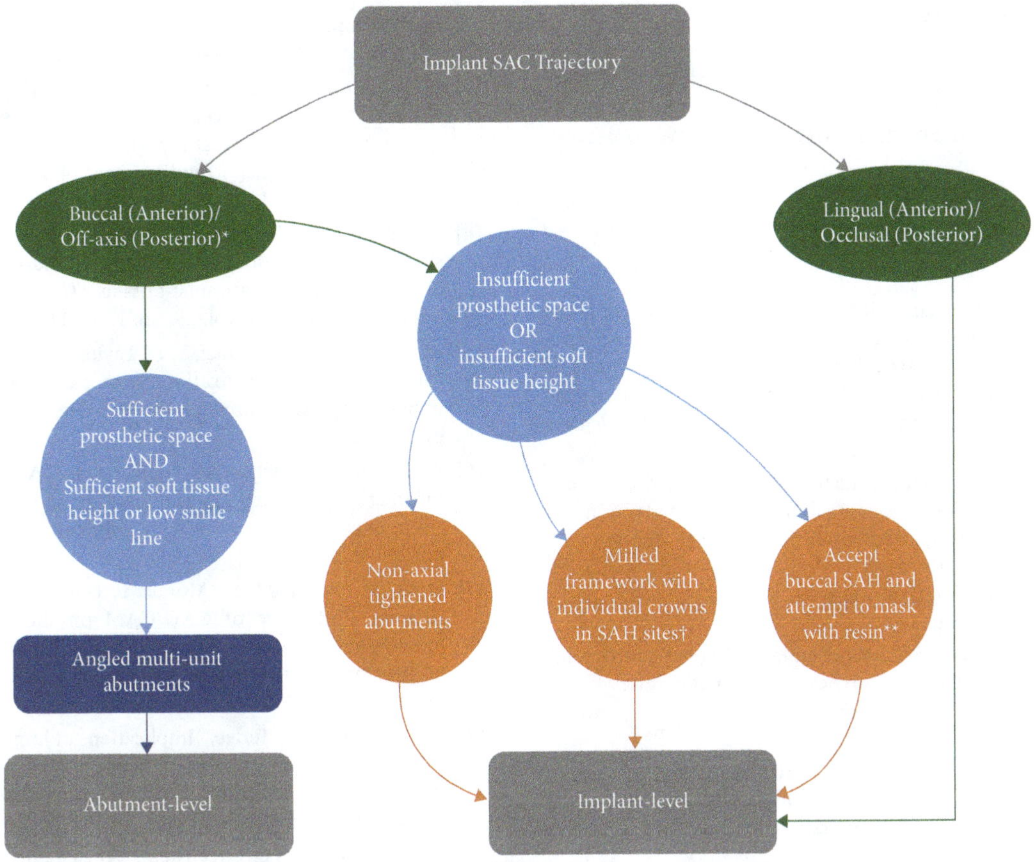

FIGURE 12: Proposed decision tree to facilitate the management of buccal SAH positioning. SAC: screw access channel; SAH: screw access hole. *Including tilted implants; **only recommended for provisional prostheses or cases where the SAH is masked by the lip line during maximum smiling; †can also be performed for abutment-level prostheses. In addition, can be used if DAs cannot be used due to a needed angulation correction exceeding 28°.

to minimize the number of visits because patient's older age and complex medical history implied significant physical restrictions; indeed, if the multi-unit abutments were replaced, the prosthetic workflow would need to be reexecuted, involving three or four additional visits. Therefore, the author opted to use an abutment-level splinted milled zirconia framework with individual lithium disilicate crowns in buccal SAH sites. Although this approach aids in masking buccal SAHs, the crowns in the respective sites are damaged in the process of prosthesis retrieval. However, the extent of damage is limited to the two crowns, which can be easily replaced in the future, instead of damaging the entire prosthesis.

The use of milled frameworks with individual crown designs has gained popularity for several reasons. In this paper, the author recommends the use of this option for abutment-level or implant-level prostheses; however, as previously mentioned, only if the screw access channel (SAC) trajectory leads to a buccally positioned SAH in individual sites. The proposed solution includes a framework that can be milled for a screw-retained implant; in sites where the SAH is positioned buccally, the lab can be instructed to design the framework in a way that can accommodate individual crowns by digitally designing and milling the abutments accordingly. Then, the fabricated individual crowns are to be cemented in the mouth after the delivery of the screw-retained prosthesis. Hence, masking the SAHs still results in a screw-retained prosthesis. If the prosthesis needs to be retrieved in the future, then only those sites' crowns are damaged, which can then be individually replaced, and the remaining prosthesis can be retrieved by accessing the screws through the SAHs. Furthermore, this method can be used if DAs cannot be used due to a needed angulation correction exceeding 28°.

Regarding the masking of buccal SAHs, various resin materials may be used; however, potential staining at the sites of interest is to be expected. Hence, the author recommends using resin materials strictly in the case of provisional restorations or when the SAH is masked by the lips during maximum smiling. Based on the presented report, a decision tree is proposed to facilitate the clinical decision-making process when faced with similar scenarios (Figure 12).

Acknowledgments

The author would like to thank and acknowledge the work of laboratory technicians Tobias Baars and Joscha Knauth for their work and efforts in treating the two presented patient cases.

References

[1] S. Barootchi, H. Askar, A. Ravidà, J. Gargallo-Albiol, S. Travan, and H. L. Wang, "Long-term clinical outcomes and cost-effectiveness of full-arch implant-supported zirconia-based and metal-acrylic fixed dental prostheses: a retrospective analysis," *The International Journal of Oral & Maxillofacial Implants*, vol. 35, no. 2, pp. 395–405, 2020.

[2] N. Ferrigno, M. Laureti, S. Fanali, and G. Grippaudo, "A long-term follow-up study of non-submerged ITI implants in the treatment of totally edentulous jaws. Part I: ten-year life table analysis of a prospective multicenter study with 1286 implants," *Clinical Oral Implants Research*, vol. 13, no. 3, pp. 260–273, 2002.

[3] M. Rohlin, K. Nilner, T. Davidson et al., "Treatment of adult patients with edentulous arches: a systematic review," *The International Journal of Prosthodontics*, vol. 25, no. 6, pp. 553–567, 2012.

[4] T. J. Balshi, G. J. Wolfinger, R. W. Slauch, and S. F. Balshi, "A retrospective analysis of 800 Brånemark System implants following the All-on-Four™ protocol," *Journal of Prosthodontics*, vol. 23, no. 2, pp. 83–88, 2014.

[5] K. Michalakis, H. Hirayama, and P. Garefis, "Cement-retained versus screw-retained implant restorations: a critical review," *The International Journal of Oral & Maxillofacial Implants*, vol. 18, no. 5, pp. 719–728, 2003.

[6] K. Gotfredsen and A. Wiskott, "Consensus report - reconstructions on implants. The third EAO consensus conference 2012," *Clinical Oral Implants*, vol. 23, Supplement 6, pp. 238–241, 2012.

[7] W. Martin, A. Pollini, and D. Morton, "The influence of restorative procedures on esthetic outcomes in implant dentistry: a systematic review," *The International Journal of Oral & Maxillofacial Implants*, vol. 29, Supplement, pp. 142–154, 2014.

[8] S. Sherif, H. K. Susarla, T. Kapos, D. Muñoz, B. M. Chang, and R. F. Wright, "A systematic review of screw- versus cement-retained implant-supported fixed restorations," *Journal of Prosthodontics*, vol. 23, no. 1, pp. 1–9, 2014.

[9] J. Wittneben, T. Joda, H. P. Weber, and U. Bragger, "Screw retained vs. cement retained implant-supported fixed dental prosthesis," *Periodontology 2000*, vol. 73, no. 1, pp. 141–151, 2017.

[10] W. Chee, D. A. Felton, P. F. Johnson, and D. Y. Sullivan, "Cemented versus screw-retained implant prostheses: which is better?," *The International Journal of Oral & Maxillofacial Implants*, vol. 14, no. 1, pp. 137–141, 1999.

[11] T. G. Wilson Jr., "The positive relationship between excess cement and periimplant disease: a prospective clinical endoscopic study," *Journal of Periodontology*, vol. 80, no. 9, pp. 1388–1392, 2009.

[12] C. Wadhwani, D. Rapoport, S. La Rosa, T. Hess, and S. Kretschmar, "Radiographic detection and characteristic patterns of residual excess cement associated with cement-retained implant restorations: a clinical report," *The Journal of Prosthetic Dentistry*, vol. 107, no. 3, pp. 151–157, 2012.

[13] N. Pauletto, B. J. Lahiffe, and J. N. Walton, "Complications associated with excess cement around crowns on osseointegrated implants: a clinical report," *The International Journal of Oral & Maxillofacial Implants*, vol. 14, no. 6, pp. 865–868, 1999.

[14] M. Korsch, B. P. Robra, and W. Walther, "Cement-associated signs of inflammation: retrospective analysis of the effect of excess cement on peri-implant tissue," *The International Journal of Prosthodontics*, vol. 28, no. 1, pp. 11–18, 2015.

[15] M. Karl, S. Rosch, F. Graef, T. D. Taylor, and S. M. Heckmann, "Strain situation after fixation of three-unit ceramic veneered implant superstructures," *Implant Dentistry*, vol. 14, no. 2, pp. 157–165, 2005.

[16] A. Scarano, B. Assenza, M. Piattelli et al., "A 16-year study of the microgap between 272 human titanium implants and their abutments," *The Journal of Oral Implantology*, vol. 31, no. 6, pp. 269–275, 2005.

[17] D. G. de França, M. H. Morais, F. D. das Neves, and G. A. Barbosa, "Influence of CAD/CAM on the fit accuracy of implant-supported zirconia and cobalt-chromium fixed dental prostheses," *The Journal of Prosthetic Dentistry*, vol. 113, no. 1, pp. 22–28, 2015.

[18] J. Abduo and R. B. Judge, "Implications of implant framework misfit: a systematic review of biomechanical sequelae," *The International Journal of Oral & Maxillofacial Implants*, vol. 29, no. 3, pp. 608–621, 2014.

[19] J. Cavallaro Jr. and G. Greenstein, "Angled implant abutments: a practical application of available knowledge," *Journal of the American Dental Association (1939)*, vol. 142, no. 2, pp. 150–158, 2011.

[20] A. Sethi, T. Kaus, and P. Sochor, "The use of angulated abutments in implant dentistry: five-year clinical results of an ongoing prospective study," *The International Journal of Oral & Maxillofacial Implants*, vol. 15, no. 6, pp. 801–810, 2000.

[21] T. Brosh, R. Pilo, and D. Sudai, "The influence of abutment angulation on strains and stresses along the implant/bone interface: comparison between two experimental techniques," *The Journal of Prosthetic Dentistry*, vol. 79, no. 3, pp. 328–334, 1998.

[22] J. Goldberg, T. Lee, J. H. Phark, and W. Chee, "Removal torque and force to failure of non-axially tightened implant abutment screws," *The Journal of Prosthetic Dentistry*, vol. 121, no. 2, pp. 322–326, 2019.

[23] R. S. Swamidass, J. Y. Kan, M. T. Kattadiyil, C. J. Goodacre, and J. Lozada, "Abutment screw torque changes with straight and angled screw-access channels," *The Journal of Prosthetic Dentistry*, vol. 125, no. 4, pp. 675–681, 2021.

[24] E. Berroeta, I. Zabalegui, T. Donovan, and W. Chee, "Dynamic abutment: a method of redirecting screw access for implant-supported restorations: technical details and a clinical report," *Journal of Prosthetic Dentistry*, vol. 113, no. 6, pp. 516–519, 2015.

[25] I. Abrahamsson, T. Berglundh, and J. Lindhe, "The mucosal barrier following abutment dis/reconnection: an experimental study in dogs," *Journal of Clinical Periodontology*, vol. 24, no. 8, pp. 568–572, 1997.

4

Immediate Implant Placement and Provisionalization in the Esthetic Zone: A 6.5-Year Follow-Up and Literature Review

Hsiu-Wan Meng,[1] **Esther Yun Chien**,[2] **and Hua-Hong Chien**[3]

[1]*Department of Periodontics and Dental Hygiene, The University of Texas Health Science Center School of Dentistry, Houston TX, USA*
[2]*Private Practice, Columbus OH, USA*
[3]*Division of Periodontology, College of Dentistry, The Ohio State University, Columbus OH, USA*

Correspondence should be addressed to Hsiu-Wan Meng; hsiu-wan.meng@uth.tmc.edu

Academic Editor: Konstantinos Michalakis

The success of dental implant therapy in the esthetic zone requires not only functional osseointegration but also a satisfactory esthetic outcome. To establish harmony, balance, and continuity of gingival architecture between an implant restoration and the adjacent natural dentition is challenging. Immediate implant placement and provisionalization following tooth extraction have been documented as a predictable treatment modality, with fewer surgical interventions needed, to replace a missing tooth in the esthetic zone. This case report illustrates immediate implant placement and provisionalization to replace a failing maxillary right central incisor while maintaining optimal gingival esthetics. The maxillary right central incisor was extracted without flap elevation to minimize soft and hard tissue trauma. Immediately afterwards, the implant was installed using a surgical stent and restored with a provisional crown that had no occlusal contacts. During healing, no significant adverse effects were observed clinically or radiographically. This proposed treatment modality provided the patient with immediate esthetics, function, and comfort without any complications during a follow-up period of 6.5 years.

1. Introduction

Dental implants have become a viable treatment option for completely and partially edentulous patients. Since 1968 when Dr. Branemark first introduced the concept of osseointegration, a vast amount of clinical investigation with long-term follow-up has been conducted on the effectiveness and predictability of implant-supported restorations [1–3].

Implants can be placed using a two-stage or one-stage procedure. Traditionally, they are placed using a two-stage procedure, where they are initially completely submerged under mucosal tissue during the healing process to avoid any functional loading and then later uncovered in a second minor surgery. Two-stage implants installed using a one-stage procedure have been demonstrated to be as predictable as those placed following the traditional two-stage procedure [4]. Furthermore, a prospective clinical study on two-stage implants placed using a one-stage procedure versus one-stage implants has shown comparable clinical and radiographic outcomes during the healing period [5]. Therefore, more and more implants are now placed using a one-stage procedure, in which the healing abutment is connected to the implant fixture at the time of implant surgery. A systematic review by Esposito et al. [6] looked at 5 randomized controlled trials of adults with a minimum follow-up of 6 months after loading. They found no significant differences in measured outcomes between one- and two-stage implant placement techniques. Moreover, the development of implant surface characteristics has increased bone-to-implant contact and implant stability at earlier stages in the healing process. Ultimately, the conventional protocol of including a healing period of 6 months for the maxilla and 4 to 6 months for the mandible has been reduced significantly. Some specific implant surface characteristics allowed functional loading 6 weeks after implant placement, which is a major breakthrough in surface technology [7].

Immediate implant placement in a fresh extraction socket has been reviewed extensively in the literature [8, 9]. Traditionally, a 3-month waiting period after tooth extraction is required for soft and hard tissue healing before placing a dental implant. The protocol of placing an implant in a healed socket and subsequently restoring the implant with a prosthesis is recognized as a highly predictive treatment modality for partially edentulous patients [10]. Recently, the traditional protocol has been increasingly replaced by a faster protocol in which an implant is placed immediately in a fresh extraction socket in combination with immediate restoration [11].

Immediate implant placement and restoration of a single implant in the esthetic zone have several proposed benefits, including reduced overall treatment time, fewer surgical procedures, less traumatic surgery, and greater patient satisfaction [12]. On the other hand, this treatment protocol also has inherent disadvantages, such as difficulty in achieving implant stability, higher risk of implant failure, unpredictable soft and hard tissue levels, and the need for bone grafts [13]. The placement of a provisional restoration on a single implant in the esthetic zone has been advocated for creating a good soft tissue contour, especially in conjunction with immediate implant placement [14]. Immediate implant placement and provisionalization can be a predictable treatment modality to replace a hopeless tooth in the esthetic zone when primary implant stability can be achieved, and the provisional restoration can be adjusted to clear all centric and eccentric contacts.

2. Case Presentation

A 38-year-old Caucasian female reported to the Graduate Periodontics Clinic at the College of Dentistry, The Ohio State University, for a single tooth extraction and implant therapy. A nonrestorable maxillary right central incisor with external root resorption (Figure 1) was observed at the initial examination and was confirmed by a periapical film. The patient reported a history of trauma around the upper anterior teeth resulting in endodontic treatment of teeth 12, 11, and 21. She reported no significant medical history except an allergy to penicillin. She had no history of smoking and was classified as American Society of Anesthesiologists (ASA) Physical Status Classification System I. A comprehensive periodontal exam revealed no probing depths greater than 3 mm, and the embrasure spaces between the maxillary incisors were completely filled with interdental papilla. Neither tooth mobility nor percussion/palpation pain was detected in teeth 12 to 22. Radiographic examination illustrated external root resorption on the distal aspect of tooth 11 at the CEJ level with no apical radiolucency. After clinical and radiographic preoperative analysis to assess the patient risk profile for immediate implant placement, four treatment options (immediate implant placement, early implant placement with soft tissue healing, early implant placement with partial bone healing, and late implant placement) [15] were reviewed with the patient. Immediate implant placement with provisionalization after tooth extraction was recommended, and the patient accepted the treatment plan.

One hour before the surgery, the patient was given 600 mg of Clindamycin for surgical prophylaxis to enhance the success rate of the implant [16]. Under local anesthesia, an intrasulcular incision was placed 360° around tooth 11 using a 15C blade to cut the connective tissue fibers above the bone. An anterior periotome was used to sever the periodontal ligament to facilitate the removal of tooth 11 with minimal damage of the surrounding alveolar bone. The tooth was then removed using extraction forceps with controlled rotational force without flap elevation. Extreme care was taken to avoid fracturing the socket walls, especially the buccal plate, so the gingival and bone architecture would be preserved. The external root resorption was also confirmed on the tooth removed (Figure 2). The extraction socket was thoroughly debrided using a serrated excavator to remove any granulation tissue and then irrigated with sterile saline before osteotomy. A periodontal probe was used to confirm the integrity of the socket walls and to verify that the distance from the alveolar crest to the gingival margin was less than 3 to 4 mm as recommended for immediate implant placement. A sharp precision drill (Nobel Biocare, Yorba Linda, CA) was used to penetrate the palatal wall of the extraction socket that guided the initial preparation of an osteotomy. The osteotomy was prepared under the guidance of a surgical stent and extended about 3 to 5 mm beyond the root apex to ascertain implant primary stability [17]. A periapical radiograph was taken with a twist drill to verify the angulation (Figure 3). An OsseoSpeed 4.0 × 15 mm implant (Astra Tech Dental) was placed immediately into the fresh extraction socket following the rule of restorative-driven 3-dimensional placement [18, 19], and the implant shoulder was positioned at least 3 mm apical to an imaginary line connecting the cementoenamel junctions of the adjacent teeth [20, 21] (Figure 4). The primary stability of the implant was confirmed by achieving a torque resistance of 40 Ncm. Hydrated freeze-dried bone allograft was placed in the gap between the labial bony wall and the implant. A customized screw-retained provisional crown was made so its subgingival contour supported the soft tissue emergence profile and protected the blood clot and graft particles (Figure 5). The temporary crown was torqued to 25 Ncm and left to heal for 9 months. The occlusion of the provisional crown was adjusted to ensure that it was free from any contact during articulation. The patient was informed that she should not place any pressure on the provisional crown during the healing period. Postoperatively, Clindamycin 300 mg was given four times a day for 7 days and ibuprofen 600 mg every 4 to 6 hours for the control of infection and pain, respectively. Chlorhexidine gluconate 0.12% oral rinses were prescribed twice daily for 2 weeks. The patient was advised to adhere to a soft diet and avoid forces on the anterior teeth.

The patient received regular check-ups at 2, 4, and 7 weeks and 3 and 4 months after the implant placement surgery with no tenderness reported or adverse events observed. During the postoperative follow-up appointments, the gingival margin around the implant provisional crown appeared stable and there was functional attachment (Figure 6). After a 9-month healing period, the provisional crown was

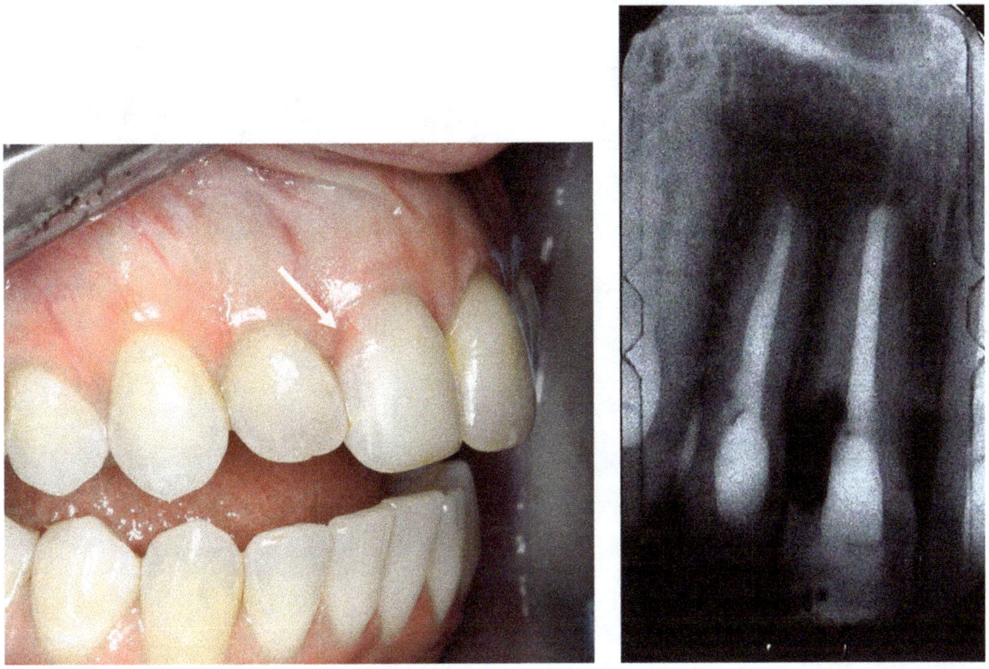

(a) (b)

FIGURE 1: (a) Upper right central incisor with external root resorption (white arrow) was confirmed by (b) a periapical radiograph.

replaced by a definitive restoration. The patient was followed for 6.5 years after final crown restoration.

Recall appointments were made every 6 months after implant loading. At these recall appointments, the implant remained stable and functioned well without any problems. The peri-implant gingiva was pink and healthy with probing depths all within 4 mm without bleeding on probing. In addition, a periapical radiograph was taken every year for the assessment of marginal bone level on the mesial and distal sides of the implant. The radiograph revealed a stable marginal bone level around the implant (Figure 7) compared to the radiograph taken at final crown delivery, without any peri-implant radiolucency noted. An excellent esthetic outcome with patient satisfaction through immediate implant placement and provisionalization was observed during the 6.5-year follow-up period (Figure 8).

3. Discussion and Conclusion

Immediate implant placement refers to the placement of an implant on the day of tooth extraction and within the same surgical procedure [22]. Wohrle was the first to report the protocol for immediate implant placement and provisionalization in the esthetic zone [23], which subsequently has been adopted in numerous studies and found to be an excellent treatment modality with high success/survival rate and stable gingival architecture [17]. A systematic review on immediate implant placement indicated that most studies evaluated the success/survival rate and radiographic marginal bone levels around immediate implant placement and provisionalization [9]. However, few studies assessed soft tissue parameters such as proximal papilla levels and facial gingival levels [14, 24–36]. Lang et al. [9] reported that the estimated 2-year survival rate of implants placed immediately in fresh extraction sockets was 98.4%. Another systemic review conducted by Slagter et al. specifically investigated immediately placed single-tooth implants in the esthetic zone and also found a similar survival rate of 97.1% [37].

An extraction socket classification system for the maxillary anterior teeth, based on the soft and hard tissue components, was introduced in 2008 [38]. According to this classification system, the extraction socket in the present case was graded type I, which was suitable for immediate implant placement. Immediate implant placement and provisionalization in a fresh extraction socket is challenging and requires careful case selection [39]. In general, the soft tissue contour of the extraction socket should closely mimic that of adjacent natural teeth without vertical soft tissue deficiency [40, 41]. Furthermore, the keratinized gingival width on the midbuccal aspect of the socket should be ≥2 mm, with a thick gingival biotype (≥2 mm). The apical bone beyond the extraction socket should be ≥4 mm to achieve primary stability of the implant. The tip of the mesial and distal papillae should lie between the interdental contact and the most coronal extent of interproximal CEJ. In other words, the papilla appearance should be categorized as Class I based on the classification system described by Nordland and Tarnow [42]. Regarding the hard tissue in the fresh extraction socket, the distance between the osseous crest and the gingival margin should be ≤3 mm on the midfacial and ≤4.5 mm on the proximal aspects [39]. In addition, the distance from the facial bone of the extraction socket to the implant should be ≥2 mm to maintain the implant soft tissue profile for ideal esthetics.

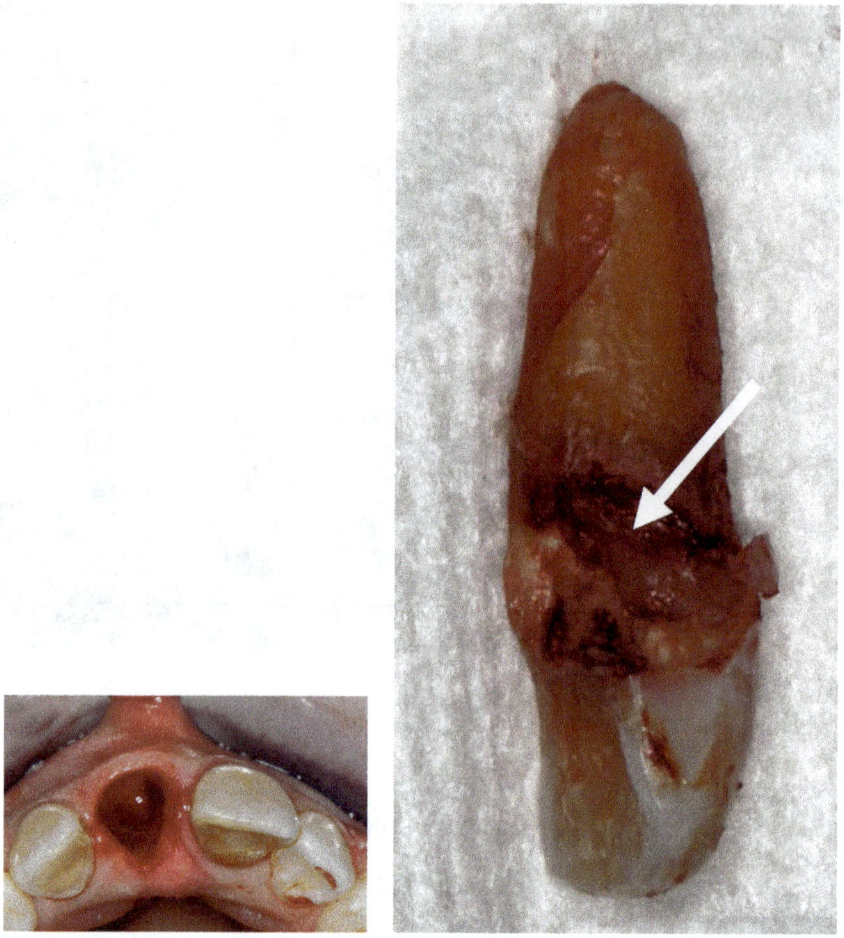

(a) (b)

FIGURE 2: (a) Extraction socket of tooth 11 after minimally invasive tooth extraction without flap elevation. (b) External root resorption was observed on the distal surface of the extracted upper right central incisor (white arrow).

In the present case, the implant was positioned at the center of the final restoration with a clearance of ≥1.5 mm between the implant fixture and the adjacent teeth to minimize the risk of damaging adjacent natural teeth. Furthermore, the implant was also placed in the cingulum position with ≥2 mm between the facial bone and the implant fixture. A recent animal study on dogs suggested a critical buccal bone wall thickness of at least 1.5 mm to compensate for the dimensional changes occurring after implant placement and the progression of peri-implantitis [43]. To obtain a better emergence profile, the implant platform should be located apicocoronally at least 3 mm from the cementoenamel junction of the adjacent tooth [39]. According to the classification system described by Kan et al. [44] on sagittal root position in relation to the anterior maxillary osseous housing, the sagittal root position in the present case was classified as Class I, where a considerable amount of bone was present on the palatal aspect, indicating a favorable setting for immediate implant placement. About 81% of teeth were classified as Class I in Kan et al.'s study.

Placing the implant in the cingulum position often results in a gap between the implant and the labial cortical plate. Dramatic changes in ridge dimension following tooth extraction have been demonstrated in clinical and histological studies, and bone augmentation has been effective in promoting bone fill and defect resolution at immediate implant sites [45, 46]. Clinical and histologic studies have shown that an esthetic hard tissue contour can be maintained both vertically and horizontally when the implant-socket gap is filled with bone grafting materials [47, 48]. Therefore, the implant-socket gap was filled with freeze-dried bone allograft in this case and the marginal bone level changes were negligible as indicated by periapical radiographs taken 6.5 years after loading.

Chu et al. proposed the dual-zone concept where bone grafts were placed in the bone and tissue zones to serve as a scaffold to maintain hard and soft tissue volume and the blood clot to facilitate initial healing [49]. Xenografts were placed in the gap between the implant and buccal bone until the gap was filled to the most coronal aspect of the free gingival margin. The authors suggested that xenograft particles incorporated into the soft tissue when placing the provisional restoration can minimize ridge collapse and increase peri-implant soft tissue thickness [50, 51]. These studies

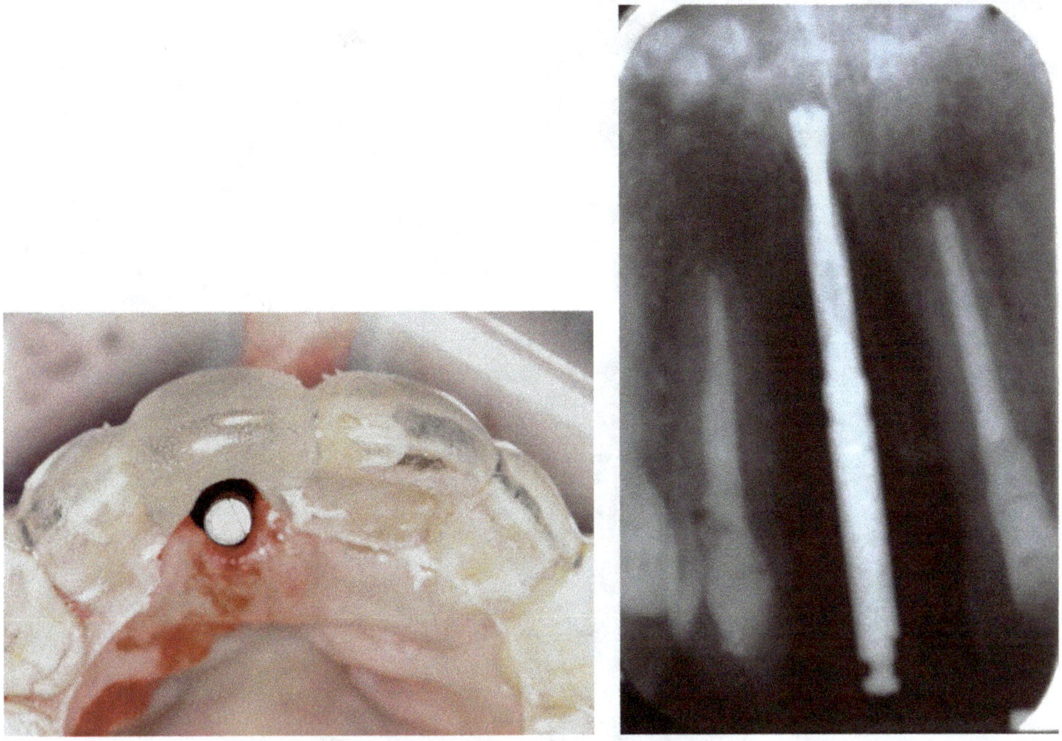

(a) (b)

FIGURE 3: (a) Initial implant osteotomy was made at the cingulum region using a precision drill under the guidance of a surgical stent. (b) A periapical radiograph was taken with a 2 mm twist drill to verify the depth and angulation for implant placement.

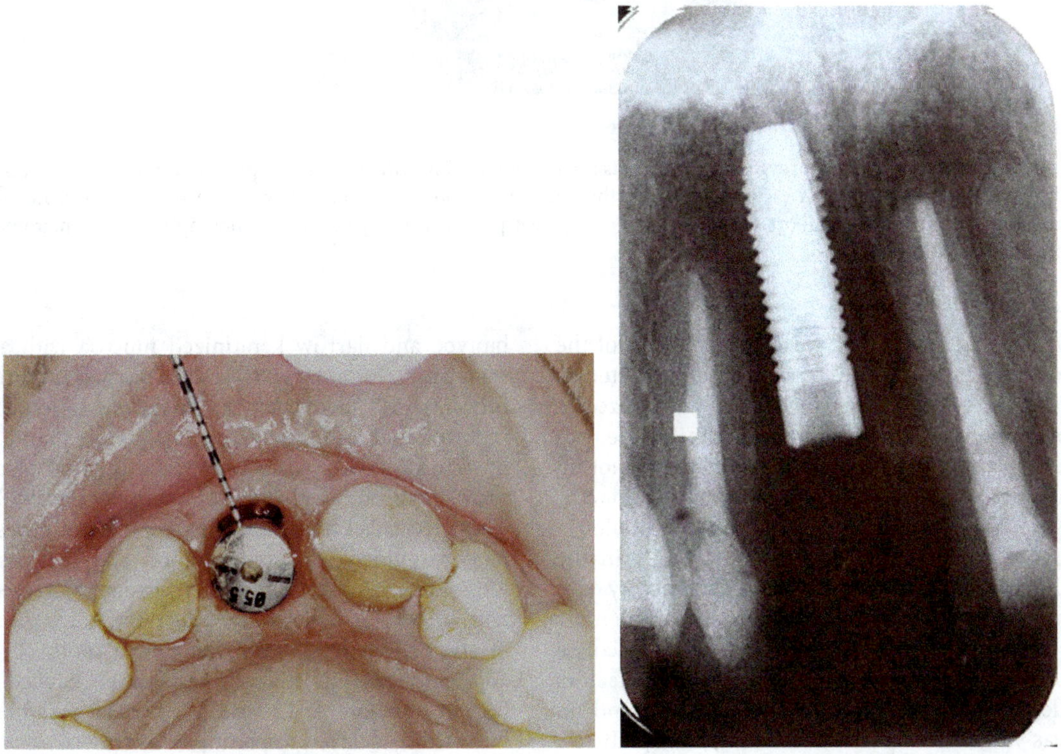

(a) (b)

FIGURE 4: (a) A 5.5 mm diameter healing abutment was connected to an OsseoSpeed 4.0 × 15 mm implant at the position of tooth 11. (b) A periapical radiograph was taken to validate that the implant shoulder was located at least 3 mm apical to the CEJ of the adjacent teeth.

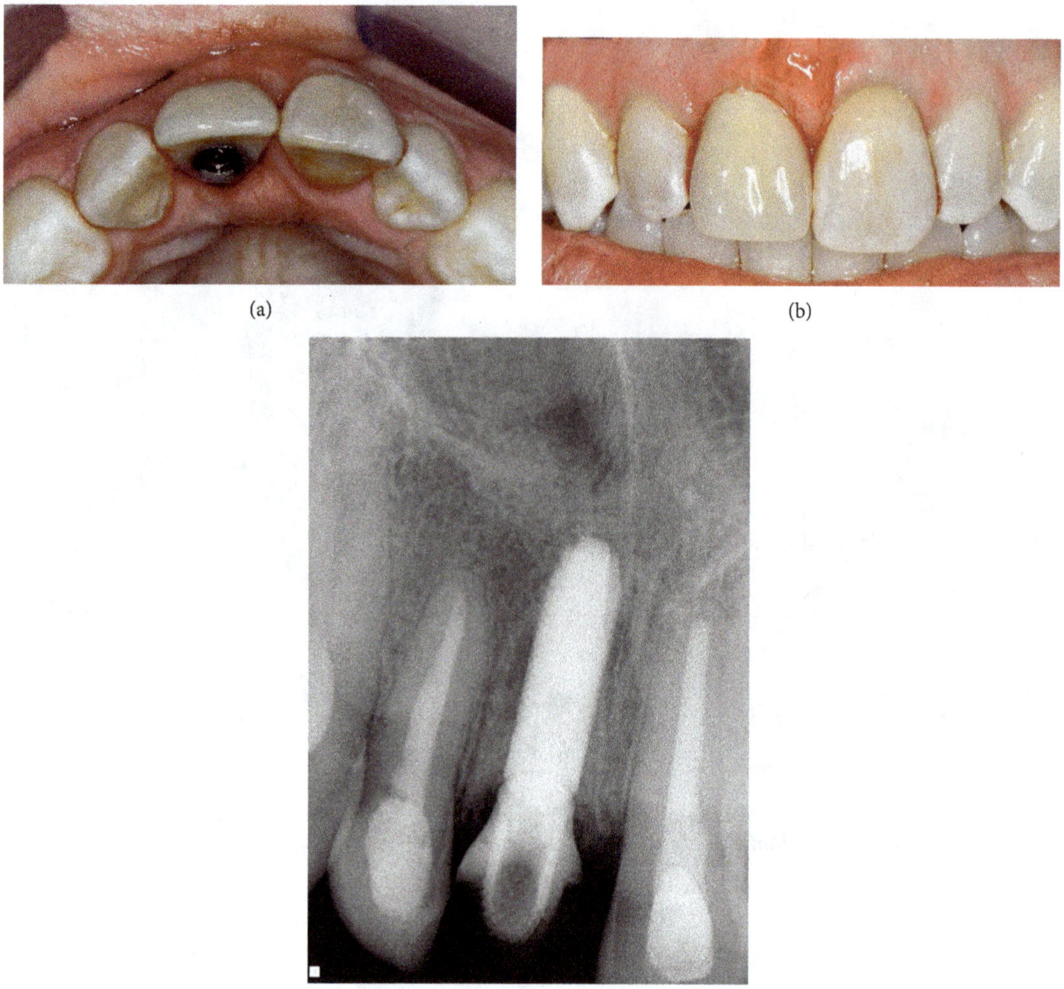

(a) (b) (c)

FIGURE 5: A customized screw-retained provisional crown was made chairside immediately after implant placement. (a) Occlusal view of the provisional crown showing the location of the implant at the cingulum region. (b) Facial view of the provisional crown displaying its subgingival contour conformed to support the soft tissue emergence profile. (c) A periapical radiograph was taken immediately after provisional crown restoration.

were followed for 6 months to 4 years after delivery of the definitive tooth restoration, and further long-term studies are still needed. In our case, the concept was not utilized at the time of surgery. We placed bone grafts in the gap between the implant fixture and buccal plate but did not fill it all the way up to the soft tissue level; nevertheless, our 6.5-year follow-up showed stable hard and soft tissue results.

The most challenging goal for implant therapy in the esthetic region is achieving soft and hard tissue stability over time. Midfacial mucosal recession has been one of the most commonly reported complications following immediate implant placement [52]. In the present case, multiple factors were considered to avoid a compromised outcome, and no recession was noted during 6.5 years of follow-up. It has been documented in the literature that anatomic factors associated with midfacial recession following immediate implant placement are the gingival biotype and the width of the keratinized mucosa [53]. More recession has been observed on implants placed in patients with a thin gingival biotype and narrow keratinized mucosa with a width less than 2 mm. A damaged facial bone wall also represents a significant risk factor for midfacial recession. Kan et al. reported that midfacial recessions greater than 1.5 mm were observed one year after immediate implant placement and provisionalization in 8.3% of tooth sockets with a narrow V-shaped facial bony defect exceeding 3 mm despite simultaneous guided bone regeneration and soft tissue grafting [26]. Furthermore, midfacial recession increased to 42.8% and 100% when the bony defect extended wider onto the mesial or distal aspect of the failing tooth (U-shaped) or adjacent teeth (UU-shaped), respectively. Staged reconstruction of unfavorable U- and UU-shaped facial bony defects followed by delayed implant placement was strongly recommended. Additionally, the position of the implant has consistently played an important role in the midfacial mucosal level [54]. Placing implants too buccally has been associated with more recession of the midbuccal mucosa. Immediate implant placement using a flapless approach also

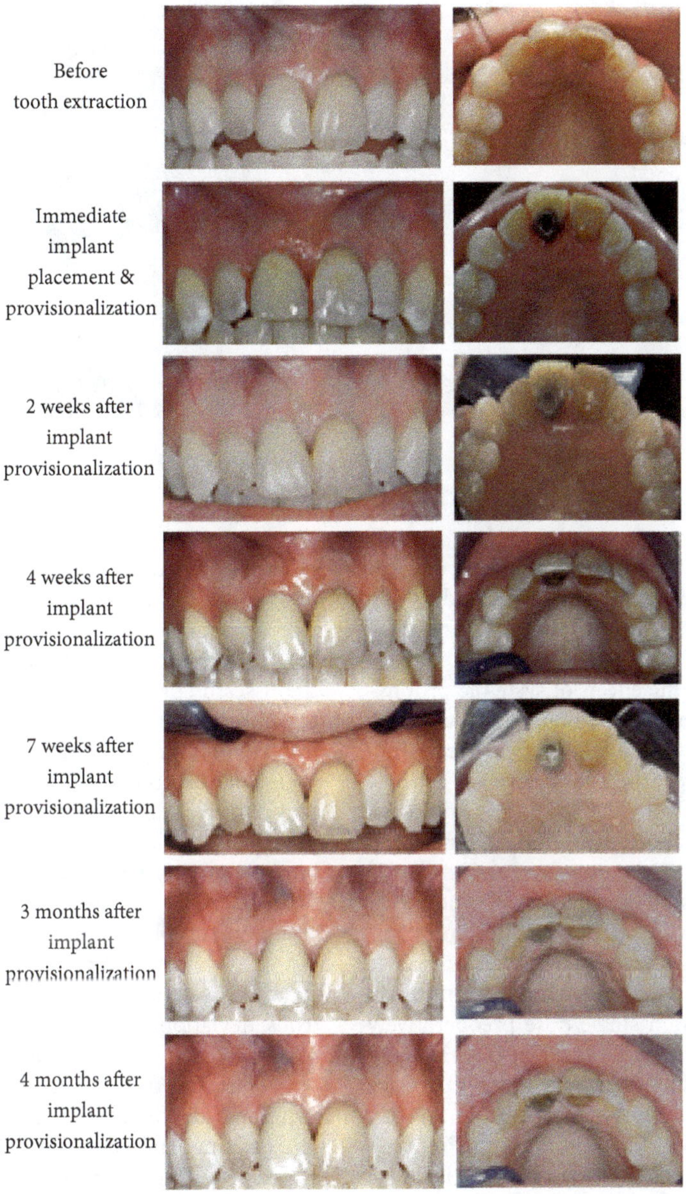

FIGURE 6: Clinical photos of tooth 11 before and after immediate implant provisionalization. During the 4-month follow-up period, the gingival tissue around implant was pink and healthy. The patient was satisfied with the esthetic outcome of the immediate implant provisionalization.

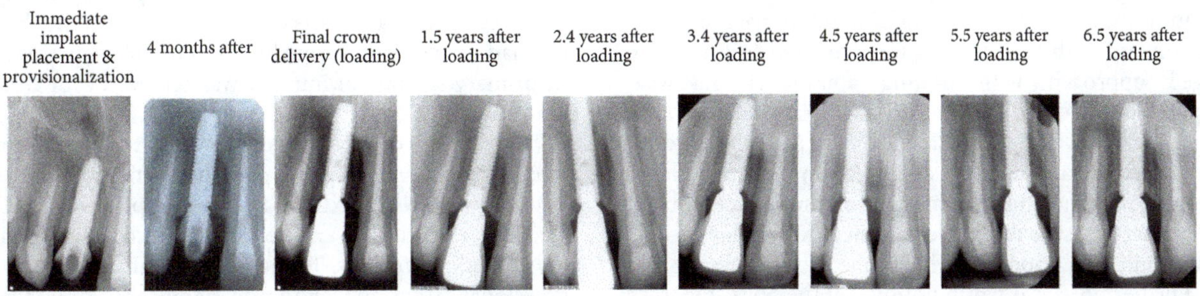

FIGURE 7: Periapical radiographs taken at immediate implant provisionalization and at various times during the 6.5-year recall period.

demonstrated an average of 0.89 mm less midfacial mucosal recession at 1 year after implant placement [55] compared to open-flap implant placement. Instant provisionalization of immediate single-tooth implants has also been shown to have 0.75 mm less midfacial recession in comparison with delayed restoration after 1 year [29].

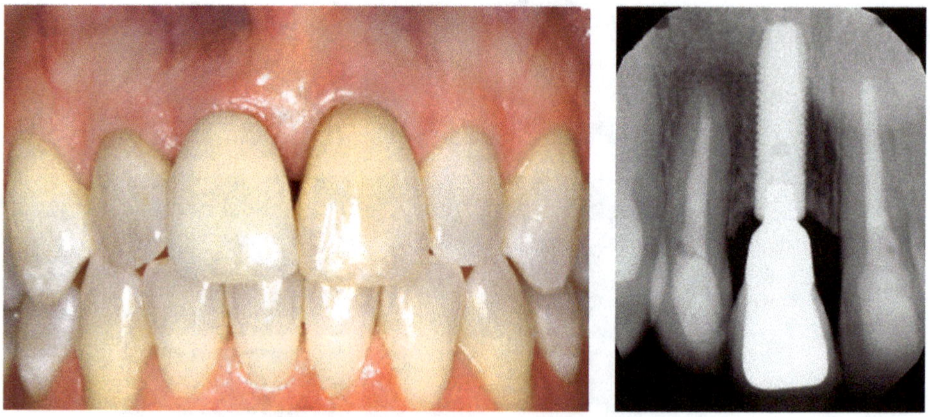

(a) (b)

Figure 8: (a) Clinical photo and (b) periapical radiograph of the implant at 6.5 years after loading.

In the present case, the patient was given 600 mg of Clindamycin one hour preoperatively followed by Clindamycin 300 mg four times a day postoperatively for 7 days. A Cochrane systemic review, including 6 randomized controlled clinical trials, assessed the effects of systemic prophylactic antibiotics at dental implant placement and found that there was no clear evidence whether postoperative antibiotics were beneficial. However, the routine use of a single dose of 2 g or 3 g prophylactic amoxicillin one hour preoperatively significantly reduces failure of dental implants [56]. On the other hand, a systematic review by Lang et al. [9] investigated 33 prospective studies where antibiotics were prescribed in immediate implant placement cases and compared subjects who had received a preoperative single dose of antibiotic prophylaxis (PreOP), postoperative antibiotic use of 5-7 days (PostOP), and a single dose preoperatively plus 5-7 days of postoperative antibiotics (PreOP + PostOP). Lower estimated annual failure rates were found in groups that were provided with a course of postoperative 5-7-day antibiotics (0.51% and 0.75% in PostOP and PreOP + PostOP, respectively, compared to 1.87% in PreOP). It was concluded that the regimen of antibiotic use affected the survival rate significantly as the duration of usage might have played an important role.

Similar clinical outcomes were found for submerged and nonsubmerged implants placed in fresh extraction sockets [57], indicating that there is no need to submerge the immediate implant with primary closure compared to a nonsubmerged approach with healing abutments. Likewise, comparable outcomes with regard to implant success rates and radiographic bone level stability were also observed for both immediate and delayed loading of immediately placed implants [58]. Therefore, submerging an immediate implant with primary closure did not lead to significant benefits over a nonsubmerged approach with immediate provisionalization. Furthermore, it is worth noting that the nonsubmerged approach demonstrated better attached gingiva and mucogingival junction (MGJ) harmony and fewer soft tissue adverse effects [57, 58]. Because primary closure results in coronal displacement of the MGJ and a decrease in the amount of buccal attached gingiva, apically positioned flaps at implant uncovering or further mucogingival surgery may be necessary to correct this problem.

Although only two-dimensional radiographs (periapical and panoramic) were taken before implant placement for the assessment of bone quantity, we strongly recommend the utilization of state-of-the-art technology such as virtual implant planning systems that integrate CBCT data to assess bone quantity and allow for greater predictability and accuracy of implant placement in the esthetic zone. Current technology also includes a digital workflow for computer-guided implant surgery which improves diagnostic capabilities and provides more precise and prosthetically driven planning and implant placement [59]. However, substantial errors can occur at each individual step and can accumulate, significantly impacting the final accuracy with potentially disastrous deviations from ideal implant placement [60]. It is always crucial to mitigate these risks through complete understanding of the guided implant surgery process, thorough and careful surgical technique, advanced comprehensive training, and adequate case preparation.

Above all, primary stability of the implant is the most important factor for immediate implant provisionalization. The torque at time of implant placement can be used as an indicator of initial stability. Ottoni et al. reported that an insertion torque greater than 32 Ncm is necessary for an implant restored with an immediate provisional crown [61]. They found that 9 out of 46 implants failed because they had an insertion torque of 20 Ncm. In the present case, the primary stability of implant was achieved with an insertion torque > 35 Ncm.

The purpose of this case report was to review the surgical steps of immediate implant placement and provisionalization following tooth extraction. Careful planning and case selection are critical to ensure implant success with satisfactory esthetic outcomes. Immediate implant placement and provisionalization appear to add significant advantages for the esthetically driven replacement of anterior teeth. This treatment strategy helps to preserve physiologic soft and hard tissue architecture and, therefore, predictably leads to excellent esthetic outcomes and patient satisfaction. The long-term success of this approach depends on the achievement of primary stability, and the immediate provisionalization must be designed to avoid any centric and eccentric contact during healing. Extraction using a flapless procedure followed by immediate implant placement and provisionalization without functional loading offers a predictable therapeutic option for single-tooth replacement in the esthetic zone.

References

[1] P. I. Brånemark, U. Breine, R. Adell, B. O. Hansson, J. Lindström, and Å. Ohlsson, "Intra-osseous anchorage of dental prostheses. I. Experimental studies," *Scandinavian Journal of Plastic and Reconstructive Surgery*, vol. 3, no. 2, pp. 81–100, 1969.

[2] P. I. Brånemark, B. O. Hansson, R. Adell et al., "Osseointegrated implants in the treatment of the edentulous jaw. Experience from a 10-year period," *Scandinavian Journal of Plastic and Reconstructive Surgery. Supplementum*, vol. 16, pp. 1–132, 1977.

[3] T. Lindh, J. Gunne, A. Tillberg, and M. Molin, "A meta-analysis of implants in partial edentulism," *Clinical Oral Implants Research*, vol. 9, no. 2, pp. 80–90, 1998.

[4] K. Heydenrijk, G. M. Raghoebar, H. J. A. Meijer, W. A. van der Reijden, A. J. van Winkelhoff, and B. Stegenga, "Two-part implants inserted in a one-stage or a two-stage procedure. A prospective comparative study," *Journal of Clinical Periodontology*, vol. 29, no. 10, pp. 901–909, 2002.

[5] H. J. Meijer, K. Heijdenrijk, and G. M. Raghoebar, "Mucosal and radiographic aspects during the healing period of implants placed in a one-stage procedure," *The International Journal of Prosthodontics*, vol. 16, no. 4, pp. 397–402, 2003.

[6] M. Esposito, M. G. Grusovin, Y. S. Chew, P. Coulthard, and H. V. Worthington, "Interventions for replacing missing teeth: 1- versus 2-stage implant placement," *Cochrane Database of Systematic Reviews*, vol. 3, article CD006698, 2009.

[7] M. Scacchi, B. R. Merz, and A. R. Schar, "The development of the ITI DENTAL IMPLANT SYSTEM. Part 2: 1998-2000: steps into the next millennium," *Clinical Oral Implants Research*, vol. 11, Supplement 1, pp. 22–32, 2000.

[8] M. Esposito, M. G. Grusovin, I. P. Polyzos, P. Felice, and H. V. Worthington, "Interventions for replacing missing teeth: dental implants in fresh extraction sockets (immediate, immediate-delayed and delayed implants)," *Cochrane Database of Systematic Reviews*, vol. 9, article CD005968, 2010.

[9] N. P. Lang, L. Pun, K. Y. Lau, K. Y. Li, and M. C. M. Wong, "A systematic review on survival and success rates of implants placed immediately into fresh extraction sockets after at least 1 year," *Clinical Oral Implants Research*, vol. 23, Supplement 5, pp. 39–66, 2012.

[10] B. E. Pjetursson, K. Tan, N. P. Lang, U. Bragger, M. Egger, and M. Zwahlen, "A systematic review of the survival and complication rates of fixed partial dentures (FPDs) after an observation period of at least 5 years," *Clinical Oral Implants Research*, vol. 15, no. 6, pp. 625–642, 2004.

[11] M. A. Atieh, A. G. T. Payne, W. J. Duncan, and M. P. Cullinan, "Immediate restoration/loading of immediately placed single implants: is it an effective bimodal approach?," *Clinical Oral Implants Research*, vol. 20, no. 7, pp. 645–659, 2009.

[12] N. Khzam, H. Arora, P. Kim, A. Fisher, N. Mattheos, and S. Ivanovski, "Systematic review of soft tissue alterations and esthetic outcomes following immediate implant placement and restoration of single implants in the anterior maxilla," *Journal of Periodontology*, vol. 86, no. 12, pp. 1321–1330, 2015.

[13] R. U. Koh, I. Rudek, and H. L. Wang, "Immediate implant placement: positives and negatives," *Implant Dentistry*, vol. 19, no. 2, pp. 98–108, 2010.

[14] J. Y. Kan, K. Rungcharassaeng, and J. Lozada, "Immediate placement and provisionalization of maxillary anterior single implants: 1-year prospective study," *The International Journal of Oral & Maxillofacial Implants*, vol. 18, no. 1, pp. 31–39, 2003.

[15] D. Buser, V. Chappuis, U. C. Belser, and S. Chen, "Implant placement post extraction in esthetic single tooth sites: when immediate, when early, when late?," *Periodontol 2000*, vol. 73, no. 1, pp. 84–102, 2017.

[16] D. M. Laskin, C. D. Dent, H. F. Morris, S. Ochi, and J. W. Olson, "The influence of preoperative antibiotics on success of endosseous implants at 36 months," *Annals of Periodontology*, vol. 5, no. 1, pp. 166–174, 2000.

[17] T. De Rouck, K. Collys, and J. Cosyn, "Single-tooth replacement in the anterior maxilla by means of immediate implantation and provisionalization: a review," *The International Journal of Oral & Maxillofacial Implants*, vol. 23, no. 5, pp. 897–904, 2008.

[18] D. Buser, W. Martin, and U. C. Belser, "Optimizing esthetics for implant restorations in the anterior maxilla: anatomic and surgical considerations," *The International Journal of Oral & Maxillofacial Implants*, vol. 19, Supplement, pp. 43–61, 2004.

[19] M. Al-Sabbagh, "Implants in the esthetic zone," *Dental Clinics of North America*, vol. 50, no. 3, pp. 391–407, 2006.

[20] W. Becker and M. Goldstein, "Immediate implant placement: treatment planning and surgical steps for successful outcome," *Periodontol 2000*, vol. 47, pp. 79–89, 2008.

[21] A. P. Saadoun and C. J. Landsberg, "Treatment classifications and sequencing for postextraction implant therapy: a review," *Practical Periodontics and Aesthetic Dentistry*, vol. 9, no. 8, pp. 933–941, 1997.

[22] C. H. Hammerle, S. T. Chen, and T. G. Wilson Jr., "Consensus statements and recommended clinical procedures regarding the placement of implants in extraction sockets," *The International Journal of Oral & Maxillofacial Implants*, vol. 19, Supplement, pp. 26–28, 2004.

[23] P. S. Wohrle, "Single-tooth replacement in the aesthetic zone with immediate provisionalization: fourteen consecutive case reports," *Practical Periodontics and Aesthetic Dentistry*, vol. 10, no. 9, pp. 1107–1114, 1998.

[24] H. de Bruyn, F. Raes, L. F. Cooper et al., "Three-years clinical outcome of immediate provisionalization of single Osseospeed™implants in extraction sockets and healed ridges," *Clinical Oral Implants Research*, vol. 24, no. 2, pp. 217–223, 2013.

[25] P. Mura, "Immediate loading of tapered implants placed in postextraction sockets: retrospective analysis of the 5-year clinical outcome," *Clinical Implant Dentistry and Related Research*, vol. 14, no. 4, pp. 565–574, 2012.

[26] J. Y. Kan, K. Rungcharassaeng, A. Sclar, and J. L. Lozada, "Effects of the facial osseous defect morphology on gingival dynamics after immediate tooth replacement and guided bone regeneration: 1-year results," *Journal of Oral and Maxillofacial Surgery*, vol. 65, no. 7, 7 Supplement 1, pp. 13–19, 2007.

[27] J. Y. Kan, K. Rungcharassaeng, J. L. Lozada, and G. Zimmerman, "Facial gingival tissue stability following immediate placement and provisionalization of maxillary anterior single implants: a 2- to 8-year follow-up," *The International Journal of Oral & Maxillofacial Implants*, vol. 26, no. 1, pp. 179–187, 2011.

[28] L. F. Cooper, F. Raes, G. J. Reside et al., "Comparison of radiographic and clinical outcomes following immediate provisionalization of single-tooth dental implants placed in healed alveolar ridges and extraction sockets," *The International Journal of Oral & Maxillofacial Implants*, vol. 25, no. 6, pp. 1222–1232, 2010.

[29] T. de Rouck, K. Collys, I. Wyn, and J. Cosyn, "Instant provisionalization of immediate single-tooth implants is essential to optimize esthetic treatment outcome," *Clinical Oral Implants Research*, vol. 20, no. 6, pp. 566–570, 2009.

[30] T. De Rouck, K. Collys, and J. Cosyn, "Immediate single-tooth implants in the anterior maxilla: a 1-year case cohort study on hard and soft tissue response," *Journal of Clinical Periodontology*, vol. 35, no. 7, pp. 649–657, 2008.

[31] P. Palattella, F. Torsello, and L. Cordaro, "Two-year prospective clinical comparison of immediate replacement vs. immediate restoration of single tooth in the esthetic zone," *Clinical Oral Implants Research*, vol. 19, no. 11, pp. 1148–1153, 2008.

[32] L. Canullo and G. Rasperini, "Preservation of peri-implant soft and hard tissues using platform switching of implants placed in immediate extraction sockets: a proof-of-concept study with 12- to 36-month follow-up," *The International Journal of Oral & Maxillofacial Implants*, vol. 22, no. 6, pp. 995–1000, 2007.

[33] A. Barone, L. Rispoli, I. Vozza, A. Quaranta, and U. Covani, "Immediate restoration of single implants placed immediately after tooth extraction," *Journal of Periodontology*, vol. 77, no. 11, pp. 1914–1920, 2006.

[34] I. J. De Kok, S. S. Chang, J. D. Moriarty, and L. F. Cooper, "A retrospective analysis of peri-implant tissue responses at immediate load/provisionalized microthreaded implants," *The International Journal of Oral & Maxillofacial Implants*, vol. 21, no. 3, pp. 405–412, 2006.

[35] R. Cornelini, F. Cangini, U. Covani, and Wilson TG Jr, "Immediate restoration of implants placed into fresh extraction sockets for single-tooth replacement: a prospective clinical study," *The International Journal of Periodontics & Restorative Dentistry*, vol. 25, no. 5, pp. 439–447, 2005.

[36] M. Groisman, W. M. Frossard, H. M. Ferreira, L. M. de Menezes Filho, and B. Touati, "Single-tooth implants in the maxillary incisor region with immediate provisionalization: 2-year prospective study," *Practical Procedures & Aesthetic Dentistry*, vol. 15, no. 2, pp. 115–22, 124; quiz 126, 2003.

[37] K. W. Slagter, L. den Hartog, N. A. Bakker, A. Vissink, H. J. A. Meijer, and G. M. Raghoebar, "Immediate placement of dental implants in the esthetic zone: a systematic review and pooled analysis," *Journal of Periodontology*, vol. 85, no. 7, pp. e241–e250, 2014.

[38] G. Juodzbalys, D. Sakavicius, and H. L. Wang, "Classification of extraction sockets based upon soft and hard tissue components," *Journal of Periodontology*, vol. 79, no. 3, pp. 413–424, 2008.

[39] J. Y. K. Kan, K. Rungcharassaeng, M. Deflorian, T. Weinstein, H. L. Wang, and T. Testori, "Immediate implant placement and provisionalization of maxillary anterior single implants," *Periodontol 2000*, vol. 77, no. 1, pp. 197 212, 2018.

[40] C. E. Nemcovsky, Z. Artzi, O. Moses, and I. Gelernter, "Healing of marginal defects at implants placed in fresh extraction sockets or after 4-6 weeks of healing. A comparative study," *Clinical Oral Implants Research*, vol. 13, no. 4, pp. 410–419, 2002.

[41] G. Juodzbalys, "Instrument for extraction socket measurement in immediate implant installation," *Clinical Oral Implants Research*, vol. 14, no. 2, pp. 144–149, 2003.

[42] W. P. Nordland and D. P. Tarnow, "A classification system for loss of papillary height," *Journal of Periodontology*, vol. 69, no. 10, pp. 1124–1126, 1998.

[43] A. Monje, V. Chappuis, F. Monje et al., "The critical peri-implant buccal bone wall thickness revisited: an experimental study in the beagle dog," *The International Journal of Oral & Maxillofacial Implants*, vol. 34, no. 6, pp. 1328–1336, 2019.

[44] J. Y. Kan, P. Roe, K. Rungcharassaeng et al., "Classification of sagittal root position in relation to the anterior maxillary osseous housing for immediate implant placement: a cone beam computed tomography study," *The International Journal of Oral & Maxillofacial Implants*, vol. 26, no. 4, pp. 873–876, 2011.

[45] M. G. Araujo and J. Lindhe, "Dimensional ridge alterations following tooth extraction. An experimental study in the dog," *Journal of Clinical Periodontology*, vol. 32, no. 2, pp. 212–218, 2005.

[46] M. G. Araujo, F. Sukekava, J. L. Wennstrom, and J. Lindhe, "Ridge alterations following implant placement in fresh extraction sockets: an experimental study in the dog," *Journal of Clinical Periodontology*, vol. 32, no. 6, pp. 645–652, 2005.

[47] M. G. Araujo, E. Linder, and J. Lindhe, "Bio-Oss collagen in the buccal gap at immediate implants: a 6-month study in the dog," *Clinical Oral Implants Research*, vol. 22, no. 1, pp. 1–8, 2011.

[48] S. T. Chen, I. B. Darby, and E. C. Reynolds, "A prospective clinical study of non-submerged immediate implants: clinical outcomes and esthetic results," *Clinical Oral Implants Research*, vol. 18, no. 5, pp. 552–662, 2007.

[49] S. J. Chu, M. A. Salama, H. Salama et al., "The dual-zone therapeutic concept of managing immediate implant placement and provisional restoration in anterior extraction sockets," *The Compendium of Continuing Education in Dentistry*, vol. 33, no. 7, pp. 524–632, 2012.

[50] D. P. Tarnow, S. J. Chu, M. A. Salama et al., "Flapless postextraction socket implant placement in the esthetic zone: part 1. The effect of bone grafting and/or provisional restoration on facial-palatal ridge dimensional change-a retrospective cohort study," *The International Journal of Periodontics & Restorative Dentistry*, vol. 34, no. 3, pp. 323–331, 2014.

[51] S. J. Chu, M. A. Salama, D. A. Garber et al., "Flapless postextraction socket implant placement, part 2: the effects of bone grafting and provisional restoration on peri-implant soft tissue height and thickness- a retrospective study," *The International Journal of Periodontics & Restorative Dentistry*, vol. 35, no. 6, pp. 803–809, 2015.

[52] G. H. Lin, H. L. Chan, and H. L. Wang, "Effects of currently available surgical and restorative interventions on reducing midfacial mucosal recession of immediately placed single-tooth implants: a systematic review," *Journal of Periodontology*, vol. 85, no. 1, pp. 92–102, 2014.

[53] C. D. Evans and S. T. Chen, "Esthetic outcomes of immediate implant placements," *Clinical Oral Implants Research*, vol. 19, no. 1, pp. 73–80, 2008.

[54] S. T. Chen, I. B. Darby, E. C. Reynolds, and J. G. Clement, "Immediate implant placement postextraction without flap elevation," *Journal of Periodontology*, vol. 80, no. 1, pp. 163–172, 2009.

[55] F. Raes, J. Cosyn, E. Crommelinck, P. Coessens, and H. de Bruyn, "Immediate and conventional single implant treatment in the anterior maxilla: 1-year results of a case series on hard and soft tissue response and aesthetics," *Journal of Clinical Periodontology*, vol. 38, no. 4, pp. 385–394, 2011.

[56] M. Esposito, M. G. Grusovin, and H. V. Worthington, "Interventions for replacing missing teeth: antibiotics at dental implant placement to prevent complications," *Cochrane Database of Systematic Reviews*, vol. 7, article CD004152, 2013.

[57] L. Cordaro, F. Torsello, and M. Roccuzzo, "Clinical outcome of submerged vs. non-submerged implants placed in fresh extraction sockets," *Clinical Oral Implants Research*, vol. 20, no. 12, pp. 1307–1313, 2009.

[58] O. Shibly, A. Kutkut, N. Patel, and J. M. Albandar, "Immediate implants with immediate loading vs. conventional loading: 1-year randomized clinical trial," *Clinical Implant Dentistry and Related Research*, vol. 14, no. 5, pp. 663–671, 2012.

[59] L. Rutten and P. Rutten, "Creating high-end esthetic results in implantology using a digital workflow and interdisciplinary planning - from a master technician viewpoint," *The International Journal of Esthetic Dentistry*, vol. 15, no. 4, pp. 402–426, 2020.

[60] D. N. Tatakis, H. H. Chien, and A. O. Parashis, "Guided implant surgery risks and their prevention," *Periodontol 2000*, vol. 81, no. 1, pp. 194–208, 2019.

[61] J. M. Ottoni, Z. F. Oliveira, R. Mansini, and A. M. Cabral, "Correlation between placement torque and survival of single-tooth implants," *The International Journal of Oral & Maxillofacial Implants*, vol. 20, no. 5, pp. 769–776, 2005.

5

Soft Tissue Dehiscence Associated with a Titanium Patient-Specific Implant: A Prosthetic Solution as an Alternative to Soft Tissue Grafting

Sharaf Eldeen M. Abbas and Mohamed A. ElKhashab

Department of Prosthodontics, Faculty of Dentistry, Cairo University, Cairo, Egypt

Correspondence should be addressed to Sharaf Eldeen M. Abbas; sharafeldeen.m.abbas@gmail.com

Academic Editor: Konstantinos Michalakis

Patients. This clinical report describes the detailed prosthodontic management of a 23-year-old male patient suffering from soft tissue complication following the placement of a 3d-printed titanium patient-specific implant. This implant was implemented simultaneously with the resection of a calcifying cystic odontogenic tumor related to the maxillary arch. Later, soft tissue dehiscence and implant exposure were encountered with subsequent food impaction, infection, and pus discharge. The treatment plan was to fabricate removable partial denture. The prosthesis was planned to be retained by bar and clip attachment on the patient-specific implant side, while on the other side, the removable prosthesis was allowed to engage two abutments with an embrasure clasp assembly in addition to covering the palatal tissues to offer protection for the soft tissue dehiscence against food impaction. *Discussion.* Soft tissue dehiscence and implant exposure are among the frequently reported complications associated with the patient-specific implant. The resulting infection complicates the prognosis of the implemented implant and necessitates, in some occasions, its removal. The selection of the removable prosthesis to cover soft tissue dehiscence was a conservative alternative to the implant removal as it protects the exposed titanium surface from food impaction while maintaining the implant functionality. *Conclusion.* Three-year follow-up showed complete resolution of the patient's complaints while fulfilling the patient's aesthetic and functional demands and indicates that the use of detachable overlay prosthesis could be one of the proposed treatment options.

1. Introduction

For the past decade, facially anchored osseointegrated implants [1] and free flaps [2] have been universally accepted for maxillofacial reconstruction after surgical resection. Such advances in surgical reconstruction techniques have brought up the possibility of complete defect closure and provide a good foundation for further intraoral implant placement, allowing the patients to experience more life-like restorations [3–5]. Unfortunately, because of the insufficient bone after tumor ablation surgeries, these reconstructive procedures often require demanding surgeries which are associated with distant site morbidity and prolonged healing period [3].

Thanks to the advances in imaging modalities and manufacturing techniques, patient-specific implants (PSIs) have been proposed to overcome the pitfalls associated with the previously mentioned treatment options [6]. Initially, PSI was fabricated by the prebending of metal plates over 3d-printed models [7]. Unfortunately, with this technique, PSI suffered from metal plate weakness following bending [8, 9]. Recently, patient-specific implants have been manufactured by 3d printing of metals with remarkable improvement in their strength and adaptation [6, 10–12].

Ciocca and his colleagues in 2012 [10] were the first to use 3d-printed PSI manufactured by direct laser metal sintering for mandibular reconstruction in conjunction with a free flap. Since then, several authors have reported the utilization of 3d-printed PSI for the restoration of maxillary and mandibular defects, alone or in conjunction with free flaps [12–14], using different materials such as titanium and polyether ether ketone (PEEK) [15].

Despite all attempts to enhance bone and soft tissue healing around PSI restorations, soft tissue dehiscence and recurrent infection have been reported in multiple studies [12, 16, 17]. The problem with these complications is the difficulty in management and recurrence that may necessitate, in some cases, the removal of the whole assembly [12]. In this case report, the authors describe a prosthetic solution to salvage a successfully anchored PSI associated with extensive soft tissue dehiscence.

2. Methodology

A 23-year-old male patient was referred to F.G. Maxillofacial Prosthodontics Unit, Faculty of Dentistry, Cairo University, after undergoing surgical installation of patient-specific implant (PSI) following surgical resection of calcifying cystic odontogenic tumor CCOT related to the left maxillary arch extending to the orbital floor. The patient was complaining of hygiene-related complications as a result of extensive soft tissue exposure of PSI.

Upon reviewing the patient's records, it was revealed that the patient was scheduled for total maxillary resection with simultaneous reconstruction using patient-specific implant prosthesis. With the aid of digital software (Materialise Mimics, Leuven, Belgium), the lesion was virtually resected, and the patient-specific implant was designed with maximum extensions engaging the whole maxillary surfaces superiorly, medially, and laterally. Finally, the implant was printed with an EBM machine (Arcam AB, Stockholm, Sweden) into medical grade 23 titanium Ti–6Al–4V, after then it was subjected to several procedures of surface treatment and sterilization.

At the time of tumor ablation surgery, the implant was installed and stabilized using 2 mm grade 5 titanium fixation screws on the facial bones extending from the orbital floor to the palate. The palatal soft tissue on the tumor side was preserved and used as a soft tissue drape to cover the implant surface. The patient did not receive any adjunctive treatment before or after the surgery. Three months after the surgery, the patient received a five-unit fixed partial denture restoration cemented on the extruding metal posts.

Six months later, the patient presented with soft tissue dehiscence and complained of frequent food impaction and persistent foul odor. The patient was instructed to rinse daily with antiseptic mouthwash till the condition subsides in addition to strict routine oral hygiene measures. By the age of 23, implant surface exposure has become more extensive, and the patient suffered further hygiene-related complications. Accordingly, the surgical team decided to remove the PSI. However, based on the patient's desire not to get involved in further surgical interventions, he was referred to our team for possible prosthetic management.

Data collected from patient interviewing, clinical examination, and radiographic imaging revealed that PSI was stable, functioning, and pain-free. Titanium surface was exposed and extending along the buccal and palatal surfaces of PSI (Figure 1).

Diagnostic impressions were made for both arches by using irreversible hydrocolloid impression material (Cavex CA37 normal set, Haarlem, Netherlands). A customized maxillary tray was fabricated by using cold cure acrylic resin (Acrostone, cold cure special tray material, Cairo, Egypt) over which the definitive impression was made by using a two-step impression technique with rubber base impression material (Zhermack, Zetaplus & Oranwash VL, Badia Polesine RO, Italy). Inlay pattern resin (Duralay, Reliance, Edmonton, Canada) supported with metal wires was used to pour the metal posts portion of the impression while the rest was completed with a hard stone. Modeling wax (Cavex, Set Up Hard, Haarlem, Netherlands) occlusion rims were adjusted intraorally over cold-cured acrylic resin record bases, and the interocclusal record was made at maximum intercuspation. Casts were mounted on a semiadjustable articulator with a face bow transfer. Wax-up of acrylic teeth was done for diagnostic and treatment planning purposes.

A condensation silicon putty index was adapted on the buccal aspect of the diagnostic wax-up to determine the prosthetic space available occlusocervically and buccolingually, the size of the artificial teeth, and its relation to the metal posts. A 20 mm interocclusal distance was revealed with sufficient space between the metal posts and the buccal aspect of the future teeth. Surveying of the cast was carried out to determine the amount of natural teeth undercuts, guiding planes, and the potential path of insertion.

Accordingly, the plan was to exclude the middle post and fabricate a bar and clip attachment connecting the two distant metal posts to support a partial overdenture. Embrasure clasp assembly was planned on the maxillary right first molar and maxillary right second premolar to aid for retention, support, and bracing in addition to a palatal plate extending over the palatal surfaces of the maxillary right first premolar, canine, lateral incisor, and central incisor and maxillary left central incisor to the areas of soft tissue dehiscence at the patient-specific implant. Before the execution of the planned prosthetic management, the patient was instructed to follow comprehensive oral hygiene measures. These instructions included rinsing with chlorhexidine mouthwash twice daily and brushing the PSI with soft toothbrush and chlorhexidine gel. Besides that, he was encouraged to use dental floss between the remaining teeth and tooth brushing by soft toothbrush twice daily. Empirical antibiotics were prescribed to the patient to manage any possible infection at the exposure site.

The planned mouth preparation was executed as follows: cutting the middle post by using a transmetal bur under copious irrigation, preparation of a mesial occlusal rest seat on the maxillary right first molar, and preparation of a distal occlusal rest seat on the maxillary right second premolar. Additionally, there is a mesial guiding plane on the proximal surface of the maxillary left central incisor. The definitive impression and mounting procedures were performed with the same techniques mentioned earlier. OT Bar multiuse (Rhein83, Bologna, Italy) was waxed, cast into Co-Cr, and then cemented on the metal posts (Figure 2). Metal

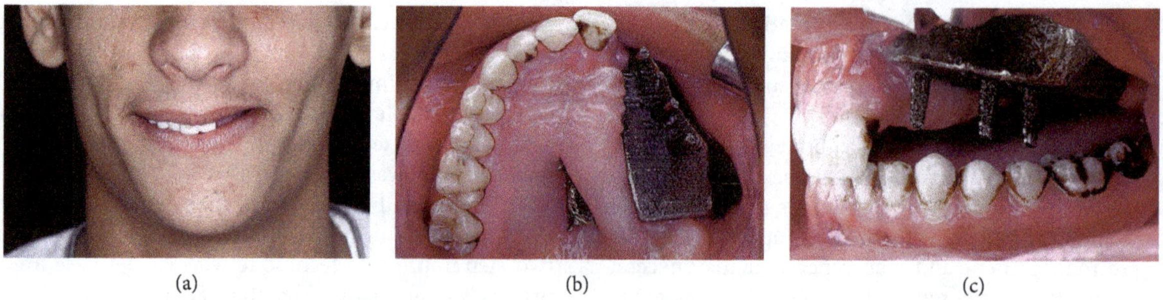

FIGURE 1: Initial situation when the patient presented to the prosthodontic clinic: (a) extraoral frontal view, (b) intraoral occlusal view, and (c) intraoral left side view.

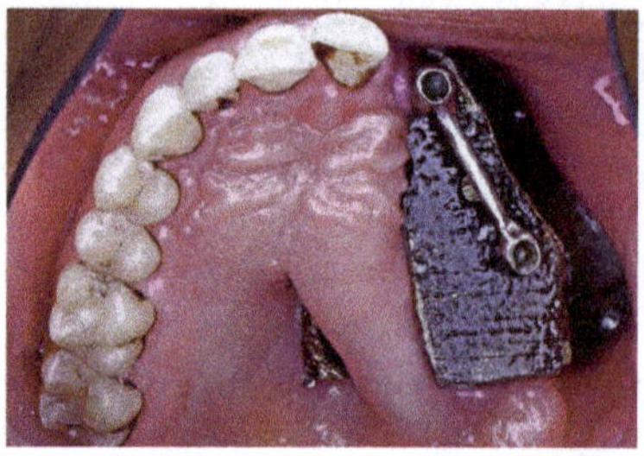

FIGURE 2: Intraoral occlusal view showing the bar after cementation.

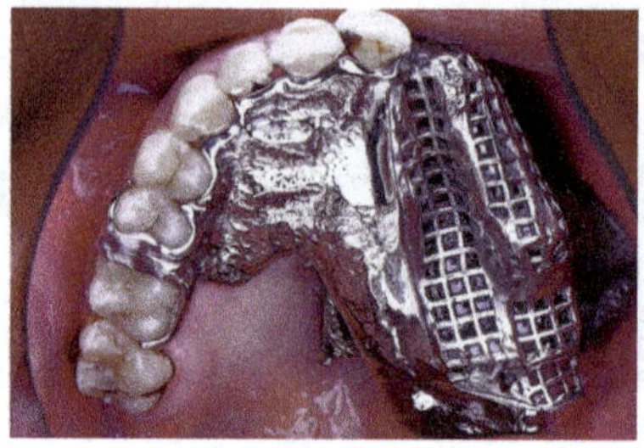

FIGURE 3: Intraoral occlusal view showing metal framework try-in.

framework partial denture was cast and tried intraorally to check for the fit, stability, support, retention, and path of insertion (Figure 3).

The trial setting of artificial acrylic teeth guided with the diagnostic wax-up was done and tried intraorally. The approved wax trial tooth arrangement was flasked and packed by using heat-cured acrylic resin (Acrostone, heat cure denture base material, Cairo, Egypt). At the time of bar and clip attachment pickup, the undercut beneath the bar was blocked out using a putty consistency rubber base to avoid the unnecessary flow of the pickup material. After insulating the polished surface of the prosthesis, a doughy mix of cold-cure acrylic resin was added to the intaglio surface, and a medium retention clip was picked up under maximum intercuspation.

The prosthesis was finished and polished, and the patient received instructions regarding prosthesis insertion, removal, and maintenance (Figure 4). Additionally, strict daily oral hygiene measures were instructed to the patient. These instructions include tooth brushing with soft toothbrush daily, cleaning the prosthesis and PSI immediately after food ingestion, and rinsing with chlorhexidine for 14 consecutive days monthly.

The patient was recalled monthly for the first year and every three months during the following years. During this period, the patient received professional intraoral cleaning and debridement every 3 months. After 3 years of follow-up, no signs or symptoms of hygiene-related complications were observed clinically or radiographically (Figure 5). Additionally, the patient reported complete resolution of previously mentioned complaints as well as significant satisfaction with the aesthetics and function of the prosthesis.

3. Discussion

Surgical reconstruction is nowadays considered a well-accepted treatment modality for the rehabilitation of oral defects, and it is achieved either by using free grafts, zygomatic implants, or patient-specific implants. Advances in volumetric imaging and 3d planning before the ablation surgery allow the surgeons to make more accurate decisions regarding the procedure and give the chance to manufacture personalized implants with the help of additive manufacturing technology to fit more readily during surgery.

In this patient, the implant was 3d printed from Ti6Al4V. The surfaces of PSI facing the bone were subjected to sandblasting and chemical treatment procedures in an attempt to enhance osseointegration, while the surfaces facing the soft tissue were left unpolished after the 3d printing procedure. Although it was hypothetically claimed that the unpolished surface facing the soft tissue would decrease the possibility of its dehiscence [11], our patient suffered from extensive soft tissue dehiscence with subsequent food impaction and bad odor. This sort of complication has been documented previously by several authors [12, 16, 17]. Rendenbach et al. [17] studied the placement of PSI in conjunction with free flaps and reported plate exposure in 29.7% of CAD/CAM plates. Similarly, Mounir et al. [12] described the removal of three mandibular PSIs placed immediately following benign tumor removal due to failure of management and resolution of infection.

Despite the several attempts to manage the condition by medication, debridement, and daily oral hygiene measures, the soft tissue complications were persistent and bothersome to the patient. Custom implant removal was the first line of treatment proposed by the surgical team. Accordingly, an

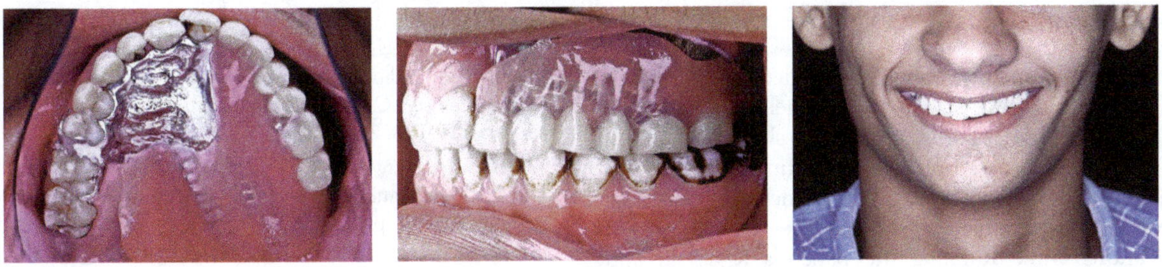

(a) (b) (c)

FIGURE 4: After prosthesis insertion: (a) intraoral occlusal view, (b) intraoral left side view, and (c) extraoral frontal view.

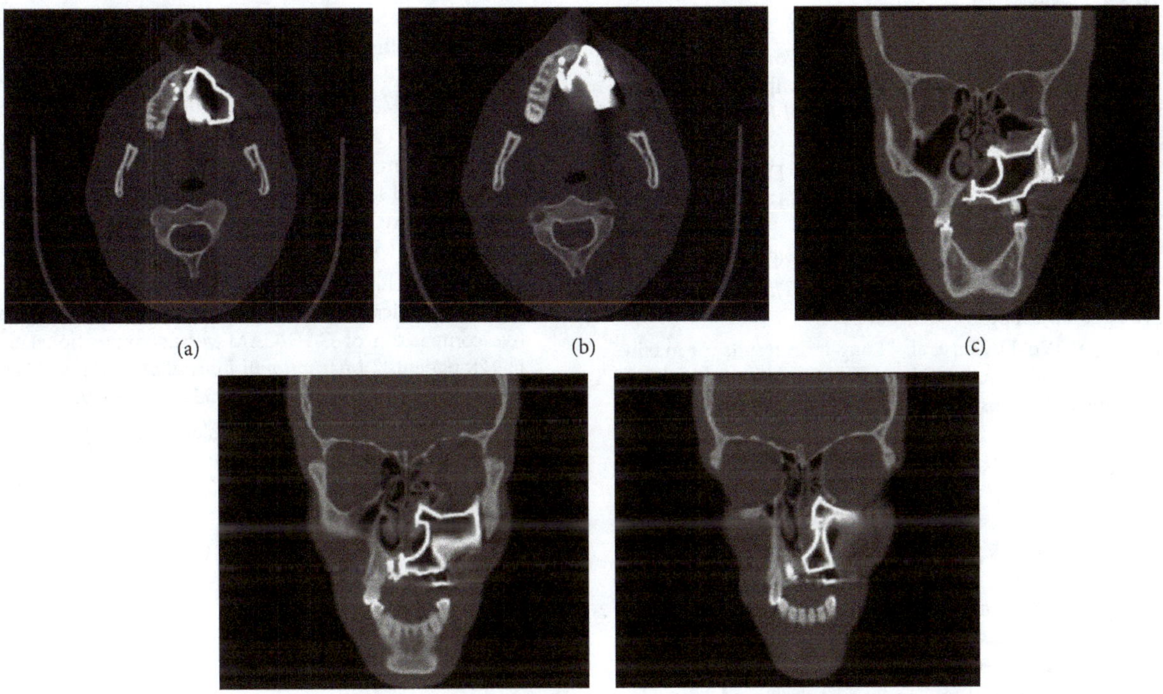

(a) (b) (c)

(d) (e)

FIGURE 5: Computed tomography after 3 years of follow-up: (a, b) axial cuts and (c–e) coronal cuts.

immediate restoration of the resultant surgical defect was addressed either using immediate surgical obturator or surgical reconstruction. Several authors [5] have suggested the use of osteomyocutaneous free graft with subsequent implant placement as a reliable option which allows implant insertion using flapless or open flap technique. An alternative conservative prosthetic option was recommended by the prosthetic team based on the patient preference to overcome the soft tissue dehiscence problem and eliminate the need for implant removal. The removable prosthesis was selected for this case to fully cover the remaining palatal tissues and the area of soft tissue defect at the implant site to avoid food impaction during function and to allow full access for proper oral cleaning procedures. Retention and support of the prosthesis were primarily derived from PSI and the remaining teeth with no support derived from the soft tissue.

On the intact side, the removable prosthesis was allowed to engage two abutments with an embrasure clasp assembly in addition to covering the palatal tissues to offer cross arch stabilization. On the implant side, the presence of enough prosthetic space enabled the use of a bar and clip attachment, which fulfilled the high retention demands in comparison to other attachment systems [18].

The main limitation associated with the chosen treatment option is the lack to provide a permanent soft tissue closure but rather preventing food impaction which is highly dependent on the patient compliance. The patient was instructed to follow strict oral hygiene measures; however, it was not anticipated to experience significant food impactions beneath this rigid design unlike soft tissue-supported ones. Another addressed concern is the need for continuous follow-up clinically and radiographically to ensure the patient's compliance and to detect early signs of possible complications. The possibility of discarding the prosthesis and the removal of the PSI was also discussed with the patient in case of the development of persistent infection, which could be life threatening.

4. Conclusion

Patient-specific implants may be regarded successful in terms of fixation and stability; nevertheless, soft tissue dehiscence is a serious complication that should be anticipated and managed early during the treatment. The use of detachable overlay prosthesis can be considered a promising solution to conservatively overcome the hygiene-related complications while fulfilling the patient's aesthetic and functional demands.

References

[1] S. Hackett, B. El-Wazani, and C. Butterworth, "Zygomatic implant-based rehabilitation for patients with maxillary and mid- facial oncology defects: a review," *Oral Diseases*, vol. 27, no. 1, pp. 27–41, 2021.

[2] A. Vincent, J. Burkes, F. Williams, and Y. Ducic, "Free flap reconstruction of the maxilla," *Seminars in Plastic Surgery*, vol. 33, no. 1, pp. 30–37, 2019.

[3] J. S. Brown and R. J. Shaw, "Reconstruction of the maxilla and midface: introducing a new classification," *The Lancet Oncology*, vol. 11, no. 10, pp. 1001–1008, 2010.

[4] W. Huang, Y. Wu, D. Zou et al., "Long-term results for maxillary rehabilitation with dental implants after tumor resection," *Clinical Implant Dentistry and Related Research*, vol. 16, no. 2, pp. 282–291, 2014.

[5] S. M. Meloni, M. Tallarico, G. De Riu et al., "Guided implant surgery after free-flap reconstruction: four-year results from a prospective clinical trial," *Journal of Cranio-Maxillo-Facial Surgery*, vol. 43, no. 8, pp. 1348–1355, 2015.

[6] M. F. Huang, D. Alfi, J. Alfi, and A. T. Huang, "The use of patient-specific implants in oral and maxillofacial surgery," *Oral and Maxillofacial Surgery Clinics of North America*, vol. 31, no. 4, pp. 593–600, 2019.

[7] J. T. Lambrecht and F. Brix, "Individual skull model fabrication for craniofacial surgery," *The Cleft Palate Journal*, vol. 27, no. 4, pp. 382–385, 1990.

[8] F. Wilde, K. Winter, K. Kletsch, K. Lorenz, and A. Schramm, "Mandible reconstruction using patient-specific pre-bent reconstruction plates: comparison of standard and transfer key methods," *International Journal of Computer Assisted Radiology and Surgery*, vol. 10, no. 2, pp. 129–140, 2015.

[9] M. J. H. Witjes, R. H. Schepers, and J. Kraeima, "Impact of 3D virtual planning on reconstruction of mandibular and maxillary surgical defects in head and neck oncology," *Current Opinion in Otolaryngology & Head and Neck Surgery*, vol. 26, no. 2, pp. 108–114, 2018.

[10] L. Ciocca, S. Mazzoni, M. Fantini, F. Persiani, C. Marchetti, and R. Scotti, "CAD/CAM guided secondary mandibular reconstruction of a discontinuity defect after ablative cancer surgery," *Journal of Cranio-Maxillo-Facial Surgery*, vol. 40, no. 8, pp. e511–e515, 2012.

[11] M. Mounir, M. Atef, A. Abou-Elfetouh, and M. M. Hakam, "Titanium and polyether ether ketone (PEEK) patient-specific sub-periosteal implants: two novel approaches for rehabilitation of the severely atrophic anterior maxillary ridge," *International Journal of Oral and Maxillofacial Surgery*, vol. 47, no. 5, pp. 658–664, 2018.

[12] M. Mounir, A. Abou-ElFetouh, W. ElBeialy, and R. Mounir, "Patient-specific alloplastic endoprosthesis for reconstruction of the mandible following segmental resection: a case series," *Journal of Cranio-Maxillo-Facial Surgery*, vol. 48, no. 8, pp. 719–723, 2020.

[13] A. Sutradhar, J. Park, D. Carrau, T. H. Nguyen, M. J. Miller, and G. H. Paulino, "Designing patient-specific 3D printed craniofacial implants using a novel topology optimization method," *Medical & Biological Engineering & Computing*, vol. 54, no. 7, pp. 1123–1135, 2016.

[14] W. W. Wong and M. C. Martin, "Reconstruction of extended orbitomaxillectomy and hemimandibulectomy defects with fibula flaps and patient-specific implants," *The Journal of Craniofacial Surgery*, vol. 27, no. 2, pp. 380–384, 2016.

[15] S. Järvinen, J. Suojanen, E. Kormi et al., "The use of patient specific polyetheretherketone implants for reconstruction of maxillofacial deformities," *Journal of Cranio-Maxillo-Facial Surgery*, vol. 47, no. 7, pp. 1072–1076, 2019.

[16] M. Rana, S. J. Chin, T. Muecke et al., "Increasing the accuracy of mandibular reconstruction with free fibula flaps using functionalized selective laser-melted patient-specific implants: a retrospective multicenter analysis," *Journal of Cranio-Maxillo-Facial Surgery*, vol. 45, no. 8, pp. 1212–1219, 2017.

[17] C. Rendenbach, C. Steffen, H. Hanken et al., "Complication rates and clinical outcomes of osseous free flaps: a retrospective comparison of CAD/CAM versus conventional fixation in 128 patients," *International Journal of Oral and Maxillofacial Surgery*, vol. 48, no. 9, pp. 1156–1162, 2019.

[18] T. Trakas, K. Michalakis, K. Kang, and H. Hirayama, "Attachment systems for implant retained overdentures: a literature review," *Implant Dentistry*, vol. 15, no. 1, pp. 24–34, 2006.

6

Guided Bone Regeneration of an Atrophic Maxilla using Heterologous Cortical Lamina

Carlos Polis-Yanes,[1] Carla Cadenas-Sebastián,[1] Patricia Gual-Vaqués,[1] Raúl Ayuso-Montero,[1,2] Antoni Marí-Roig,[2,3] and José López-López[2,4]

[1]*School of Dentistry, University of Barcelona, University Campus of Bellvitge, Barcelona, Spain*
[2]*Oral Health and Masticatory System Group (Bellvitge Biomedical Research Institute) IDIBELL, University of Barcelona, L'Hospitalet de Llobregat, Barcelona, Spain*
[3]*Department of Maxillofacial Surgery, University Hospital of Bellvitge, Catalonia, Spain*
[4]*Department of Odontostomatology, Faculty of Medicine and Health Sciences (Dentistry), Odontological Hospital University of Barcelona, University of Barcelona, Spain*

Correspondence should be addressed to José López-López; 18575jll@gmail.com

Academic Editor: Jamil Awad Shibli

Alloplastic dental implants are currently the best way to replace lost teeth. In order to achieve good function and prognosis of dental implants, having bone and soft tissue to support them is necessary. When the amount of bone left is not enough to ensure the outcome of the implant, techniques such as shorts implants, zygomatic implants, or guided bone regeneration have been used. Even though autologous bone is mostly the "gold standard," other biomaterials such as xenografts have led to the reduction of the morbidity of treatments and to the improvement of the regeneration technique outcomes. We present a clinical case of severe atrophy of the maxilla in which we used different types of biomaterials: heterologous cortical lamina, xenograft and autologous bone, and microscrews.

1. Introduction

Teeth are necessary organs for the development of a normal life that take part in different functions such as the mastication, phonation, and maintenance of a functional orofacial anatomy. In the absence of the teeth, dental implants have proved to be efficient to replace lost teeth. In order to ensure the long-term function of dental implants, most studies confirm the importance of having and maintaining a good peri-implant bone and enough soft tissue (gingiva) [1].

When the amount of bone is not enough to place dentals implants, sometimes the professional has to use techniques of guided bone regeneration (GBR), bone distraction, sinus elevation technique, block grafts, or implant alternatives (short implants, zygomatic implants, etc.) [1]. Throughout the years, several techniques have been proposed to regenerate the alveolar bone. The type of bone defect or the prosthetic rehabilitation and the preferences of the clinician and the patient will lead the professional to choose one technique or the other. In terms of bone condition, the ideal material for bone regeneration should be osteoconductive, osteoinductive, and osteogenic. Autologous bone is still nowadays the gold standard because of its osteogenic property [2, 3]. Besides the bone condition, other bone properties that should be expected from a regeneration biomaterial are (i) osteoconduction; (ii) stimulation of neoangiogenesis; (iii) absence of antigenic, teratogenic, or carcinogenic reactions; (iv) boundless source; (v) satisfactory and stable structure; (vi) minimum morbidity and complications; (vii) hydrophilic nature; (viii) easy handling; and (ix) low cost [3].

GBR uses barrier membranes, including resorbable and nonresorbable membranes, in order to avoid certain types of nonosteogenic, rapidly proliferating cells, such as epithelial and connective tissue cells. And on the contrary, these barriers promote the growth of slow-maturing tissue made by osteoforming cells. These membranes are considered an essential part of the GBR treatment [3]. Among the different membrane systems and materials that have been proposed, any membrane should meet the following criteria: biocompatibility, integration by the soft tissues, clinical manageability, ability to isolate the bone graft, and adequate mechanical and physical properties [4, 5].

2. Objective

The aim of this study is to report a clinical case that deals with bone regeneration, using as a bone graft a mixture of autogenous and xenogenic bone and as a membrane a cortical bone lamina fixed with microscrews.

3. Case Presentation

A 45-year-old man presented mobility of a metal-ceramic fixed bridge in the second quadrant after ten years of function (Figure 1). After the exploration, the bridge and the pillar teeth were considered nonrestorable, and in the Cone Beam Computed Tomography (CBCT), a severe loss of the alveolar bone of the second quadrant is evidenced (Figure 2). Extraction of the teeth, regeneration of the lost bone, and following rehabilitation with dental implants were the agreed treatment.

After the teeth extraction, we decided to wait a month to make sure the healing and stabilization of the soft tissues (Figure 3). In a second surgery stage, we performed a regenerative surgery. A heterologous cortical lamina (OsteoBiol Lamina® from Tecnoss®) was decided to be used instead of other barrier techniques, such as a titanium mesh, because of its resorbable condition. The surgical procedure was as follows: (i) mucoperiosteal flap with vertical discharges (Figures 4, 5(a), and 5(b)); (ii) periosteoplasty techniques; (iii) decorticalization and bone collection with a bone scraper (Figure 6); (iv) palatal fixation of the cortical lamina with two microscrews—no previously hydration is needed—(Figure 7); (v) filling of the defect with mixture of autologous bone and heterologous bone (OsteoBiol Apatos® from Tecnoss®) (Figures 8 and 9); (vi) vestibular fixation with two microscrews; (vii) mesial sealing with heterologous collagen membrane and resorbable polyglycolic acid suture (Serapid® from Serag-Wiessner®) (Figure 10); (viii) hydration with physiological serum prior to suture; and (ix) closure by first intention, without tensions, using monofilament suture, with simple and mattress stiches that relieve stress when inflamed (Figure 11). Immediately after the surgery, a control orthopantomography was taken (Figure 12).

The treatment was performed under antibiotic coverage with amoxicillin 750 mg (1 comp/8 h) 24 h before and 7 days later. 11.4 mg of postoperative intramuscular (gluteus) betamethasone was administered right after the surgery and dexketoprofen 25 mg (1 comp/8 h) was prescribed for 5 days. An antiseptic topical gel based on 0.2% chlorhexidine (one application every 8 hours) for 10 days was given to the patient. After 10 days, the suture was removed. During the bone healing period, the patient was told not to use any removable prostheses.

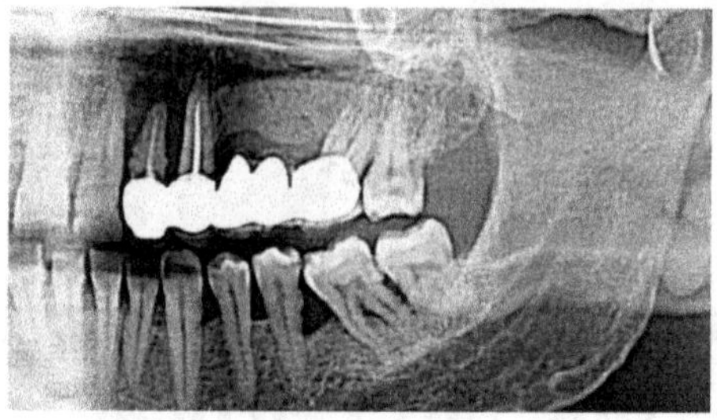

FIGURE 1: Orthopantomography previous to dental extractions.

Six months after the surgery, a new CBCT was performed (Figure 13) for implant planning and three internal conical connection implants (Galimplant® Sarria, Lugo, Spain) were placed in positions 22, 24, and 25 (3.5 × 12 mm, 4 × 12 mm, and 4.5 × 8 mm, respectively), with an insertion torque of 30 N/cm (Figures 14 and 15). During this surgery, the microscrews that blocked the implant placement were removed.

After four months, prosthetic rehabilitation was made by another clinician in another dental office, and thus, the follow-up was not possible.

4. Discussion

During the first 24 hours after regenerative surgery, the spaces are filled by a blood clot that is then resorbed by macrophages and neutrophils and replaced by granulation tissue rich in mesenchymal stem cells and blood vessels, allowing nutrients and cells to reach the site, forming the osteoid tissue [5]. Following this, there is a deposit of minerals and then bone tissue is formed, around which the bone continues to mature into lamellar bone. We will find bone neoformation about four weeks after the GBR. The main role of the membranes is to exclude connective and epithelial tissue cells from the area of the wound to be regenerated and also to create and maintain the space in which the pluripotent and osteogenic cells are free to migrate [5].

Currently, barrier membranes are considered necessary to carry out a successful GBR. Nevertheless, the potential hostage and cell activation of each membrane has not been established yet [4].

Elgali et al. [4] reported in their meta-analysis and systematic review soft tissue complications in approximately 16.8% of cases—with no significant differences between resorbable and nonresorbable membranes—concluding that the importance of the soft tissue management is essential to improve the prognosis of regenerative techniques. On the other hand, Soldatos et al. [5] concluded in their study the importance of the professional being familiar with the properties of the membranes to be used. For example, in case of height regeneration, the authors suggest the use of a nonresorbable membrane. The study concludes that the exposure of the membranes is a risk for the GBR and that the nonabsorbable membranes have a higher risk of exposure. Both membranes offer an adequate function as long as screws or the membrane itself is used to stabilize the GBR [5].

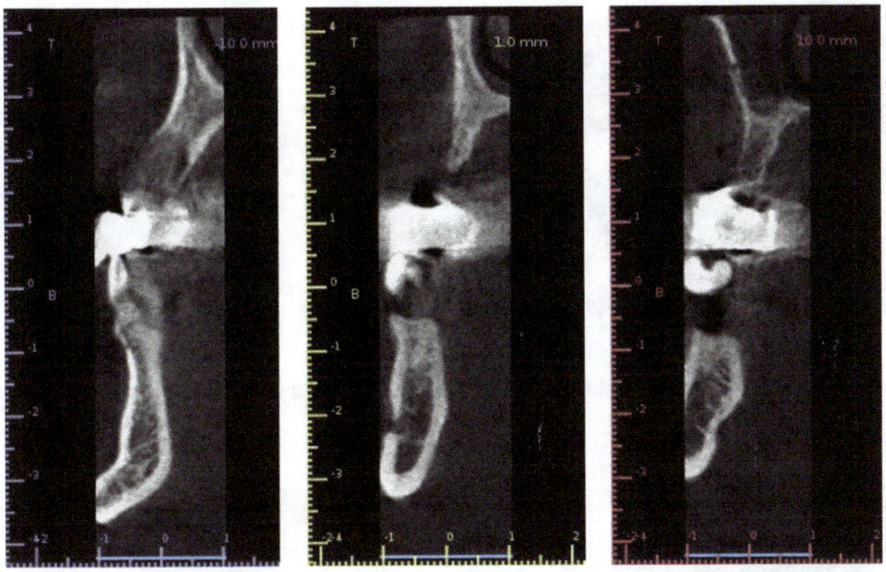

(a) (b) (c)

Figure 2: Previous CBCT.

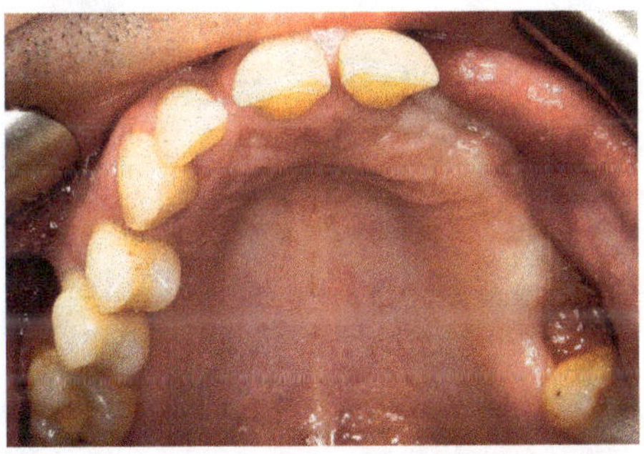

Figure 3: Intraoral view before guided bone regeneration surgery.

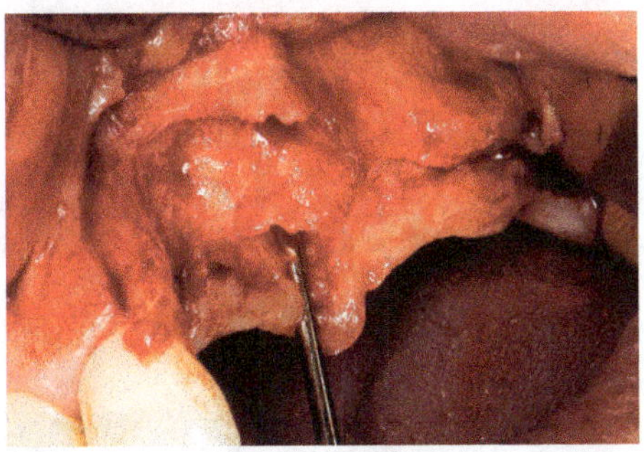

Figure 4: Appearance of the bone after the mucoperiosteal flap. There is a great defect with horizontal and vertical component, not suitable for the placement of dental implants.

Titsinides et al. [3] concluded in their review that an ideal biomaterial for bone regeneration has not yet been developed. Nevertheless, predictable results are obtained with allografts, xenografts, and alloplastic grafts, all of them with their advantages and disadvantages [3]. The use of cortical autologous bone as a scaffold has been shown to be successful in a 10-year retrospective study by Khoury and Hanser [6] with 3328 patients treated with blocks for the management of atrophic bone ridges [6].

Bone blocks, cortical laminas, and membranes of heterologous cortical bone have been used successfully in recent years in plastic and maxillofacial surgery due to their plasticity and biocompatible structure and may be a less morbid alternative to distance block grafting. Being all of them resorbable is another advantage when compared to nonresorbable membranes and barriers [7, 8].

Regarding the use of cortical laminas, Lopez et al. [9] carried out GBR techniques with heterologous cortical lamina in twenty patients with thirty implants, twenty-four of them placed in the same surgery. They suggest the use of cortical laminas as a valid alternative to conventional GBR techniques. Similarly, Amr et al. [10] did a study on 14 patients who needed horizontal ridge regeneration. The sample was divided into two groups: group 1 underwent autologous block graft surgery while group 2 underwent heterologous cortical lamina surgery. Clinically and radiographically, there were no statistically significant differences between the two groups in terms of the bucco-lingual bone gain. The histomorphometric analysis showed no statistically significant differences between the mean areas of the bone surface in the two groups and no statistically significant difference between the mean osteoblast counts in the two groups. Thus, the authors concluded that xenogenic cortical lamina can be successfully used to increase the horizontal alveolar ridge as an alternative to the autogenous block bone graft.

Showing a different application for the cortical lamina, Scarano et al. [11] performed a randomized clinical study among twenty patients in which two different techniques of maxillary sinus floor elevation with lateral window were used. In one group, heterologous cortical lamina was used and the sinus cavity was not filled up with any biomaterial.

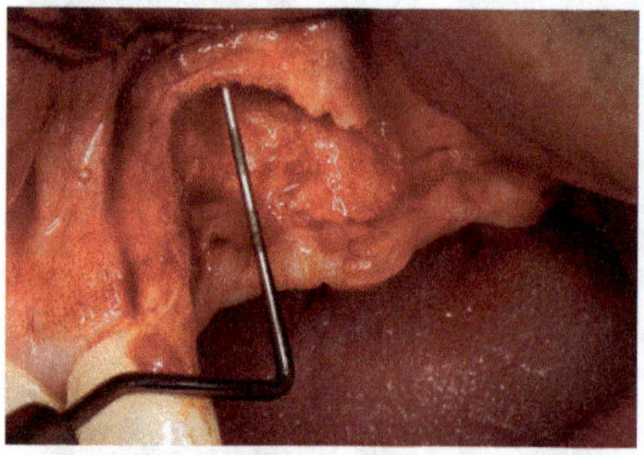

(a)

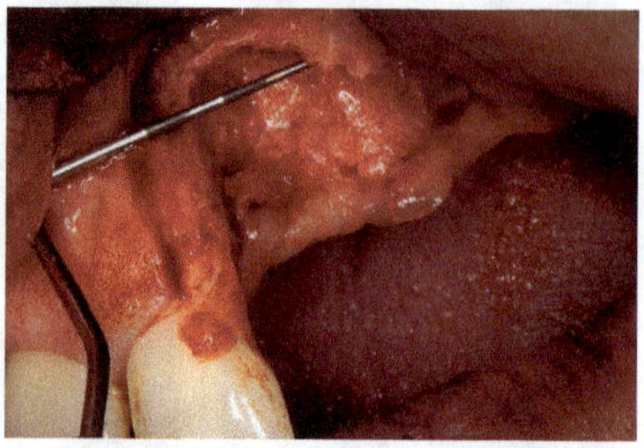

(b)

FIGURE 5: (a) Measurement of the most severe defect. (b) Measurement of the most severe defect.

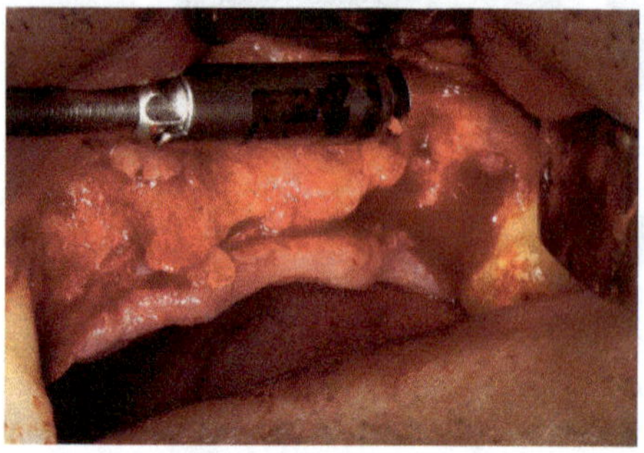

FIGURE 6: Bone scraper to decorticate and to collect autologous bone.

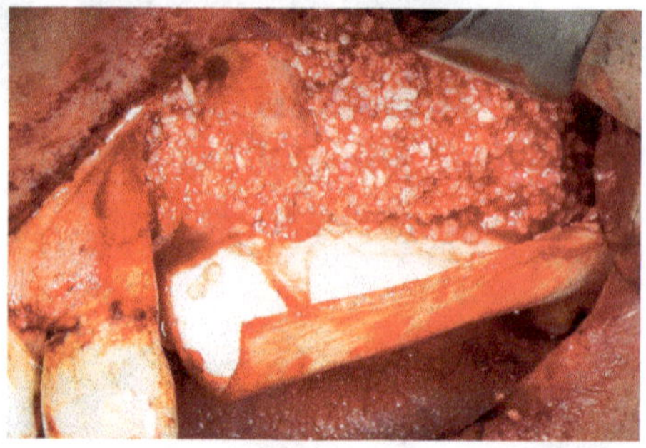

FIGURE 9: Bone graft placing taking as buccal limit the canine eminence conserved from the patient.

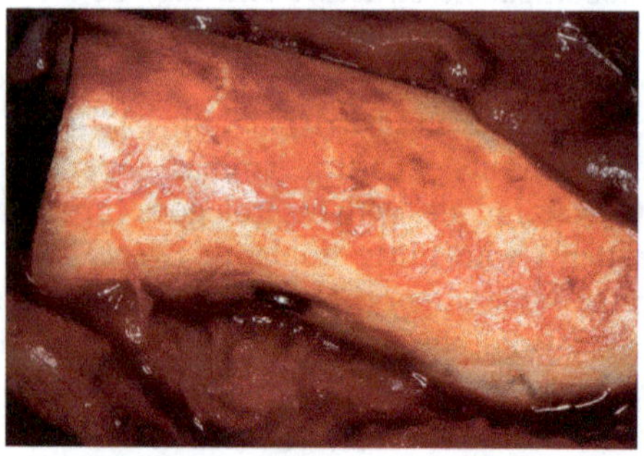

FIGURE 7: Cortical lamina fixed with microscrews in its palatal portion.

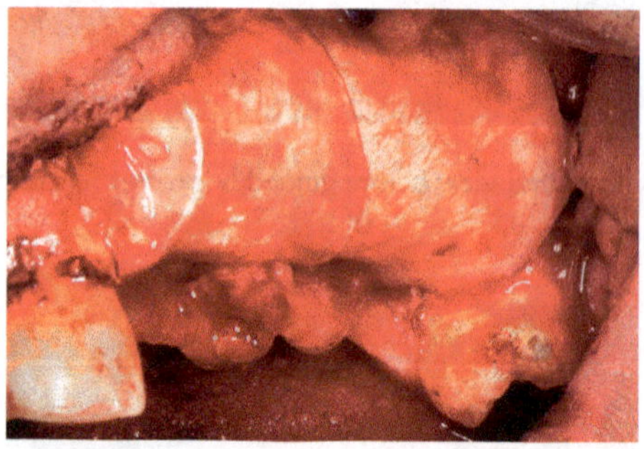

FIGURE 10: Buccal fixation of the cortical bone membrane with microscrews and covering of the mesial defect with a resorbable collagen membrane.

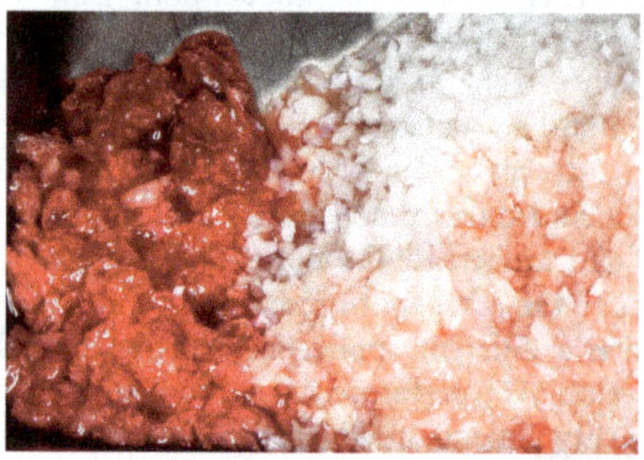

FIGURE 8: Autologous bone and xenograft.

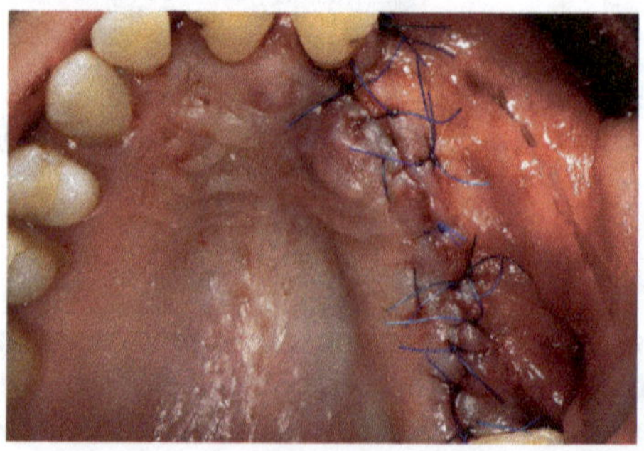

FIGURE 11: Suture without stress using monofilament suture.

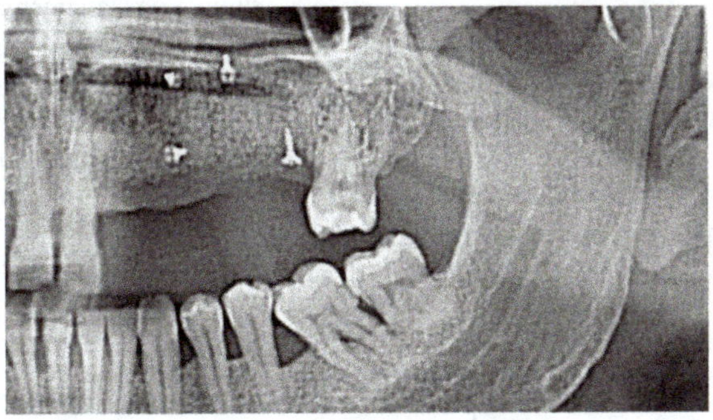

FIGURE 12: Orthopantomography after the surgery.

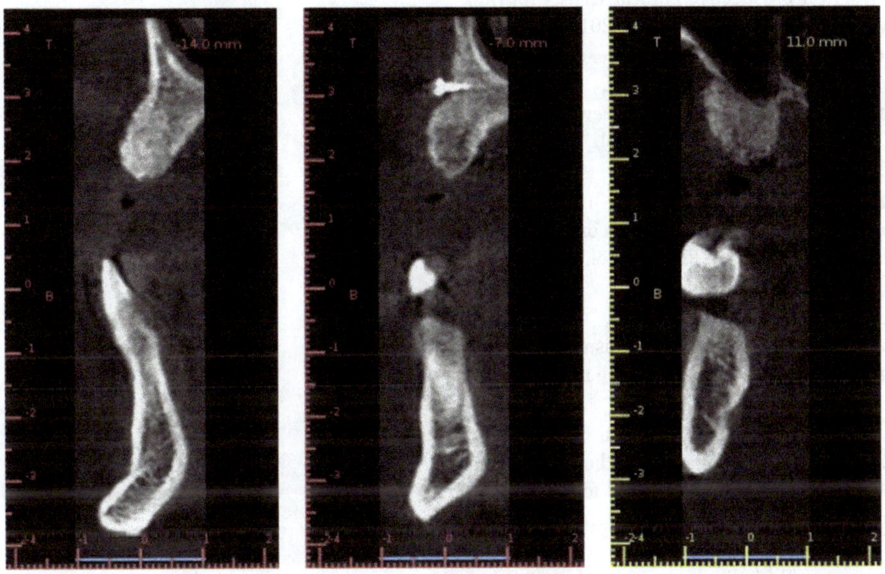

(a) (b) (c)

FIGURE 13: CBCT after healing during 6 months.

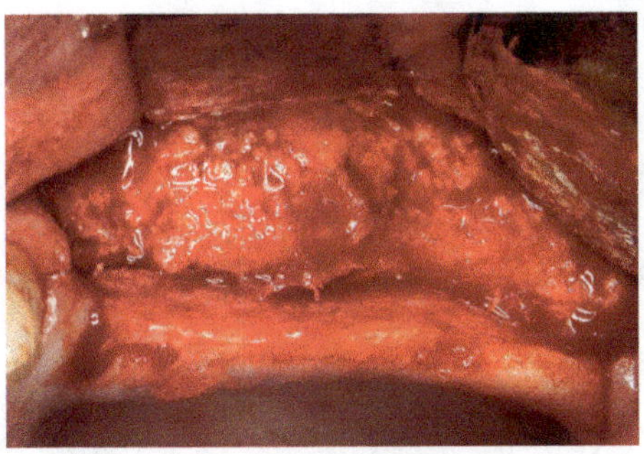

FIGURE 14: Clinical view after 6 months during dental implant placement.

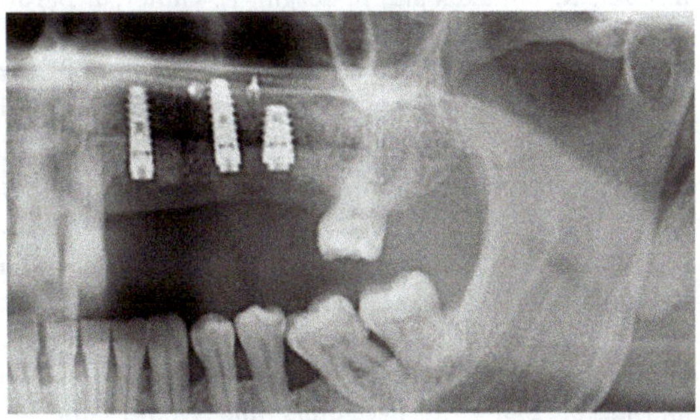

FIGURE 15: Orthopantomography after dental implant surgery.

In the second group, 100% porcine heterologous bone graft was used to fill up the sinus cavity plus a porcine heterologous collagen membrane to close the window. This study showed that the use of heterologous cortical laminas is a valid technique for the mechanical support of the sinus membrane. CBCT outcomes showed that the material was not completely resorbed after six months, although it was clearly integrated into the bone.

In another publication from the same authors, Scarano et al. [12] used the heterologous cortical lamina for the mechanical support of sinus membranes to preserve the space in sinus floor augmentation and showed the importance of Cone Beam Computed Tomography to evaluate the efficacy of this GBR technique.

5. Conclusion

Heterologous cortical laminas used as barrier membranes are a plausible biomaterial to be used in GBR, especially in medium and large bone defects. Long-term randomized studies are necessary to compare cortical lamina properties with other types of membranes that are more commercialized and well-studied.

References

[1] A. Monje, H. L. Chan, J. H. Fu, F. Suarez, P. Galindo-Moreno, and H. L. Wang, "Are short dental implants (<10 mm) effective? A meta-analysis on prospective clinical trials," *Journal of Periodontology*, vol. 84, no. 7, pp. 895–904, 2013.

[2] P. Gual-Vaqués, C. Polis-Yanes, A. Estrugo-Devesa, R. Ayuso-Montero, A. Marí-Roig, and J. López-López, "Autogenous teeth used for bone grafting: a systematic review," *Medicina Oral Patología Oral y Cirugia Bucal*, vol. 23, no. 1, pp. e112–e119, 2018.

[3] S. Titsinides, G. Agrogiannis, and T. Karatzas, "Bone grafting materials in dentoalveolar reconstruction: a comprehensive review," *Japanese Dental Science Review*, vol. 55, no. 1, pp. 26–32, 2019.

[4] I. Elgali, O. Omar, C. Dahlin, and P. Thomsen, "Guided bone regeneration: materials and biological mechanisms revisited," *European Journal of Oral Sciences*, vol. 125, no. 5, pp. 315–337, 2017.

[5] N. K. Soldatos, P. Stylianou, V. P. Koidou, N. Angelov, R. Yukna, and G. E. Romanos, "Limitations and options using resorbable versus nonresorbable membranes for successful guided bone regeneration," *Quintessence International*, vol. 48, no. 2, pp. 131–147, 2017.

[6] F. Khoury and T. Hanser, "Mandibular bone block harvesting from the retromolar region: a 10-year prospective clinical study," *International Journal of Oral and Maxillofacial Implants*, vol. 30, no. 3, pp. 688–697, 2015.

[7] B. Ozel, K. Findikcioglu, B. Sezgin, K. Guney, I. Barut, and S. Ozmen, "A new option for the reconstruction of orbital floor defects with heterologous cortical bone," *Journal of Cranio-Maxillo-Facial Surgery*, vol. 43, no. 8, pp. 1583–1588, 2015.

[8] C. Rinna, G. Reale, E. Foresta, and M. C. Mustazza, "Medial orbital wall reconstruction with swine bone cortex," *Journal of Craniofacial Surgery*, vol. 20, no. 3, pp. 881–884, 2009.

[9] M. A. Lopez, M. Andreasi Bassi, L. Confalone, F. Carinci, Z. Ormianer, and D. Lauritano, "The use of resorbable cortical lamina and micronized collagenated bone in the regeneration of atrophic crestal ridges: a surgical technique. Case series," *Journal of Biological Regulators and Homeostatic Agents*, vol. 30, 2 Suppl 1, pp. 81–85, 2016.

[10] A. E. H. Amr, K. A. Abdel Ghaffar, H. A. Abuel-Ela, and E. S. Abd Elhamid, "Xenogenic flexible bone lamina graft: a successful alternative to the autogenous onlay bone block graft in alveolar ridge augmentation: a clinical, radiographic and histological evaluation," *Journal of Dental Treatment and Oral Care*, vol. 1, p. 104, 2017.

[11] A. Scarano, P. S. de Oliveira, T. Traini, and F. Lorusso, "Sinus membrane elevation with heterologous cortical lamina: a randomized study of a new surgical technique for maxillary sinus floor augmentation without bone graft," *Materials*, vol. 11, no. 8, article 1457, 2018.

[12] A. Scarano, G. Murmura, F. Mastrangelo, F. Lorusso, A. Greco Lucchina, and F. Carinci, "A novel technique to prevent sinus membrane collapse during maxillary sinus floor augmentation without bone graft: technical note," *Journal of Biological Regulators and Homeostatic Agents*, vol. 32, no. 6, pp. 1589–1592, 2018.

7

Stability of Tissue Augmented with Deproteinized Bovine Bone Mineral Particles Associated with Implant Placement in Anterior Maxilla

David Buntoro Kamadjaja[1,2] **Ni Putu Mira Sumarta,**[1] **and Andra Rizqiawan**[1]

[1]*Department of Oral and Maxillofacial Surgery, Faculty of Dental Medicine, Universitas Airlangga, Surabaya, Indonesia*
[2]*Stem Cell Research and Development Center, Universitas Airlangga, Surabaya, Indonesia*

Correspondence should be addressed to David Buntoro Kamadjaja; david-b-k@fkg.unair.ac.id

Academic Editor: Luis M. J. Gutierrez

Background. Implant placement in defective anterior maxilla poses a great challenge regarding functional and aesthetic outcomes. Therefore, it requires predictable alveolar ridge augmentation. Deproteinized bovine bone mineral (DBBM) particle has commonly been used for bone grafting. However, it is associated with low resorption rates which potentially compromise the outcome of horizontal augmentation in conjunction with implant placement. *Aims.* This study is aimed at evaluating the stability of tissue augmented with DBBM particle associated with implant placement in the anterior maxilla. *Materials and Methods.* The inclusive criteria consist of patients being treated with guided bone regeneration (GBR) incorporating the use of DBBM particles with either a simultaneous or staged approach. The parameters analyzed include the implant survival rate, post-GBR clinical stability based on tissue resorption level, and the tissue stability between simultaneous and staged approaches. Statistical analysis using Mann-Whitney test is performed with significance determined at p value < 0.05. *Results.* Seventeen patients with 23 implant placements satisfy the criteria for this study. Simultaneous approach is adopted in 18 (78.3%) implants and a staged approach in 5 (21.7%) implants. The implant survival rate is 100%. The evaluation of horizontal tissue stability reveals a low resorption level in 19 (82.6%) implants, while moderate and high resorption levels are found in 3 (13.0%) and 1 (4.3%) implants, respectively. The statistical analysis shows that the simultaneous approach produces significantly ($p = 0.005$) lower resorption level compared to the staged approach. *Conclusion.* Horizontal ridge augmentation using DBBM particles associated with implant placement in the anterior maxilla produces good clinical stability. The stability appears to be higher in the simultaneous approach compared to the staged approach.

1. Introduction

Nowadays, increasing numbers of patients are seeking dental implant treatment due to its high success rate which poses significant challenges to clinicians dealing with such treatment. One such challenge in implant placement is tissue deficiency in the anterior maxilla leading to functional, structural, and aesthetic compromises which require horizontal ridge augmentation [1, 2].

Guided bone regeneration technique has been widely employed in horizontal augmentation [3] for which autogenous bone graft has represented the gold standard graft material. However, autogenous bone graft has been associated with limited donor sources and donor site morbidity [4]. Therefore, bone substitutes are now preferred since they permit minimally invasive surgery.

Deproteinized bovine bone mineral (DBBM) particle is a natural bone substitute with good osteoconductive properties which has been shown to achieve impressive results in various experimental and clinical studies [5–8]. However, DBBM has also been associated with very low degradation rates with the result that defect healing is characterized by graft particles being integrated within the new bone, rather than by complete replacement with new bone or bone regeneration

[9]. This clinical study attempts to evaluate the stability of tissue augmented with DBBM particle in conjunction with implant placement in the anterior maxilla.

2. Subjects and Methods

This retrospective study evaluates patients treated with bone grafting procedures in conjunction with implant placement at the Outpatient Clinic, Dental Hospital, Universitas Airlangga, Surabaya, between July 2010 and August 2018. The study is certified to be ethically cleared by Health Research Ethical Clearance, Faculty of Dental Medicine, Universitas Airlangga (number 288/HRECC. FODM/VIII/2018). The inclusion criteria for the study are as follows. Patients present with reduced horizontal dimension of the alveolar ridge after extraction of the anterior maxillary teeth requiring implant replacement (Figure 1(a)). The augmentation procedure for alveolar defects consists of guided bone regeneration using DBBM particles and resorbable membrane through either a simultaneous approach in which the bone grafting procedure and implant placements are performed at the same time or a staged approach in which the bone grafting procedure is conducted prior to implant placement. Excluded from this study are patients with poorly controlled diabetes mellitus who fail to return for review or whose cases involve the application of bone graft other than DBBM. Informed consent forms are signed by all patients regarding the use of bone substitutes and implant placement.

Data collected during this study includes the distribution of sample sex and age, the duration of treatment in the simultaneous and staged approaches, the length of observation, and the distribution of the number of implant placement related with augmentation approaches. The parameters analyzed comprise the implant survival rate and the stability of alveolar tissue width post augmentation procedure involving the use of resorption level. The tissue resorption is established by measuring clinically the difference in alveolar width between the immediate post augmentation procedure (Figure 1(b)) and the follow-up at the end of the study period (Figure 1(c)). The data collected is then categorized into such scores as *low* if the difference is less than 1 mm, *moderate* = 1-2 mm, and *high* = more than 2 mm.

The surgical procedure within the simultaneous approach uses trapezoidal incision and mucoperiosteal flap in order to expose the defective bone. Bone preparation is performed in a slightly palatal direction as a means of achieving initial implant stability. An osseointegrated implant (Axiom®, Anthogyr, France) is inserted until an initial stability of 35 Ncm torque is achieved leaving implant threads exposed, at least, labially (Figure 2(a)). The peri-implant gap is filled and the horizontal bone defect augmented with DBBM particle (Cerabone®, Botiss GmbH, Germany) (Figure 2(b)). A resorbable membrane (Jason Membrane®, Botiss biomaterials GmbH, Germany) is then placed over the bone graft particle. Healing abutments are installed in the immediate loading, while a cover screw is placed in the delayed loading. Primary closure is facilitated with a periosteal releasing incision. In the staged approach, the bone defects are filled with bone substitute particle, covered with membrane and primarily closed. The graft is allowed to heal for at least 6 months before implant placement is conducted.

In immediate loading cases, implant impression is undertaken approximately 2 months after implant placement. In delayed loading cases, phase 2 is initiated around 6 months post implant placement. Crestal incision is made to expose the implant platform and insert the healing abutment (Figure 2(c)). Approximately one month thereafter, when the soft tissue remodelling around the healing abutment is completed (Figure 2(d)), implant impression is undertaken with closed tray technique for final restoration (Figure 2(e)).

3. Results

A total of 17 patients with 23 dental implant placement fulfills the inclusion criteria outlined above, consisting of 9 females and 8 males with a mean age of 43.6 years (range 18 to 66). The length of observation ranged from 8 to 90 months (average 34.9 months). The augmentation was done with simultaneous approach in 18 (78.3%) implant placements and with the staged approach in 5 (21.7%) implant placements (Table 1). Complication documented is wound dehiscence and graft particle exposure in a case treated with a staged approach. A second operation is performed in order to remove the old graft and close the wound without compromising the remainder of the grafted site. The average treatment length in the simultaneous approach was 6.6 months compared to 14.5 months in the staged approach.

The implant survival rate was 100% as no failures are documented during the observation period. Direct horizontal tissue gain is clinically achieved after the augmentation procedure in all cases. The evaluation of clinical alveolar width (horizontal) stability shows low resorption level in 19 (82.6%) implant placements, while moderate and high resorption levels are found in 3 (13.0%) and 1 (4.3%) implant placements, respectively (Table 2).

The evaluation of clinical horizontal tissue stability after GBR procedure using DBBM particle reveals that low resorption level is documented in 94.4% of implant placements augmented with simultaneous approach while moderate resorption level is found in 5.6% implants and none is associated with high resorption level. On the contrary, low and moderate resorption levels are documented both in 40% of implants and 20% of them is related with high resorption level when augmented with the staged approach (Figure 3). Mann-Whitney test result confirms that the resorption level in the simultaneous approach is significantly ($p = 0.005$) lower compared to that in the staged approach.

4. Discussion

Implant treatment in the anterior maxilla or aesthetic zone should be performed taking into account one important consideration, i.e., the aesthetic expectations of the patient [10]. One of the major problems associated with early or delayed implant placement in the anterior maxilla is horizontal tissue deficiency due to resorption

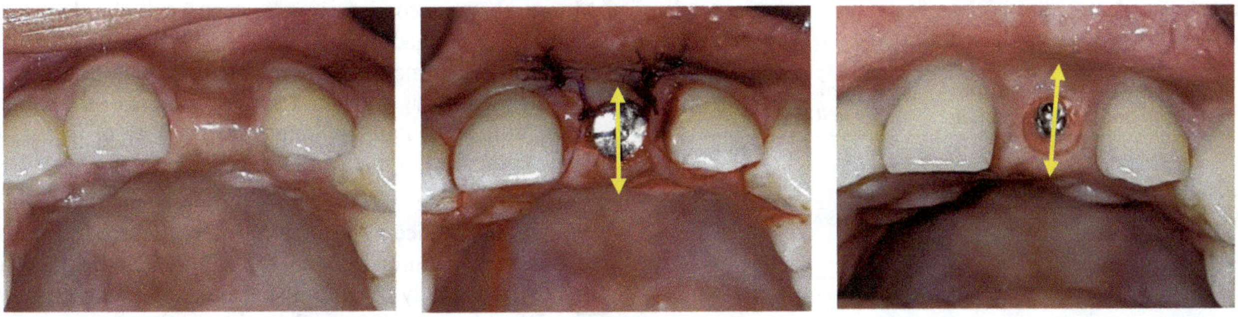

(a) (b) (c)

FIGURE 1: The measurement of augmented tissue resorption. (a) Postextraction horizontal defect of 21 alveolar ridge prior to augmentation; the tissue resorption is established by measuring clinically the difference in alveolar width between the immediate post augmentation procedure (b) and the follow-up at the end of the study period (c). The data collected is subsequently categorized into tissue resorption level as *low* if horizontal loss < 1 mm, *moderate* = 1-2 mm, and *high* > 2 mm.

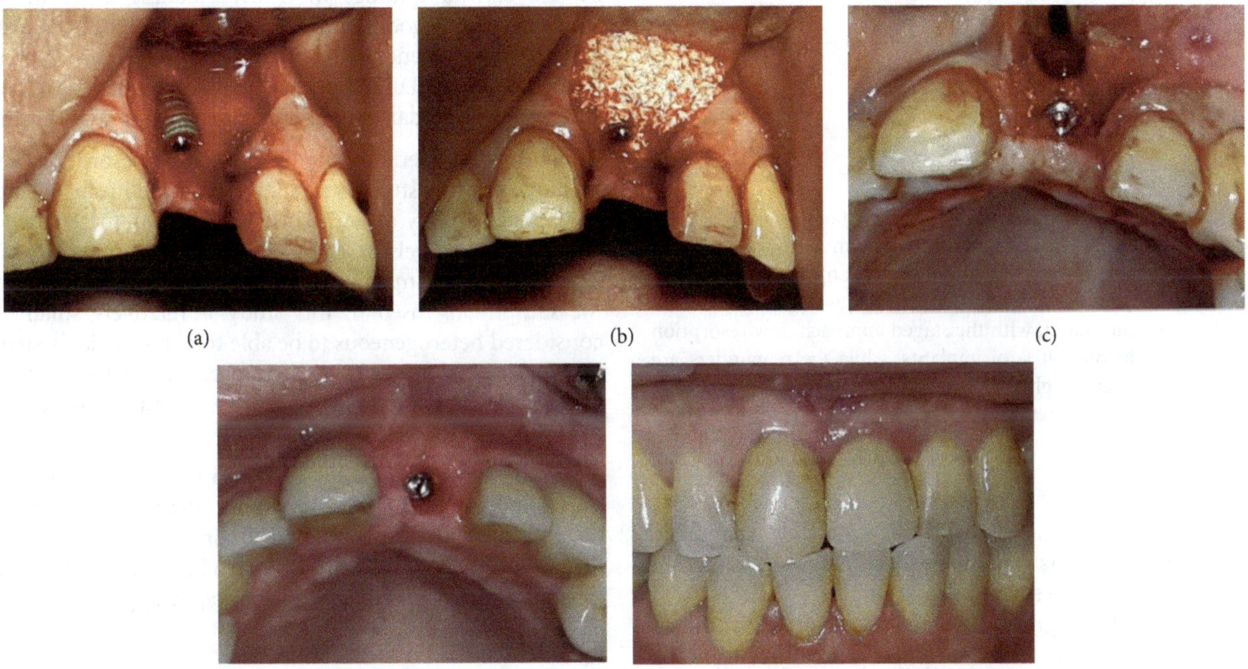

(a) (b) (c) (d) (e)

FIGURE 2: Simultaneous implant placement and horizontal augmentation in the anterior maxilla with delayed loading strategy. (a) Postextraction horizontal defect of 21 alveolar ridge, in which implant placement leaves two-thirds of the implant length exposed; (b) DBBM particle is applied to cover the implant and augment the alveolar defect; (c) at reentry six months after bone grafting, the augmented area is stable with still visible DBBM particles blended with the newly formed bone; (d) at prosthetic phase, the labial tissue width is shown to be comparable to the adjacent tissue; (e) final restoration shows healthy labial and interdental peri-implant tissue.

TABLE 1: The distribution of implant placement associated with simultaneous and staged augmentation approaches.

	Simultaneous augmentation	Staged augmentation
Male	9	2
Female	9	3
Total	**18** (78.3%)	**5** (21.7%)

of alveolar bone especially in the labial aspect. In order to achieve optimal peri-implant tissue support in the anterior maxilla, one should perform bone augmentation with bone graft or bone substitute to provide appropriate stability [11].

The results of this study showed that implant placements grafted with GBR using DBBM produce clinical stability in the horizontal dimension as the majority (82.6%) exhibits low resorption levels during the follow-up review (Table 2). This result is consistent with those of previous studies which reveal good osteoconductivity and stability of the grafted bone [6, 7]. This finding is most likely caused by the high volume stability of DBBM granules which may be associated with its poor degradability. Various studies have demonstrated that DBBM has a very slow degradation

TABLE 2: The distribution of tissue resorption level after implant placement associated with simultaneous and staged approaches.

Resorption level	Simultaneous augmentation	Staged augmentation	Total
Low	17	2	**19** (82.6%)
Moderate	1	2	**3** (13.0%)
High	0	1	**1** (4.3%)
Total	**18**	**5**	**23**

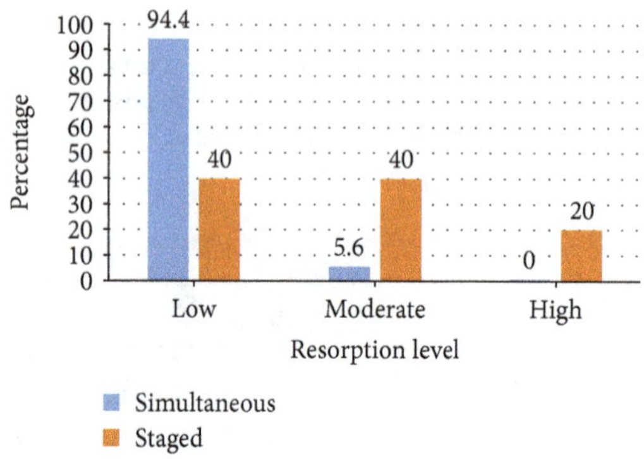

FIGURE 3: The resorption level of simultaneous and staged augmentation with DBBM particle. The majority (94.4%) of implant augmented with the simultaneous approach shows low resorption level, while only 5.6% is moderate and none is high level. On the other hand, with the staged approach, low resorption level is found in only 40% of implants, while the remainders are moderate (40%) and high (20%) levels. Mann-Whitney test result reveals significant difference ($p = 0.005$) in tissue resorption level between the two approaches.

rate, up to 3 to 4 years, or may not be completely degradable [12, 13]. Moreover, its stability as graft material can last up to 1.5 years in the absence of dental implants [14].

Alveolar ridge augmentation can be performed at different time points during treatment and is generally categorized as staged or simultaneous approach. The simultaneous approach is obviously the technique preferred by both patients and clinicians since it reduces both the time and cost of treatment [15]. This finding is in accordance with the results of our study in which the treatment duration of the staged approach is more than twice than that of the simultaneous approach.

The result of this study reveals that GBR with the simultaneous approach produces significantly lower resorption level compared to the staged approach. Furthermore, moderate and high resorption levels are predominantly found in the staged approach (Figure 3). This result is noteworthy since DBBM is supposed to be mechanically stable. One plausible explanation would be that the staged augmentation approach is applied to cases with larger tissue deficit which precludes simultaneous implant placement. Larger deficit may have caused a certain degree of instability of the graft particles due to mucosal pressure or mechanical load exerted by provisional prosthesis or mastication [10] resulting in reduced horizontal dimension during the follow-up period. Moreover, the second surgery performed for implant placement in the staged approach might have caused a certain degree of inflammation subsequently inducing bone resorption. These findings highlight the advantages of the simultaneous approach, namely, long-term stability of the grafted tissue compared to that of the staged approach.

The sole use of DBBM to promote augmentation of implant dehiscence might, theoretically, reduce the amount of bone regeneration around the exposed implant surface, thereby potentially compromising implant osseointegration. The DBBM particulate used in this study was made from bovine cancellous bone which demonstrates much higher porosity compared to cortical bone granules. The higher the porosity, the more effective the osteoconductivity of the graft material since it promotes faster bone formation around the exposed implant surface [16]. This is supported by the clinical findings in delayed-loading cases in this study in which good integration between DBBM particle and the new regenerated bone is evident (Figure 2). This suggests that the DBBM particle promotes osteoconduction supporting secondary implant stability during graft healing.

The novel method to measure tissue resorption level employed in this study is a relatively simple means of measuring the stability of grafted tissue. The parameter used in this method is purely based on clinical dimensions not taking into account the magnitude of grafted bone. Furthermore, the sample size used in this study is relatively small and considered heterogeneous to be able to obtain reliably strong inference. Further study is, therefore, required with bigger sample size and with imaging tools enabled to evaluate the magnitude of the grafted bone.

From the results of the study, it may be concluded that horizontal bone augmentation with deproteinized bovine bone mineral particle produces a clinically stable tissue in the anterior maxilla. Stability seems to be higher in the simultaneous approach compared to the staged approach.

Additional Points

Key Messages. Deproteinized bovine cancellous bone mineral particle represents a suitable bone substitute for guided bone regeneration of implant placement in the anterior maxilla due to its strong osteoconductive properties and structural stability. These allow for effective bone integration and stable grafted tissue leading to the effective functioning and aesthetic appeal of implant-supported prosthesis.

Acknowledgments

The author would like to thank the Faculty of Dental Medicine, Universitas Airlangga, and Dental Hospital, Universitas Airlangga, which has supported the study. The study would not have been possible without the permission from them.

References

[1] D. C. Tong, K. Rioux, M. Drangsholt, and O. R. Beirnem, "A review of survival rates for implants placed in grafted maxillary sinuses using meta-analysis," *The International Journal of Oral & Maxillofacial Implants*, vol. 13, pp. 175–182, 1998.

[2] H. L. Wang and K. Al-Shammari, "HVC ridge deficiency classification: a therapeutically oriented classification," *The International Journal of Periodontics & Restorative Dentistry*, vol. 22, pp. 335–343, 2002.

[3] B. S. McAllister and K. Haghighat, "Bone augmentation techniques," *Journal of Periodontology*, vol. 78, no. 3, pp. 377–396, 2007.

[4] G. M. Raghoebar, C. Louwerse, W. W. I. Kalk, and A. Vissink, "Morbidity of chin bone harvesting," *Clinical Oral Implants Research*, vol. 12, no. 5, pp. 503–507, 2011.

[5] M. Caneva, D. Botticelli, E. Stellini, S. L. S. Souza, A. Salata, and N. P. Lang, "Magnesium-enriched hydroxyapatite at immediate implants: a histomorphometric study in dogs," *Clinical Oral Implants Research*, vol. 22, no. 5, pp. 512–517, 2011.

[6] M. Caneva, D. Botticelli, F. Pantani, G. M. Baffone, I. G. Rangel Jr., and N. P. Lang, "Deproteinized bovine bone mineral in marginal defects at implants installed immediately into extraction sockets: an experimental study in dogs," *Clinical Oral Implants Research*, vol. 23, no. 1, pp. 106–112, 2012.

[7] A. Barone, M. Ricci, J. L. Calvo-Guirado, and U. Covani, "Retracted: bone remodelling after regenerative procedures around implants placed in fresh extraction sockets: an experimental study in Beagle dogs," *Clinical Oral Implants Research*, vol. 22, no. 10, pp. 1131–1137, 2011.

[8] J. Nart, L. Barallat, D. Jimenez et al., "Radiographic and histological evaluation of deproteinized bovine bone mineral vs. deproteinized bovine bone mineral with 10% collagen in ridge preservation. A randomized controlled clinical trial," *Clinical Oral Implants Research*, vol. 28, no. 7, pp. 840–848, 2017.

[9] N. Venkataraman, S. Bansal, P. Bansal, and S. Narayan, "Dynamics of bone graft healing around implants," *Journal of the International Clinical Dental Research Organization*, vol. 7, no. 3, pp. 40–47, 2015.

[10] U. Kuchler and T. von Arx, "Horizontal ridge augmentation in conjunction with or prior to implant placement in the anterior maxilla: a systematic review," *The International Journal of Oral & Maxillofacial Implants*, vol. 29, Supplement, pp. 14–24, 2014.

[11] P. L. Santos, J. L. Gulinelli, C. S. Telles et al., "Bone substitutes for peri-implant defects of postextraction implants," *International Journal of Biomaterials*, vol. 2013, Article ID 307136, 7 pages, 2013.

[12] T. Berglundh and J. Lindhe, "Healing around implants placed in bone defects treated with Bio-Oss®: an experimental study in the dog," *Clinical Oral Implants Research*, vol. 8, no. 2, pp. 117–124, 1997.

[13] A. Skoglund, P. Hising, and C. Young, "A clinical and histologic examination in humans of the osseous response to implanted natural bone mineral," *International Journal of Oral & Maxillofacial Implants*, vol. 12, pp. 194–199, 1997.

[14] B. McAllister, M. Margolin, A. Cogan, D. Buck, J. Hollinger, and S. Lynch, "Eighteen-month radiographic and histologic evaluation of sinus grafting with anorganic bovine bone in the chimpanzee," *International Journal of Oral & Maxillofacial Implants*, vol. 14, no. 3, pp. 361–368, 1999.

[15] P. Fairbairn and M. Leventis, "Protocol for bone augmentation with simultaneous early implant placement: a retrospective multicenter clinical study," *International Journal of Dentistry*, vol. 2015, Article ID 589135, 8 pages, 2015.

[16] A. Scarano, "Maxillary sinus augmentation with decellularized bovine compact particles: a radiological, clinical, and histologic report of 4 cases," *BioMed Research International*, vol. 2017, Article ID 2594670, 6 pages, 2017.

8

The Zygomatic Buttress as an Efficient Intraoral Donor Site for Limited Maxillary Reconstructions: A Case Series and Brief Literature Review

Joseph Bassil,[1] **Alain Abi Sleiman**,[2] **Stephanie Mrad**,[1] **and Ziad Noujeim**[3]

[1]*Department of Oral Surgery, Faculty of Dental Medicine, Saint Joseph University of Beirut, Lebanon*
[2]*Attending Oral Surgeon, Lebanese Army Dental Department, Beirut, Lebanon*
[3]*Department of Oral and Maxillofacial Surgery, Faculty of Dental Medicine, Lebanese University, Beirut, Lebanon*

Correspondence should be addressed to Stephanie Mrad; stephanie.mrad93@gmail.com

Academic Editor: Gilberto Sammartino

Limited maxillary defects are commonly grafted with bone blocks harvested from the symphysis or the ramus; harvesting a second surgical site in the mandible increases both operative time and patient's postoperative morbidity. To overcome these disadvantages, the zygomatic buttress (ZB) was suggested as an alternative maxillary source of autogenous bone. This intraoral donor site has a natural convex shape and can be accessed along with the recipient site through the same flap design. We report a case series describing this uncommon technique of bone harvesting from the zygomatic buttress to reconstruct limited alveolar defects in the maxilla.

1. Introduction

Implant placement in the correct—prosthetic and esthetic—three-dimensional position requires sufficient alveolar bone volume. However, unfavorable ridge conditions are commonly encountered, and a grafting procedure is necessary to augment alveolar bone width prior to implant placement. Several bone grafting substitutes such as allogeneic, xenogeneic, and alloplastic materials have shown successful results, yet autogenous bone remains the gold standard for alveolar bone reconstructions [1]. Two of the most common intraoral donor sites used to treat limited maxillary defects are the mandibular symphysis and ramus. This implicates the necessity of a second surgical site, more operative time, and more postoperative patient morbidity. To overcome these disadvantages, the zygomatic buttress (ZB) was suggested as a source of autogenous bone [2]. The exhaustive surgical technique describing the use of ZB graft for limited maxillary reconstructions is rarely reported in the literature.

The ZB is formed by the junction of the zygomatic process of the maxilla and the maxillary process of the zygoma. It is responsible for sustaining the forces applied to the maxilla. The quality, density, and natural convex shape of the ZB compensate for the limited bone quantity can be harvested from this region. Also, easy accessibility to the donor site and its proximity to the recipient site make it possible to perform only one flap reducing both operative time and postoperative morbidity [3, 4]. The ZB block can be fixed in direct contact to the recipient site as described in the "onlay technique" or distant from the alveolar ridge as defined in the containment and contouring "shell technique" [3, 5].

This series is aimed at describing five cases of bone harvesting from the zygomatic buttress to reconstruct limited maxillary defects.

2. Case Series

2.1. Patient Selection. Five patients who required implant placement in the maxilla and presented insufficient alveolar bone thickness, ranging from 2 to 4 mm, were enrolled in this study. Grafting procedures using bone blocks harvested from the ZB were planned to reconstruct the thin ridges before

TABLE 1: Description of each case.

Case no.	Sex	Age	Graft side(s)	Grafting technique	Implant position(s)	Implant diameter (in mm)
1	Male	21	Left	Onlay graft technique: cortico-cancellous ZB bone block	21	3.3 mm (for prosthetic and esthetic considerations only)
2	Male	49	Right	Shell technique+sinus elevation	14, 15, 16	4.1 mm
3	Male	41	Left	Shell technique: cortical ZB bone block	25, 26, 27	4.1 mm
4	Female	55	Left +right	Bilateral shell technique	17, 16, 13, 23, 25, 26	4.1 mm
5	Female	49	Right	Onlay graft technique: cortico-cancellous ZB bone block	14, 15	4.1 mm

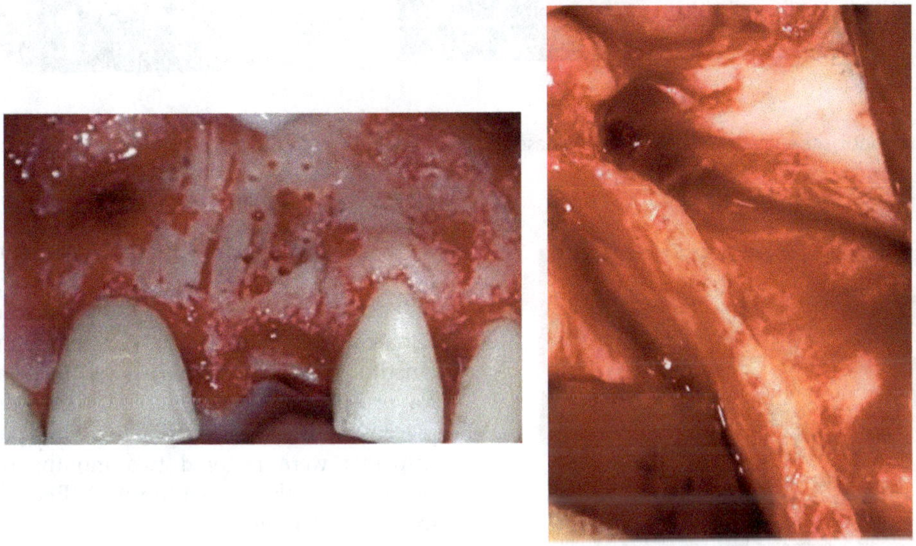

(a) (b)

FIGURE 1: Preoperative view of the deficient maxillary recipient sites: (a) case no. 1: partially edentulous anterior site; (b) case no. 2: fully edentulous posterior site.

implant placement (Table 1). All patients signed an informed consent agreement before surgery, and all work was conducted in accordance with the Declaration of Helsinki. Because the study was retrospective, it was granted a written exemption by the ethical committee of the Saint Joseph University of Beirut IRB.

Inclusion criteria were as follows: partial or complete maxillary edentulism, horizontal ridge deficiency, and noncontributory medical history.

Exclusion criteria were as follows: smoking, pregnancy, breast-feeding, systemic diseases, and poor oral hygiene.

2.2. Surgical Technique. After local anesthesia infiltrations, a linear crestal incision was made along the edentulous ridge and was continued by intrasulcular incisions around the adjacent teeth and two mesial and distal vertical release incisions. The distal vertical release was continued into a horizontal incision in the maxillary vestibule, 3 to 5 mm above the mucogingival junction. Wide trapezoidal full-thickness flaps were raised to expose the thin maxillary ridges (ranging from 2 to 4 mm) and the ZB (Figure 1).

Bone blocks of approximately 1.5 cm^2 were harvested from the ipsilateral ZB tail using Piezosurgery (Mectron®; Carasco-GE, Loreto, Italy) (Figure 2).

In 2 cases, the "Onlay graft technique" was applied (Table 1): thick cortico-cancellous bone blocks harvested from the ZB were fixed, without further shaping, in direct contact with the concave alveolar defects using two titanium osteosynthesis miniscrews (smartDrive®; KLS Martin Group, Tuttlingen, Germany) (Figure 3). Autogenous bone chips were collected from the outer cortex of the same area using a bone scraper (Safescraper® Twist; CGM SpA, Divisione Medicale META, Reggio Emilia, Italy) and were mixed with anorganic bovine bone (Bio-Oss®, Geistlich Pharma AG, Wolhusen, Switzerland) particles in equal quantities to cover the outer surface of the blocks.

In the 3 other cases, the "Shell technique" was applied (Table 1): thin cortical bone blocks were harvested from the ZB and fixed at a distance from the recipient sites with titanium screws (Figure 4). In one of these cases, a simultaneous sinus floor elevation was performed to ensure sufficient bone height for later implant placement. In another advanced fully

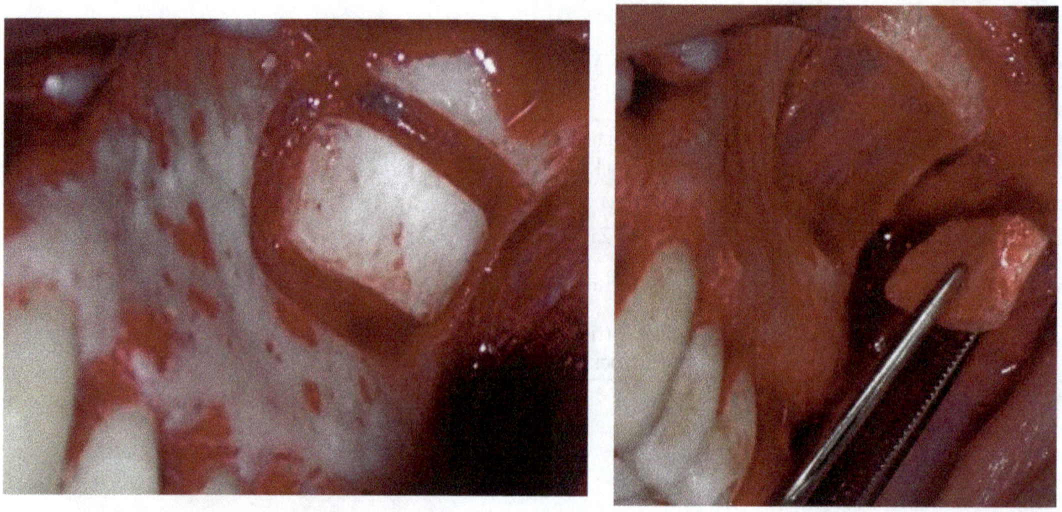

(a) (b)

FIGURE 2: View of the donor site—lower tail of the ZB—in case no. 1: (a) bone cut with the piezoelectric surgical device; (b) ZB bone block harvest.

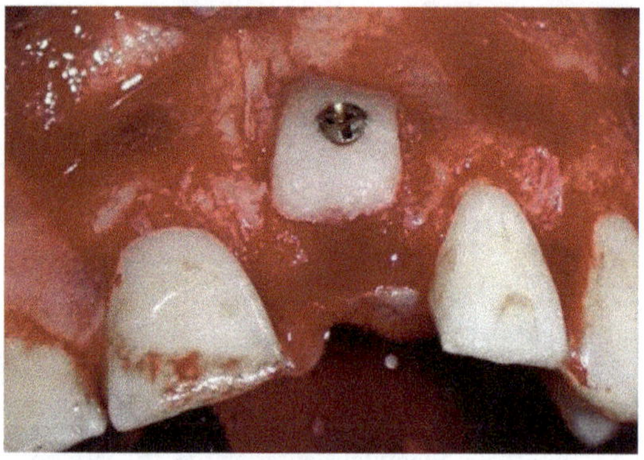

FIGURE 3: Onlay grafting procedure in case no. 1: ZB graft placed in direct contact with the recipient site and stabilized with a miniscrew.

edentulous case, bone blocks harvested from the bilateral ZB were fixed to the right and left recipient sites using the shell/-tenting technique. The 50 : 50 ratio mixture of bone particles (autogenous+xenogeneic) was used to fill the gaps between the bone blocks and the alveolar ridges.

In all cases, the grafted sector was covered with a large collagen membrane (Bio-Gide®, Geistlich Pharma AG, Wolhusen, Switzerland) to optimize bone remodeling and growth (Figure 4). Perforation of the Schneiderian membrane did not occur in any case. Periosteal releasing incisions of the full thickness flap allowed tension-free wound closure.

After six months of uneventful healing, cone beam computed tomography (CBCT) scans were taken to evaluate the amount of bone gain (Figure 5).

The grafted areas were surgically reopened for conventional implant placement. After local anesthesia, a small trapezoidal full-thickness flap was raised, and the miniscrews were removed. The grafted area showed a large amount of regenerated alveolar bone with preserved convex shape in all cases (Figure 6).

Regular-diameter (4.1 mm) Straumann® dental implants (Institut Straumann® AG, Basel, Switzerland) were placed in 4 cases according to the ideal prosthetic axis. In one case, a narrow-diameter (3.3 mm) Straumann® dental implant (Institut Straumann® AG, Basel, Switzerland) was placed for prosthetic and esthetic considerations even though the placement of a wider implant was possible (Figure 7). Implants were restored two months later with cement-retained porcelain fused to metal (PFM) crowns after abutments' tightening.

3. Discussion

Bone grafting procedures are commonly needed to ensure adequate bone volume before implant placement. Among several bone substitutes, autogenous bone remains the gold standard for alveolar bone reconstructions. The retromolar and symphysis intraoral donor sites are indicated in cases of large reconstructions in the mandible, whereas the ZB is described as a relatively novel intraoral donor site for small and limited bone augmentations in the maxilla [1, 6]. Gellrich et al. stated that 1.5 to 2 cm^2 of bone can be harvested from this site without compromising midfacial strength. This quantity of harvested bone is sufficient to reconstruct limited to medium alveolar defects (sufficient for 1 or 2 implants) [3]. Kainulainen et al. also measured the volume of 40 blocks harvested from the ZB of 20 cadavers of an elderly population. Bone was either compressed into a syringe or placed in a water displacement tube to quantify its volume. An average of 0.59 mL bone was calculated with the syringe and 0.53 mL with the water displacement. It is important to note that grafts in this study were harvested from cadavers of an elderly population with moderately atrophic facial bone [4].

The ZB technique presents several advantages. A study on ten cases reported a mean horizontal bone gain of 1.82 $\pm$ 0.16 mm, 4 months after grafting with bone harvested from the ZB. These grafted sites showed similar bone density

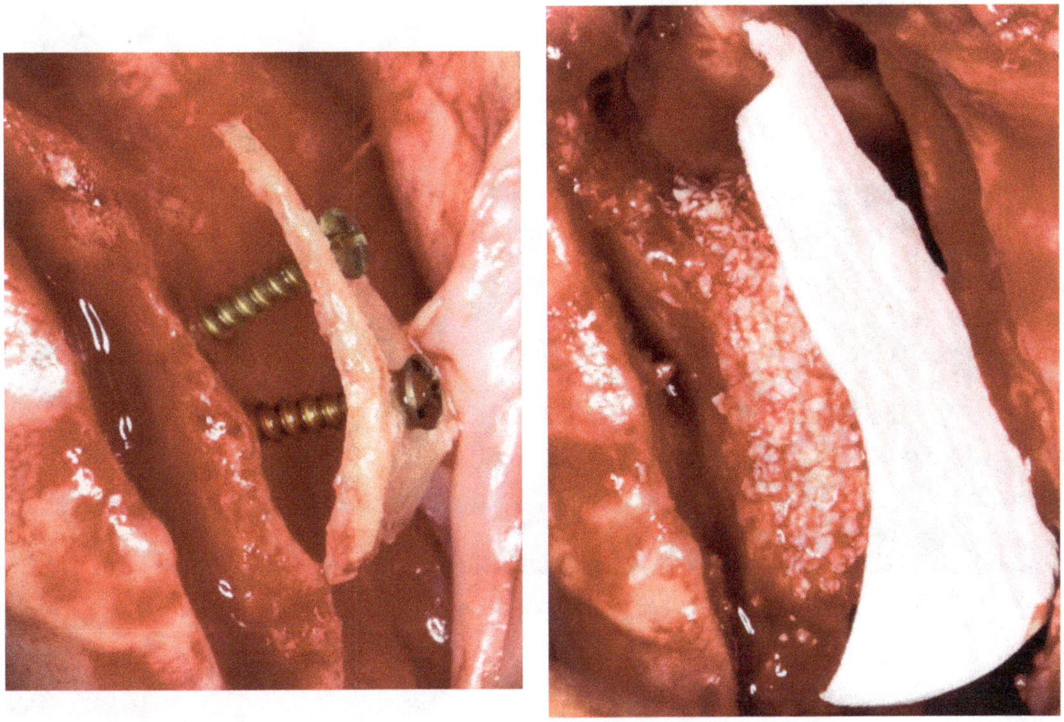

(a) (b)

Figure 4: Shell grafting procedure in case no. 2: (a) ZB graft placed at a distance from the recipient site and stabilized with two miniscrews; (b) gap filled with 50 : 50 mixture (autogenous+xenogeneic) bone particles and covered with a large collagen membrane.

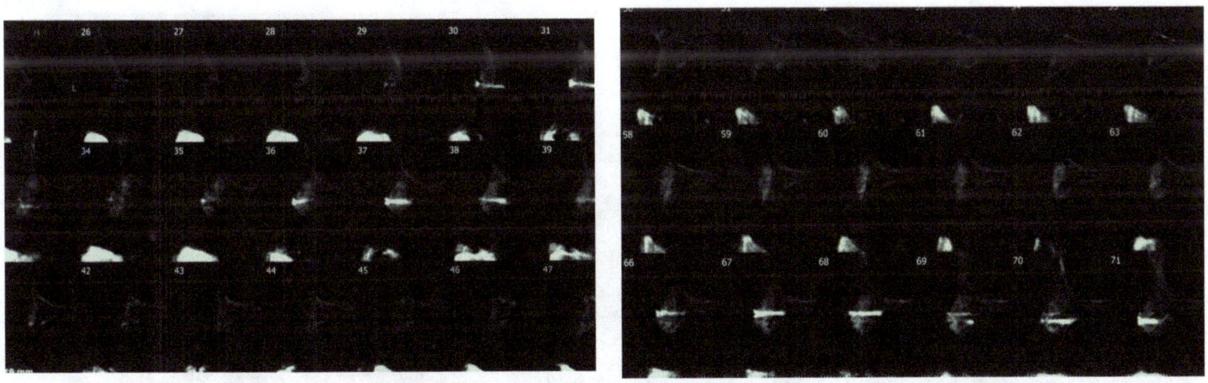

(a) (b)

Figure 5: Sagittal view of CBCT images in case no. 2: (a, b) grafted areas 6 months postoperatively.

values to those of the native alveolar bone [7]. This ZB also offers bone of good quality and correct convex morphology for maxillary defects. In several studies, bone harvested from the ZB was grafted without further shaping and successfully restored a pronounced ridge contour [5]. In this series, the form-giving zygomatic graft was used in two cases of limited maxillary defects in the anterior region and ideally restored the original convex alveolar contour without any additional need for bone or soft tissue graft. The ZB method shows minimal postoperative morbidity at the donor site for no muscles need to be detached to access this site [3]. Patients grafted from the ZB were reported to encounter few postoperative difficulties, such as pain and edema, while patients grafted from the retromolar area were reported to experience more complications including transient postoperative paresthesia of the mandibular and lingual nerves [1, 5, 8]. Also, access to the ZB area is relatively simple and provides excellent visibility compared to other intraoral donor sites such as the retromolar region. Besides, the proximity between donor and recipient sites helps to simplify the grafting steps and reduce the surgical time [4].

The main limiting factors of this bone harvesting site are its close relationship to the infraorbital foramen and to the Schneiderian sinus membrane. The use of piezo surgical devices instead of rotary instruments can reduce the risk of membrane perforation. Kainulainen et al. found 33%

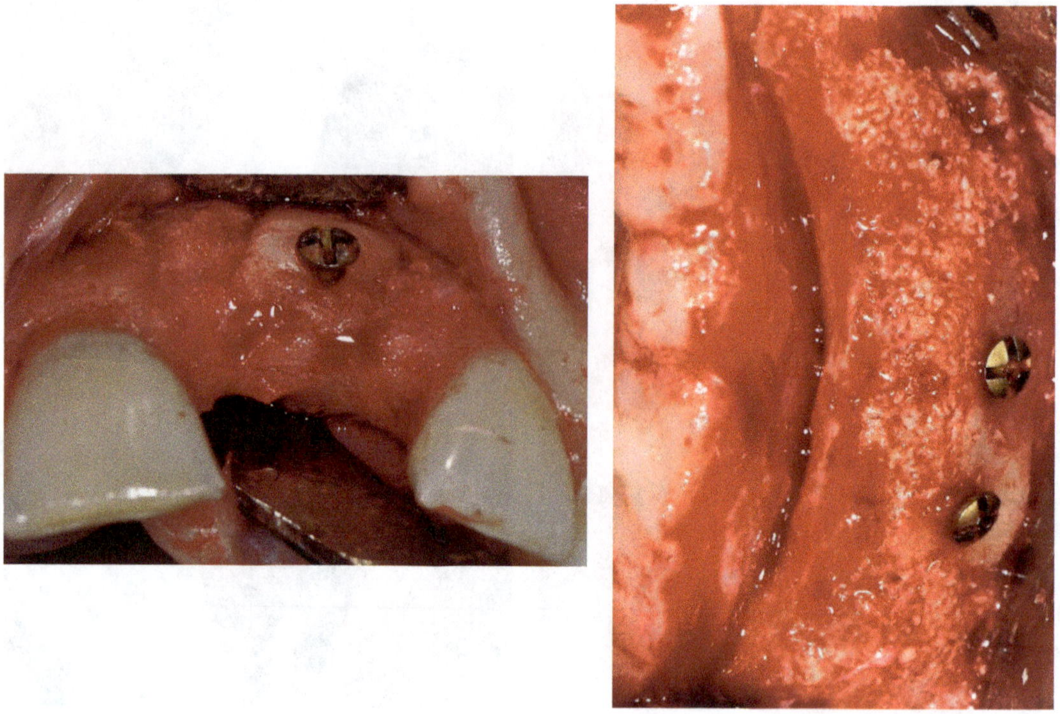

(a) (b)

Figure 6: View of the grafted sites 6 months postoperatively: (a) case no. 1; (b) case no. 2.

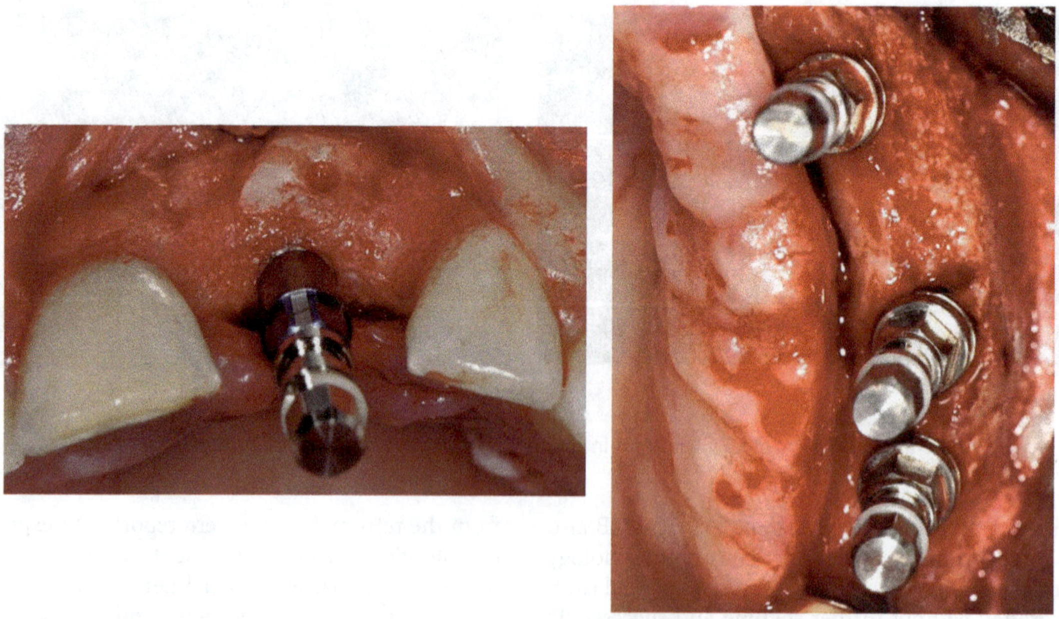

(a) (b)

Figure 7: Implant placement in the grafted sites: (a) case no. 1; (b) case no. 2.

perforated membranes among 40 surgical sites when using round burrs, while Gellrich et al. found a total of 28% perforations among 273 sites when using piezosurgery [4, 5]. However, membrane perforation did not influence the overall success of this technique. In the present series, bone harvesting was performed using a piezoelectric device to minimize the complication risk. Membrane perforation did not occur in any case.

Another key anatomic point to bear in mind when harvesting bone from the ZB is the infraorbital foramen from which the infraorbital nerve (ION) and artery (IOA) exit from the skull. Gellrich et al. propose direct visualization of the infraorbital zone to avoid any nerve injury [3]. However, this complication is rarely encountered. Sakkas et al. reported 1.7% of transient infraorbital nerve paresthesia at the time of suture removal (2 cases among 113), and all cases showed complete recovery at the time of implant placement [8]. In another retrospective study on 273 patients, no case of nerve damage was found [5]. This is in accordance with our series where no case of infraorbital nerve damage was encountered. In fact, flap retractors were positioned away from the surgical zone to avoid stretching, compressing, or lacerating the ION and IOA. Thus, the risk of bleeding or paresthesia of the ipsilateral upper lip and/or lower eyelid was minimized. The same precautions were taken when performing vertical releasing incisions that may intersect with the IOA and ION. Therefore, it is advisable not to extend the vertical incisions and to use Metzenbaum dissecting scissors for periosteum release before tension-free wound closure.

Complications related to this procedure may include infection, pus, and wound dehiscence and incision-line opening, swelling, and graft mobilization. In a study reporting complication rates of this technique, Sakkas et al. found more postoperative complications at recipient sites (17.6%) than donor sites (3.5%). Also, a significantly higher incidence of postoperative complications was found among smokers [8]. In the current report, all patients were nonsmokers and no complications were recorded confirming the previous findings. A systematic review evaluating the complications of bone harvesting from mandibular sites found high complication rates at the symphysis and the ramus [9], whereas several studies describing bone harvesting from the ZB showed very low complication and failure rates that did not significantly influence the success of this method [4, 5, 8]. Hence, the ZB appears to be a safe intraoral harvesting site.

4. Conclusion

The zygomatic buttress is a potential intraoral donor site of autogenous bone in cases of small or limited maxillary defects. The size and convex shape of these blocks are ideal to reconstruct the original contour of anterior maxillary defects. Proximity to the Schneiderian membrane and to the infraorbital nerve and artery should be taken into consideration during this surgical procedure. Still, this safe method presents very low complication and failure rates. The ZB donor site is close to the recipient site and can be accessed through the same flap design. This simple access will reduce the operating time and postoperative discomfort and morbidity.

References

[1] A. Sakkas, F. Wilde, M. Heufelder, K. Winter, and A. Schramm, "Autogenous bone grafts in oral implantology—is it still a "Gold standard"? A consecutive review of 279 patients with 456 clinical procedures," *Int J Implant Dent.*, vol. 3, no. 1, p. 23, 2017.

[2] T. Starch-Jensen, D. Deluiz, S. Deb, N. H. Bruun, and E. M. B. Tinoco, "Harvesting of autogenous bone graft from the ascending mandibular ramus compared with the chin region: a systematic review and meta-analysis focusing on complications and donor site morbidity," *Journal of Oral & Maxillofacial Research*, vol. 11, no. 3, p. e1, 2020.

[3] N.-C. Gellrich, U. Held, R. Schoen, T. Pailing, A. Schramm, and K.-H. Bormann, "Alveolar zygomatic buttress: a new donor site for limited preimplant augmentation procedures," *Journal of Oral and Maxillofacial Surgery*, vol. 65, no. 2, pp. 275–280, 2007.

[4] V. T. Kainulainen, G. K. B. Sándor, C. M. L. Clokie, A. M. Keller, and K. S. Oikarinen, "The zygomatic bone as a potential donor site for alveolar reconstruction—a quantitative anatomic cadaver study," *International Journal of Oral and Maxillofacial Surgery*, vol. 33, no. 8, pp. 786–791, 2004.

[5] N.-C. Gellrich, K.-H. Bormann, S. Tehranchian, H. Kokemüller, and M. M. Suarez-Cunqueiro, "Containment and contouring (CoCoon) technique: a biologically adequate approach to less invasive autogenous preimplant augmentation of bone," *The British Journal of Oral & Maxillofacial Surgery*, vol. 51, no. 8, pp. 880–886, 2013.

[6] L. M. Wolford and L. Cooper, "Alternative donor sites for maxillary bone grafts," *Plastic and Reconstructive Surgery*, vol. 80, no. 2, p. 328, 1987.

[7] M. M. Solaiman, A. S. EL Mahallawy, and N. E. Hassan, "Evaluation of the zygomatic buttress as a donor site for ridge augmentation prior to implant insertion in the esthetic zone," *Alexandria Dental Journal*, vol. 43, no. 1, pp. 48–54, 2018.

[8] A. Sakkas, A. Schramm, W. Karsten, N.-C. Gellrich, and F. Wilde, "A clinical study of the outcomes and complications associated with zygomatic buttress block bone graft for limited preimplant augmentation procedures," *Journal of Cranio-Maxillofacial Surgery*, vol. 44, no. 3, pp. 249–256, 2016.

[9] D. Reininger, C. Cobo-Vázquez, M. Monteserín-Matesanz, and J. López-Quiles, "Complications in the use of the mandibular body, ramus and symphysis as donor sites in bone graft surgery. A systematic review," *Medicina Oral, Patologia Oral y Cirugia Bucal*, vol. 21, no. 2, pp. e241–e249, 2016.

Guided Bilateral Transcanine Implant Placement and Implant-Supported Oral Rehabilitation in a Patient with Progressive Systemic Scleroderma

Igor Smojver,[1] **Ivan Katalinić**,[1] **Marko Vuletić**,[2] **Luka Stojić**,[3] **Dražena Gerbl**,[4] **and Dragana Gabrić**[2]

[1]*St. Catherine Specialty Hospital, Zagreb, Croatia*
[2]*Department of Oral Surgery, School of Dental Medicine, University of Zagreb, Croatia*
[3]*Private Dental Clinic, Zagreb, Croatia*
[4]*Clinic of Anesthesiology, University Hospital Clinic Zagreb, Croatia*

Correspondence should be addressed to Marko Vuletić; mvuletic@sfzg.hr

Academic Editor: Alberto Delbem

When faced with a situation where an impacted tooth is in the way of a planned implant, one approach to avoid an invasive surgical procedure and potential associated complications is to place a transcanine implant. The aim of this report was to add a new case of a transimpacted tooth dental implant placement to the existing international literature and to share our experience of transcanine implantation in the maxilla followed by implant prosthodontic rehabilitation of a patient with progressive systemic scleroderma. A 55-year-old woman attended our office for oral cavity assessment and treatment planning for complete oral rehabilitation. Digital planning software was used, and implants were positioned according to a surgical template in regions 13, 16, 23, and 26 (Straumann, Basel, Switzerland) with screw-retained metal-ceramic bridges. Placement of the dental implants through impacted canines and the creation of interfaces other than implant-bone interfaces did not lead to postoperative pain or implant failure. Clinically, overall healing was observed, and the implants were successfully used for implant-supported prosthodontic rehabilitation of the jaw. Within the limitations of this case report, transcanine implantation could represent a valuable alternative to standard implant protocols.

1. Introduction

Dental implant placement and implant-supported rehabilitation has become a widely used method for the replacement of missing teeth. Dental implants are usually placed into an edentulous jawbone but only if the three-dimensional volume is sufficient [1]. This can be a challenging task if the bone volume is insufficient or if there is an object obstructing the trajectory of the future implant, like an impacted tooth. The third mandibular molars are the most commonly impacted teeth, followed by the maxillary canines. The rate of appearance of impacted canines is 1–3% in the maxilla [2] and 0.07–1.3% in the mandible [3]. One of the fundamental implantology postulates states that the "implant surface should come into contact only with the bone" [4]. Following this rule, in a situation where an impacted tooth is in the way of a planned implant, a rather invasive surgery to remove the impacted tooth is indicated prior to implant placement. In order to avoid an invasive surgical procedure and the potential complications that may occur following such an extensive surgery, including postoperative pain, swelling, and a large residual bone defect, a staged approach to implant placement requiring two separate surgeries (the impacted tooth is firstly extracted with or without bone augmentation, then the implant is placed later) was first proposed by Davarpanah and Szmukler-Moncler in 2009 [5, 6]. These authors have conducted and published multiple successful cases of transcanine implant placement. Since then, more cases have been recorded [7, 8]; however, the total number of cases is still low as only a small number of patients are suitable for such treatment [9].

For the same reason, long-term follow-up data are also lacking [9]. Scleroderma is an autoimmune multisystem rheumatic condition that affects connective tissues. Oral and facial clinical findings are a mask-like face, thin vermilion border, radial perioral furrows, microstomia, sclerosis of the tongue-tie, and induration of the tongue. Hyposalivation, microstomia, ankyloglossia, limited mouth opening, but also minor manual skills interfere with oral hygiene ability [10, 11]. Due to these facts, the scleroderma condition represents a certain challenge for dental implant placement and/or prosthodontic rehabilitation, as the oral manifestations of scleroderma are directly relevant to the dental treatment plan and long-term management of these patients [10]. Thus, the aim of this report was to add a new case of transimpacted tooth dental implant placement to the existing international literature and to share our experience of transcanine implantation in the maxilla followed by implant prosthodontic rehabilitation of a patient with progressive systemic scleroderma.

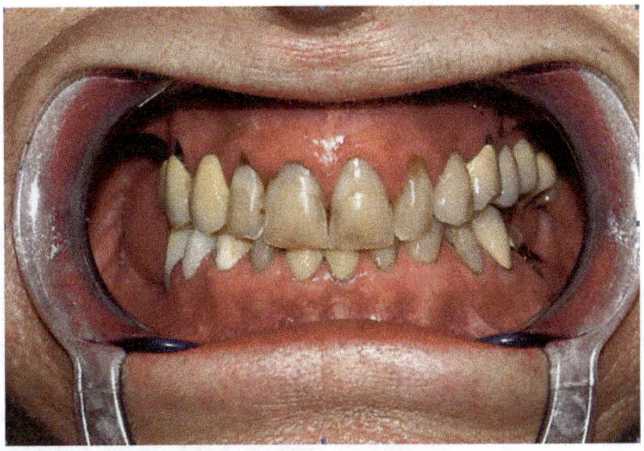

Figure 1: Preoperative intraoral status.

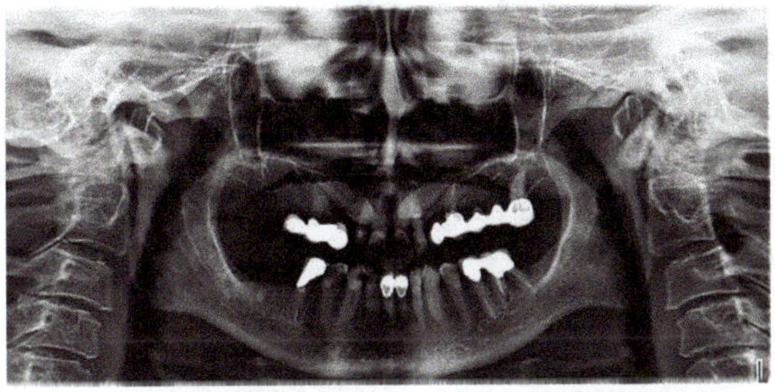

Figure 2: Preoperative panoramic image.

2. Case Report

A 55-year-old woman attended our office for oral cavity assessment and treatment planning for complete oral rehabilitation. Her medical records showed she had been diagnosed with progressive systemic sclerosis but had not been taking any medications. She complained of occasional dry mouth and inflamed gums, which is a typical oral manifestation of this disease (Figure 1). An X-ray of the jaw (digital panoramic image) revealed that teeth 14, 24, and 27 needed to be extracted or undergo root canal treatment (Figure 2). Horizontally positioned impacted upper canines were also observed, which were asymptomatic and free from any pathology. Almost all teeth had large, inadequate fillings. After thorough dental examination, an endorestorative treatment was proposed, followed by final rehabilitation of the lower jaw with full ceramic crowns. For the upper jaw, given that the impacted canines would interfere with the traditional implant-supported rehabilitation (fixed ceramic bridges), a combined prosthodontic solution was proposed (fixed ceramic crowns in the frontal region and a removable prosthesis in the back) following all necessary extractions and restorative preparations. The patient was informed that this solution for the upper jaw bares some long-term risks due to her primary diagnosis and chronically dry oral mucosa. The patient refused the removable prosthodontic solution for the upper jaw and asked for a fixed one. Two alternative options were proposed: (1) initial extraction of the impacted canines after bone augmentation, followed by later insertion of the implants, or (2) a novel, experimental approach called transdental implant insertion. The patient was informed that the second procedure was relatively new, had not been fully validated by evidence-based contemporary dentistry, and was based on several published case reports and follow-ups.

Both the benefits (avoidance of aggressive, invasive surgery including bone grafting; reduced financial cost; and increased speed of the final rehabilitation) and risks (prolonged postoperative pain due to canine pulpal tissue damage, followed by removal of the implant and the canine) of this approach were explained to the patient. In the case of failure of the experimental procedure, the conventional treatment (first proposed alternative treatment) would be provided at no additional cost for the patient. The patient chose the transcanine implantation procedure and signed the standardised dental informed consent document along with the general data protection regulation (GDPR) document.

2.1. Digital Planning Using coDiagnostiX® Software. In order to properly prepare for the implant placement procedure, coDiagnostiX® (Dental Wings Inc., Canada) digital planning software was used. Silicone impressions (ExaFast Putty and ExaFast NDS, GC Europe, Belgium) of the patient's jaws were sent to the lab, and analog models were cast out of dental stone (BriegelRock Spezial, Briegeldental, Germany). The models were scanned with an E2 lab scanner (3Shape, Copenhagen, Denmark), and a Standard Tessellation Language (STL) file of the patient's upper jaw was created. A CBCT (Cone-Beam Computed Tomography) scan (Orthophos SL, Dentsply Sirona, Bensheim, Germany) of the upper jaw in Digital Imaging and Communications in Medicine (DICOM) format was also taken and imported into the software along with the STL file of the jaw. When these two files were merged, virtual planning could begin. The implant positions were digitally planned considering the final prosthodontic solution (position of the future abutments and crowns) as well as the position of the impacted canines (i.e., avoiding hard canine enamel that could impair the drilling; Figure 3). Water cooling of the implant site was identified

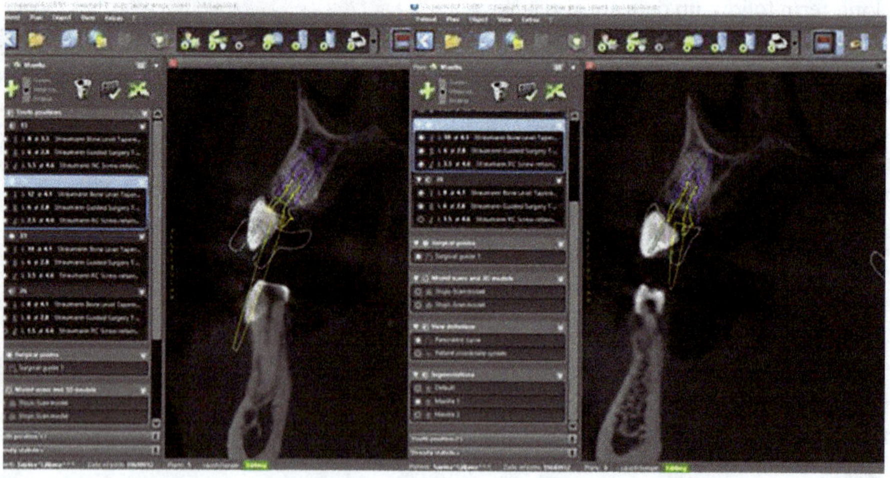

FIGURE 3: 3D planning—transcanine approach in regions 13 and 23.

as a potential problem, so a surgical guide with only pilot drill guide sleeves was created for positions 13 and 23. The guide was then 3D printed with a Straumann P20+3D printer (Rapid Shape, Heimsheim, Germany) using Pro Surgical Guide clear transparent resin material (P Pro Resin, DeltaMed, Friedberg, Germany; Figure 4).

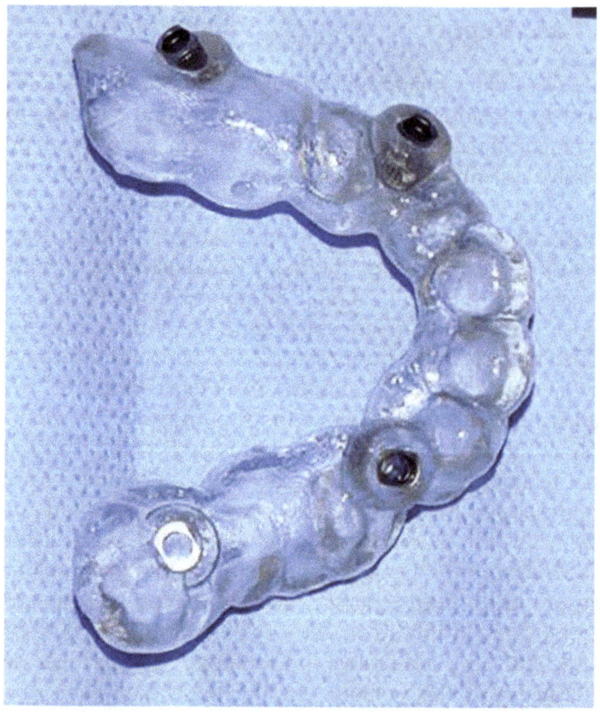

FIGURE 4: Surgical guide.

2.2. Surgical Procedure. The greatest concern associated with this guided surgery approach is the potential for excessive heat generation due to friction between the metal sleeves in the surgical template, implant drills, and corresponding guide handles [11–13]. The presence and design of a surgical template may prevent the irrigation fluid from entering the osteotomy site [13, 14]. The excessive heat generated coupled with inadequate irrigation may heat the bone higher than its biological threshold of 47°C and cause irreversible damage. Considering the CBCT measurements of the density of the dentin itself, which in some places exceeded 1000 HU, a protocol for preparation into bone density D1 [15, 16] at the positions of the impacted teeth was prepared. Therefore, we decided to use only a "partial" guided surgical approach for regions 13 and 23 and a drill up to 2.2 mm in diameter (pilot drill) to achieve the planned position of the implants in relation to the axis of the impacted teeth, bearing in mind the need to avoid the tooth enamel (Figures 5–7). A full guided surgery approach was planned at positions 16 and 26.

After raising the entire mucoperiosteal flap and setting the surgical template, osteotomies were performed in regions 16, 13, 23, and 26 with a pilot drill. Classic osteotomy without a surgical template was then done with final drills for implants at positions 13 and 23 (BLT SLActive Roxolid RC 4.1; Institut Straumann AG, Basel, Switzerland) with constant additional irrigation with 0.9% NaCl to ensure adequate cooling (Figure 6).

Implants at positions 16 (BLT SLActive Roxolid NC 3.3; Institut Straumann AG, Basel, Switzerland) and 26 (BLT SLActive Roxolid RC 4.1; Institut Straumann AG, Basel, Switzerland) were placed with a full digital approach without moving the surgical template during the whole procedure. At position 26, a transcrestal sinus lift procedure was performed without the addition of a xenograft.

After the placement of all implants, horizontal augmentation was performed with a xenograft (Xenograft 0.5 g; Institut Straumann AG, Basel, Switzerland) mixed with autologous bone, which was scraped from the nearby buccal plate, and covered with a resorbable collagen membrane (Membrane Flex; Institut Straumann AG, Basel, Switzerland) due to thickening of the residual bone, which, after implant placement, was less than the desired 2 mm buccal bone thickness at positions 16 and 26. Primary wound closure was performed with sutures.

2.3. Prosthodontic Procedure. During the healing period, the patient was provided with temporary PMMA bridges and crowns which were cemented on the remaining teeth. After 3 months of healing, screw-retained abutments, which were

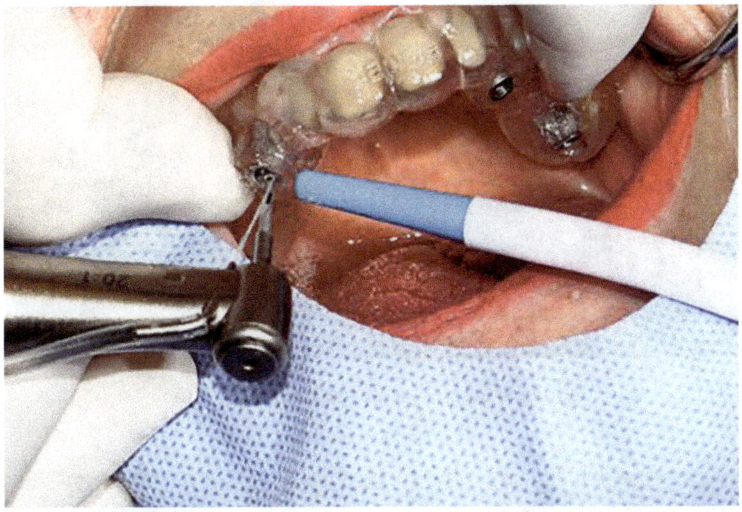

FIGURE 5: Osteotomy using a pilot drill and a surgical guide.

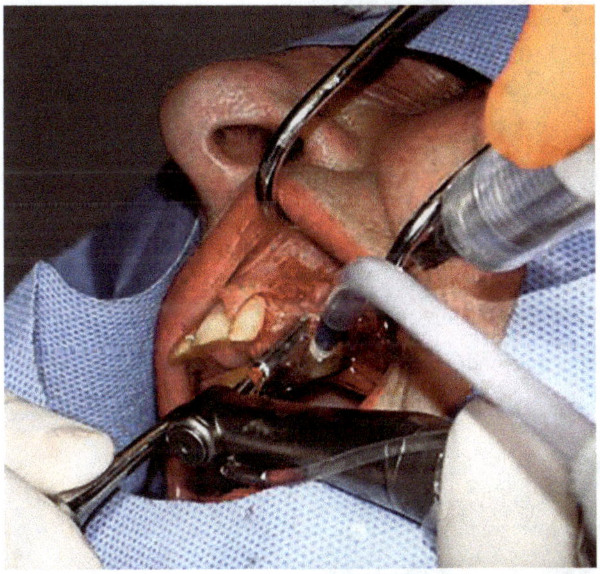

FIGURE 6: Gradual drilling with additional saline irrigation/cooling.

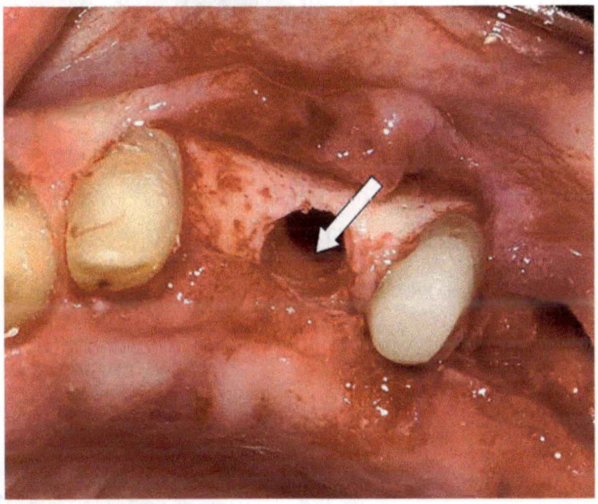

FIGURE 7: Drill hole through the bone and the impacted tooth (the white arrow).

already planned for the surgery itself, were placed and tightened to 35 N/cm according to the manufacturer's recommendation. After preparation of the remaining teeth in both jaws, impressions were taken with an individual tray using a polyether-based material (Impregum Penta Soft, 3M ESPE, Minnesota, USA). Artex Facebow was used to determine and translate intermaxillary relations to the Artex CR articulator (Amann Girrbach AG, Koblach, Austria). Zirconia ceramic crowns (Zolid Zirconia Block, Amann Girrbach, Koblach, Austria; Celtra Ceram Cladding Ceramics, Dentsply, Charlotte, USA) were produced to restore the remaining teeth. The implant crowns were made of a metal base (BEGO™ Chrome Cobalt Implant Bar, Bremen, Germany) coated with ceramics (Duceram Kiss, Dentsply, Charlotte, USA). Definite ceramic crowns were cemented using Fuji Plus cementum (GC Corp., Tokyo, Japan) on the natural teeth, and the implant crowns were tightened to SR abutments with 15 N/cm, as recommended by the manufacturer. Follow-up orthopantomogram was carried out at 3 and 6 months postoperatively (Figures 8–11). The patient was followed up for one year until now after the prosthodontic procedure was done.

3. Discussion

When an impacted tooth is in the way of an implant site, following standard implantology protocols, clinicians usually extract the tooth before placing the implant (simultaneous or delayed implantation) [17–20]. Thus, implantation in or through an impacted tooth represents a paradigm shift in the field of dental implantology. Hurzeler et al. [21] made a similar paradigm shift with the so-called "socket shield" technique, where part of the root is deliberately left inside the implant zone to support the buccal bone and prevent complications linked to postextraction bone loss. In the "socket

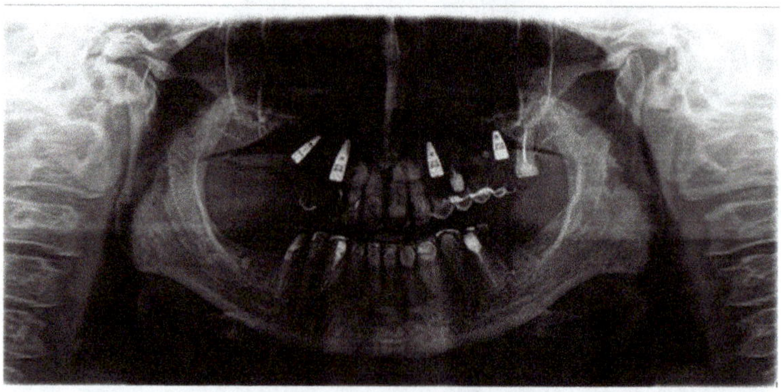

Figure 8: Panoramic image 3 months postop.

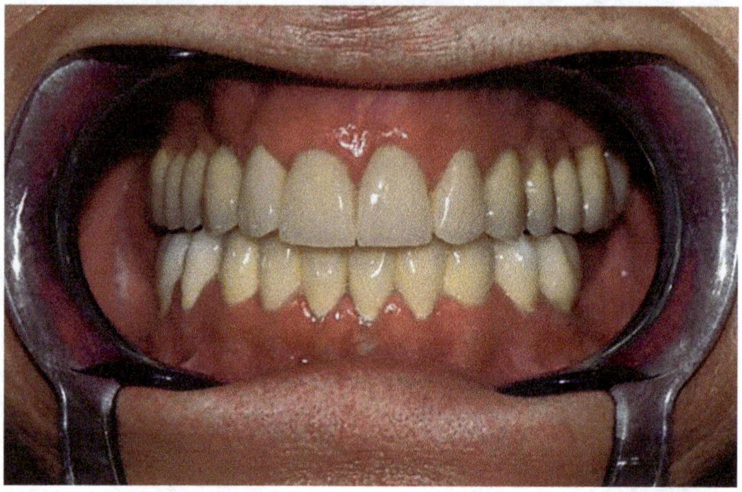

Figure 9: Intraoral status; the definite prosthodontic work.

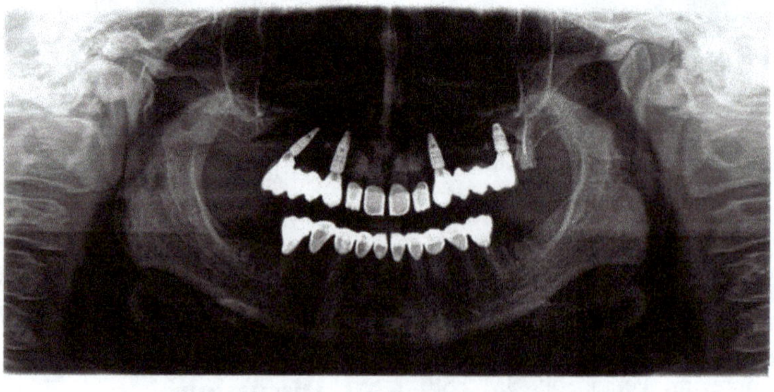

Figure 10: Panoramic image 6 months postop.

shield" approach, the implant surface comes into contact with the residual root. Histological and microscopic studies have revealed that the threads are partially filled with amorphous mineralised tissue and connective tissue. At a higher magnification, the implant threads were found to have integrated into the newly formed cementum interposed between dentin and the implant, without any fibrous tissues interposed [22]. Another unusual approach to implant placement is when the extracted tooth root is used as a bone "volume booster" in cases with an insufficient alveolar ridge volume. In this procedure, the tooth is extracted, adequately processed, and fixed laterally to the insufficient ridge in order to augment its volume. During implantation, after the healing period, the implant comes into contact with the ankylosed tooth structure, similar to the "socket shield" technique. Researchers have also confirmed the success of this approach [23].

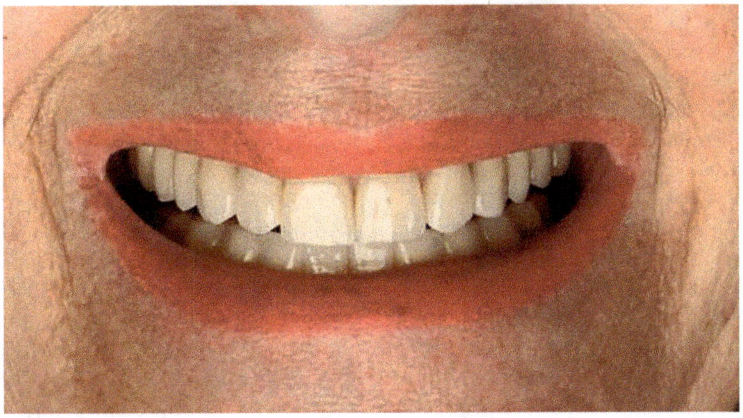

FIGURE 11: Patient's smile.

In contrast to the standard implant-tissue interface, transcanine implantation generates four "new" interfaces: (1) an implant-periodontal ligament interface, (2) an implant-cement interface, (3) an implant-dentine interface, and (4) an implant-pulp interface. We tried to avoid implant-enamel contact by using guided implant surgery and digital planning. In theory, the enamel could potentially complicate the implantation process due to its hardness, although Davarpanah et al. [9] stated that this implant-enamel contact did not jeopardize the implantation procedure or implant prognosis.

Our greatest concern was the contact between the pulp and the implant due to the potential for postoperative pain caused by pulpal damage and necrosis. However, no unusual postoperative pain was reported. A similar absence of pain was reported when coronectomy of the wisdom teeth close to the alveolar nerve was performed to avoid injuring the nerve or to move the impacted tooth away from the nerve [24, 25]. This technique was first described by Knutsson et al. [26] in 1989 and has been successfully used since then.

Results similar to ours have been reported in studies conducted by Davarpanah et al. [9] and Haddad et al. [27] in terms of an absence of postoperative pain and complications and final treatment success.

Unfortunately, we were unable to find any other studies, follow-ups or case reports, on this novel approach in the available literature. This is probably because situations where the insertion of an implant is indicated but impacted canines are in the way of the implant site are rare.

Guidelines on various implant treatments of patients with scleroderma or other autoimmune multisystem rheumatic diseases are hard to find in the available literature. Generally, in patients affected by autoimmune multisystem rheumatic diseases like scleroderma, large contact areas between oral mucosa and artificial surfaces of prosthodontic devices (especially removable ones) are less desirable, so a reduction of contact areas between prostheses and mucosa is advised [11]. Dental implants and implant-supported restorations could help achieve such requirements. Results of existing publications demonstrate encouraging outcomes regarding dental implant survival, which are comparable to those of healthy patients [11]. This is in accordance with findings of the current case report; our limited postoperative follow-up period showed no negative effects of dental implant placement on the patient suffering from scleroderma condition, both regarding oral soft tissue health and overall quality of masticatory function.

4. Conclusion

Placing dental implants through impacted canines and generating interfaces other than implant-bone interfaces did not lead to postoperative pain or implant failure. Clinically, overall healing was observed, and the implants were successfully used for implant-supported prosthodontic rehabilitation of the jaw. Within the limitations of this case report, transcanine implantation could represent a valuable alternative to standard implantation protocols.

References

[1] C. E. Misch, "Divisions of available bone," in *Contemporary Implant Dentistry*, C. E. Misch, Ed., pp. 123–155, CV Mosby, St. Louis, 1993.

[2] J. Cooke and H. L. Wang, "Canine impactions: incidence and management," *The International Journal of Periodontics & Restorative Dentistry*, vol. 26, no. 5, pp. 483–491, 2006.

[3] M. S. Yavuz, M. H. Aras, M. C. Buyukkurt, and S. Tozuglu, "Impacted mandibular canines," *The Journal of Contemporary Dental Practice*, vol. 8, no. 7, pp. 78–85, 2007.

[4] J. L. Gray and A. R. Vernino, "The interface between retained roots and dental implants. A histologic study in baboons, *Journal of Periodontology*, vol. 75, no. 8, pp. 1102–1106, 2004.

[5] M. Davarpanah and S. Szmukler-Moncler, "Unconventional implant treatment: I. implant placement in contact with ankylosed root fragments. A series of five case reports," *Clinical Oral Implants Research*, vol. 20, no. 8, pp. 851–856, 2009.

[6] M. Davarpanah and S. Szmukler-Moncler, "Unconventional implant treatment. 2: implant placed through impacted teeth. Three case reports," *The international periodontics and restorative dentistry*, vol. 29, pp. 405–413, 2009.

[7] S. Szmukler-Moncler and M. Davarpanah, "Reliability of the root-implant interface in unconventionally placed implants:

an up to 6-year follow-up of 23 implants covering 3 distinct clinical applications," *Clinical Oral Implants Research*, vol. 20, p. 814, 2009.

[8] S. Szmukler-Moncler, M. Davarpanah, K. Davarpanah, N. Capelle-Ouadah, G. Demurashvili, and P. Rajzbaum, "Unconventional implant placement part III: implant placement encroaching upon residual roots - a report of six cases," *Clinical implant dentistry and related research*, vol. 17, pp. e396–e405, 2015.

[9] M. Davarpanah, S. Szmukler-Moncler, P. Rajzbaum, K. Davarpanah, N. Capelle-Ouadah, and G. Demurashvili, "Unconventional implant placement. V: implant placement through impacted teeth; results from 10 cases with an 8- to 1-year follow-up," *International Orthodontics*, vol. 13, no. 2, pp. 164–180, 2015.

[10] H. Zigdon, Z. Gutmacher, S. Teich, and L. Levin, "Full-mouth rehabilitation using dental implants in a patient with scleroderma," *Quintessence International*, vol. 42, no. 9, pp. 781–785, 2011.

[11] F. P. Strietzel, A. M. Schmidt-Westhausen, K. Neumann, P. A. Reichart, and J. Jackowski, "Implants in patients with oral manifestations of autoimmune or muco-cutaneous diseases - a systematic review," *Medicina Oral, Patología Oral y Cirugía Bucal*, vol. 24, pp. e217–e230, 2019.

[12] S. D. Ganz, "Presurgical planning with CT-derived fabrication of surgical guides," *Journal of Oral and Maxillofacial Surgery*, vol. 63, no. 9, pp. 59–71, 2005.

[13] L. Frösch, K. Mukaddam, A. Filippi, N. U. Zitzmann, and S. Kühl, "Comparison of heat generation between guided and conventional implant surgery for single and sequential drilling protocols - an in vitro study," *Clinical Oral Implants Research*, vol. 30, no. 2, pp. 121–130, 2019.

[14] S. C. Möhlhenrich, A. Modabber, T. Steiner, D. A. Mitchell, and F. Hölzle, "Heat generation and drill wear during dental implant site preparation: systematic review," *The British Journal of Oral & Maxillofacial Surgery*, vol. 53, no. 8, pp. 679–689, 2015.

[15] Y. F. Liu, J. L. Wu, J. X. Zhang, W. Peng, and W. Q. Liao, "Numerical and experimental analyses on the temperature distribution in the dental implant preparation area when using a surgical guide," *Journal of Prosthodontics*, vol. 27, no. 1, pp. 42–51, 2018.

[16] A.'. al-Ekrish, G. Widmann, and S. A. Alfadda, "Revised, computed tomography-based Lekholm and Zarb jawbone quality classification," *The International Journal of Prosthodontics*, vol. 31, no. 4, pp. 342–345, 2018.

[17] J. J. Kruzic and R. O. Ritchie, "Fatigue of mineralized tissues: cortical bone and dentin," *Journal of the Mechanical Behavior of Biomedical Materials*, vol. 1, no. 1, pp. 3–17, 2008.

[18] Z. Mazor, M. Peleg, and M. Redlich, "IMMEDIATE PLACEMENT OF IMPLANTS IN EXTRACTION: SITES OF MAXILLARY IMPACTED CANINES," *Journal of the American Dental Association (1939)*, vol. 130, no. 12, pp. 1767–1770, 1999.

[19] D. Cardaropoli, C. Debernardi, and G. Cardaropoli, "Immediate placement of implant into impacted maxillary canine extraction socket," *The International Journal of Periodontics & Restorative Dentistry*, vol. 27, no. 1, pp. 71–77, 2007.

[20] B. García, A. Boronat, C. Larrazabal, M. Peñarrocha, and M. Peñarrocha, "Immediate implants after the removal of maxillary impacted canines: a clinical series of nine patients," *The International Journal of Oral & Maxillofacial Implants*, vol. 24, no. 2, pp. 348–352, 2009.

[21] M. B. Hurzeler, O. Zuhr, P. Schupbach, S. F. Rebele, N. Emmanouilidis, and S. Fickl, "The socket-shield technique: a proof-of-principle report," *Journal of Clinical Periodontology*, vol. 37, no. 9, pp. 855–862, 2010.

[22] D. Buser, K. Warrer, and T. Karring, "Formation of a periodontal ligament around titanium implants," *Journal of Periodontology*, vol. 61, no. 9, pp. 597–601, 1990.

[23] F. Schwarz, V. Golubovic, K. Becker, and I. Mihatovic, "Extracted tooth roots used for lateral alveolar ridge augmentation: a proof-of-concept study," *Journal of Clinical Periodontology*, vol. 43, no. 4, pp. 345–353, 2016.

[24] M. A. Pogrel, J. S. Lee, and D. F. Muff, "Coronectomy: a technique to protect the inferior alveolar nerve," *Journal of Oral and Maxillofacial Surgery*, vol. 62, no. 12, pp. 1447–1452, 2004.

[25] H. Long, Y. Zhou, L. Liao, U. Pyakurel, Y. Wang, and W. Lai, "Coronectomy vs. total removal for third molar extraction: a systematic review," *Journal of Dental Research*, vol. 91, no. 7, pp. 659–665, 2012.

[26] K. Knutsson, L. Lysell, and M. Rohlin, "Postoperative status after partial removal of the mandibular third molar," *Swedish Dental Journal*, vol. 13, no. 1-2, pp. 15–22, 1989.

[27] E. E. Haddad, R. Calcaterra, G. E. Haddad, V. Candotto, and D. Lauritano, "Treatment of maxillary retained canine with implants: new perspectives," *ORAL & implantology (Rome)*, vol. 10, no. 3, pp. 343–348, 2017.

10

Implant Prosthodontic Rehabilitation after Surgical Treatment for an Oropharyngeal Malignant Tumour using Tantalum Dental Implants

Marko Vuletić[1] **Ivica Pelivan**[2] **and Dragana Gabrić**[1]

[1]*Department of Oral Surgery, School of Dental Medicine, University of Zagreb, Zagreb, Croatia*
[2]*Department of Prosthodontics, School of Dental Medicine, University of Zagreb, Zagreb, Croatia*

Correspondence should be addressed to Marko Vuletić; mvuletic@sfzg.hr

Academic Editor: Pia L. Jornet

Oropharyngeal cancer (OPC) represents a significant portion of head and neck cancers. In most cases, it is localised in the soft palate, lingual and palatine tonsils, base of the tongue, and the surrounding tissues. Alcohol and tobacco exposure are well-known evidence-based risk factors for developing OPC; however, over the last decade, there has been a rapid increase in OPC linked to human papillomavirus (HPV). Dental implant therapy faces many challenges related to immediate and long-term success, and patients who are rehabilitated with implant prosthodontic therapy often have numerous comorbidities. Tantalum is a rare transitional metal element which has high corrosion resistance and is extremely inert. Porous tantalum trabecular metal (PTTM) has high volumetric porosity, a low modulus of elasticity, and very high friction. PTTM implant surface enhancement allows "osseoincorporation," which means the neovascularisation and formation of new bone directly onto the implant. A 65-year-old patient presented to the Department of Oral Surgery of Clinical Hospital Centre Zagreb after resection of the mandible due to OPC had oral rehabilitation. Three Zimmer Biomet Trabecular Metal™ implants (4.1 × 10 mm) were inserted in the area of lower left first incisor, lower left second premolar, and lower right second premolar, and after four months, a new upper partial denture and the bar-retained mandibular overdenture were made. Implant prosthodontic rehabilitation of head and neck cancer patients is usually challenging in terms of achieving an improvement in its main aim, quality of life; however, today it is a safe and reliable therapy. Although radiation therapy may negatively affect the patient's oral condition and influence the short- and long-term success of the implant, the presented case report showed that the excellent properties of PTTM-enhanced dental implants may give great basis for future comparative researches of using these implants in the treatment of oncologic patients.

1. Introduction

Squamous cell carcinoma affecting the head and neck is the sixth most common cancer worldwide, with 700,000 cases diagnosed per year [1]. Despite advances in multimodality therapy, the survival rate remains approximately 40–50% [2, 3]. Oropharyngeal cancer (OPC) represents a significant portion of head and neck cancers [4]. In most cases, it is localised in the soft palate, lingual and palatine tonsils, base of the tongue, and the surrounding tissues. Alcohol and tobacco exposure are well-known evidence-based risk factors for developing OPC; however, over the last decade, there has been a rapid increase in OPC linked to human papillomavirus (HPV) [5]. HPV is a DNA virus with a predilection for the squamous epithelium [6]. The epithelium covering the base of the tongue and tonsils acts as a reservoir for the virus, providing access to the basal layer for viral replication [4]. HPV infection of the oropharynx occurs five times more frequently than infection of the oral cavity, hypopharynx, and larynx because of its predilection for the reticulated crypt epithelium covering the oropharynx, which is unique to the head and neck region [7]. The majority of OPC cases related to HPV are caused by HPV-16. The recommended treatment options for OPC depend on the tumour, mode, metastasis (TNM) stage, the patient's preferences and comorbidities, and the physician's experience. Early-stage disease is often treated with single modality treatment, such as radiotherapy or surgery alone, while regionally advanced OPC is treated with dual modality treatment [8].

Dental implant therapy faces many challenges related to immediate and long-term success, and patients who are rehabilitated with implant prosthodontic therapy often have numerous comorbidities. There have been many efforts to improve dental implant performance at the point of implant-bone contact by modifying the topography and chemistry of the surface [9]. Microtopography of the surface in titanium implants was modified using sandblasting and acid-etch treatment [10]. Many studies published since the 1970s have reported that the size of the pores and percentage of porosity are the most important factors for bone healing around the dental implant [11]. In their 1999 study, Bobyn et al. [12] presented a tantalum-based, trabecular-structured biomaterial with 80% porosity, produced by coating a vitreous carbon scaffold with elemental tantalum through a chemical vapour deposition process (Trabecular Metal Material; Zimmer Biomet TMT, Parsippany, NJ, USA). Tantalum is a rare transitional metal element which has high corrosion resistance and is extremely inert such that it can only be dissolved by hydrofluoric acid and acid solutions containing fluoride and sulphur trioxide. Its inertness is ideal for the fabrication of orthopaedic implants, devices for nerve repair, electrodes for pacemakers, cranioplasty plates, and radiographic markers [13]. The development of porous tantalum metal has resulted in stronger and more biocompatible craniofacial, orthopaedic, and dental implants. Porous tantalum trabecular metal (PTTM) has high volumetric porosity, a low modulus of elasticity, and very high friction [13]. PTTM allows implant surface enhancement, not only for bone ongrowth but also bone ingrowth. This structure allows "osseoincorporation," which means the neovascularisation and formation of new bone directly onto the implant [14]. For dental applications, this PTTM biomaterial is positioned in the midsection of a conventional titanium alloy implant body (Trabecular Metal™ Dental Implants; Zimmer Biomet, Palm Beach Gardens, FL, USA), comprising the coronal, apical, and internal regions of the implant [15].

This case report presents the successful clinical use of TM dental implants in an irradiated mandible for the oral rehabilitation of an oncologic patient.

2. Case Presentation

A 65-year-old male patient presented to the Department of Oral Surgery of Clinical Hospital Centre Zagreb after resection of the mandible due to OPC that was surgically treated in April 2015 (Figures 1 and 2). He was referred by a prosthodontist due to an inability to function with a full denture. He had no history of tobacco smoking and only drank socially and did not have any other usual predisposition factors for carcinogenesis in this area. Until this disease, his medical status was remarkable. The patient's medical history revealed radical neck dissection, commando surgery, and reconstruction using an anterolateral thigh (ALT) flap due to a squamous cell carcinoma localised in the anterior palate arch with expansion into the retromolar trigonum area and lateral

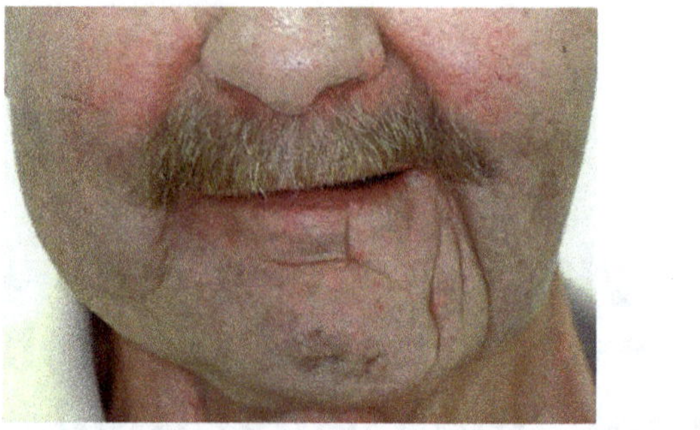

Figure 1: Frontal view of the patient.

oropharyngeal walls (T3N0M0). The patient had received postoperative chemotherapy (cisplatin i.v.) for a total of three cycles in conjunction with radiotherapy. Three-dimensional conformal radiotherapy was performed in the region of the tumour, with a total of 32 fractions using a total dose of 64 Gy. In the region of the neck lymph node bilaterally 25 fractions in a total dose of 50 Gy were performed. The patient handled the therapy well (ECOG 0), with no major side effects. The only symptom he had was the expected local side effect of mucositis. Replacement hormone therapy with 50 μg levothyroxine had also been introduced.

On initial examination, an edentulous mandible was found with a narrow zone of attached mucosa, preventing the fabrication of a satisfactory full denture (Figure 3). Three months before, the patient extracted all remained teeth, upper right molar, four mandibular incisors, and lower right canine because of impossibility of restoration due to deep caries or periapical lesions. A cone beam computed tomography (CBCT) was performed, where adequate residual alveolar ridge height and width for the insertion of dental implants were observed. After consultation with a prosthodontist, we decided to place three dental implants for future fabrication of a bar-retained overdenture.

In accordance with the ethical protocol of the School of Dental Medicine of the University of Zagreb, written consent was obtained from the patient prior to surgery in January 2019. The patient received antibiotic premedication (one day before surgery, the patient started antibiotic therapy with amoxicillin with clavulanic acid twice a day and lasted for six days postoperative). Crestal incision on the edentulous mandible was performed under local infiltration anaesthesia (4% articaine with epinephrine 1 : 200,000; 5.4 mL). The full mucoperiosteal flap was elevated to expose the residual alveolar ridge. Three Zimmer Biomet Trabecular Metal™ implants (4.1 × 10 mm) were inserted in the area of lower left first incisor, lower left second premolar, and lower right second premolar with a maximum insertion torque of 25 Ncm (Figures 4–6). Sutures were removed 7 days postoperatively without any complications. Four months after implant placement (Figure 7), the implants were reopened and gingival formers were placed (Figure 8). Two weeks later, anatomical and functional impressions of both jaws were taken for the production of a new upper partial denture and the bar-retained mandibular overdenture (Figures 9–11). The

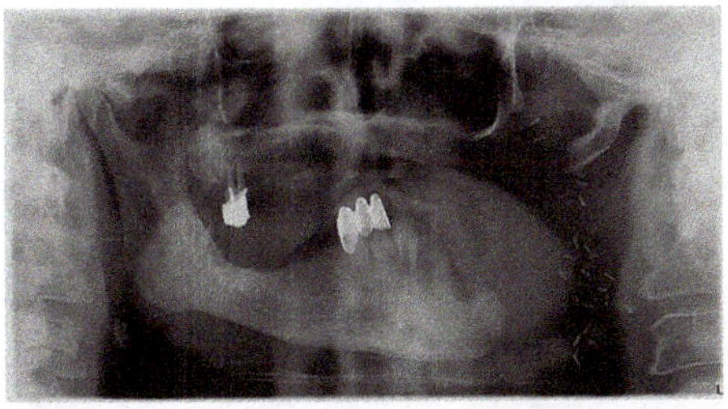

Figure 2: Panoramic image.

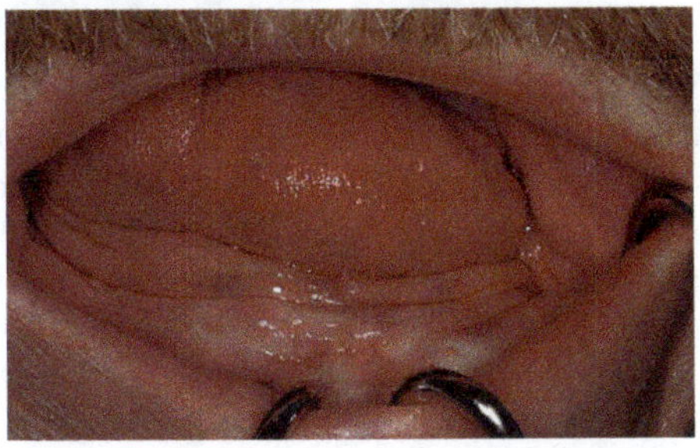

Figure 3: Intraoral situation before surgery.

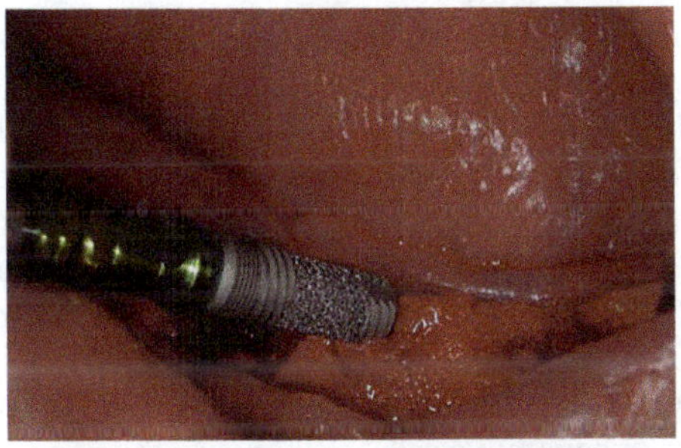

Figure 4: Insertion of Trabecular Metal™ Dental Implants (Zimmer Biomet, Palm Beach Gardens, FL, USA).

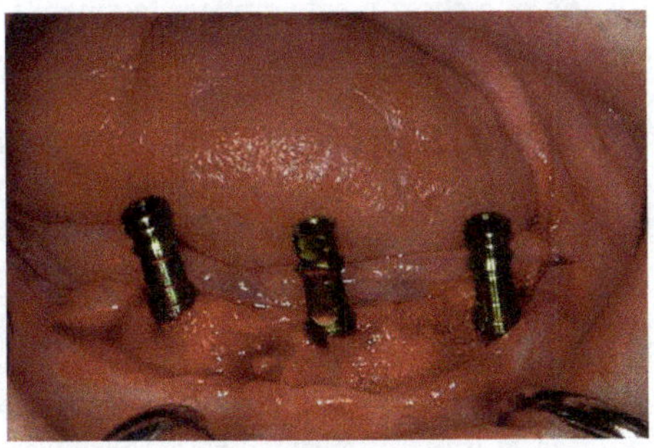

Figure 5: Clinical view after insertion.

greatest challenge was to reconcile the severely displaced maxilla mandibular relationship with an aesthetic and functional final result. Three weeks later, new dentures were given to the patient (Figure 12). No local complications of implant prosthodontic therapy were clinically observed. The patient reported a significant improvement in chewing efficiency and, consequently, quality of life in period afterwards. The patient was followed up until now for 1 year, through regular examinations every 6 months,

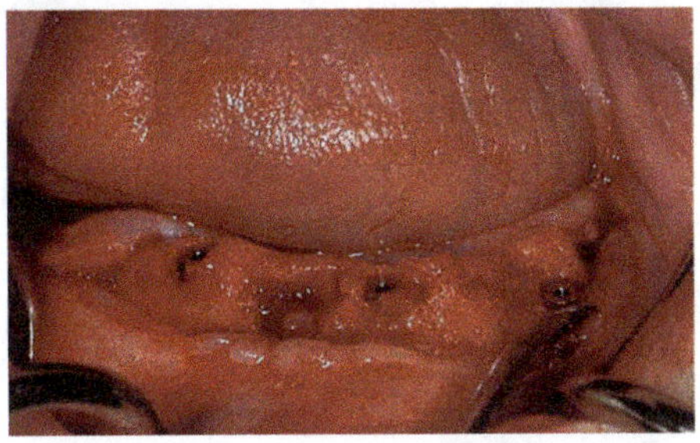

Figure 6: Situation after removing transfers.

and he did not report any problems or we did not notice any potential complications in this period.

3. Discussion

Oral rehabilitation after head and neck cancer treatment is one of the most challenging procedures in dentistry today. Patients treated with chemotherapy and radiation are predisposed to hyposalivation, mucositis, reduced angiogenesis, delayed healing, loss of taste, radiation-induced caries, trismus, and osteoradionecrosis of the jaw (ORN). ORN, which is the ischemic necrosis of bone, is the most serious complication [16]. Irradiation causes changes in the bone as a result of injury to the remodelling system (osteocytes, osteoblasts, and osteoclasts) and vascular injury, such as hyperaemia, thrombosis, endarteritis, and a progressive occlusion and obliteration of small vessels. Acellularity and avascularity with fibrosis and fatty degeneration affect the bone marrow in the postradiation period [17]. ORN occurs more frequently in the mandible than the maxilla. In 30% of cases, ORN is asymptomatic, but the remaining cases always develop fistula, pain, or bone fracture. In the literature [18, 19], the risk of developing ORN has been reported to be about 2%, but this depends on the type and invasiveness of the surgical procedure and can be much higher. The risk of trauma-induced ORN is indefinite and is related not only to the volume and radiation dose but also to the dental health of the patient [16, 18]. Because the potential risk persists throughout the patient's life, the placement of dental implants should be carefully planned. The patient in this case report only had mucositis as a side effect of head and neck treatment and showed no signs of ORN after dental extractions, which were performed three months before implant therapy.

An extensive prosthetic treatment is needed to restore function, speech, and mastication. Implant-supported prosthodontics is a challenge, but it has many advantages over conventional prostheses including improved mastication, retention, and patient acceptance [20]. Patients receiving head and neck radiation are at greater risk for dental implant failure due to the changes in hard and soft tissue mentioned earlier. Irreversible changes to the blood vessels and bone-forming cells that affect bone turnover caused by radiation therapy compromise the osseointegration of dental implants [21]. In the literature, there are no clear guidelines regarding the timing of implant placement in patients who have undergone radiotherapy of the jaw. Some authors [22] state that the

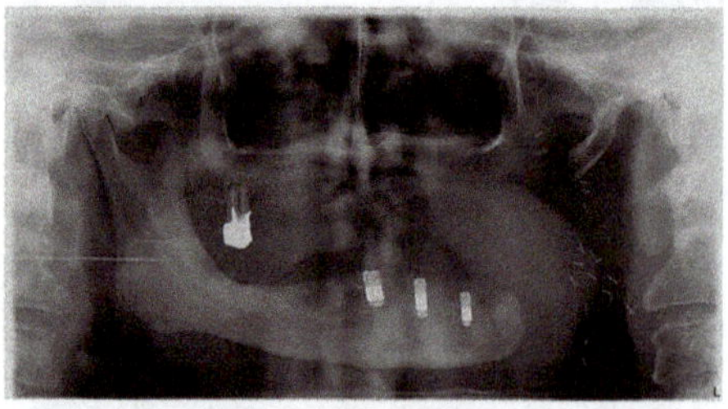

FIGURE 7: Postoperative panoramic image.

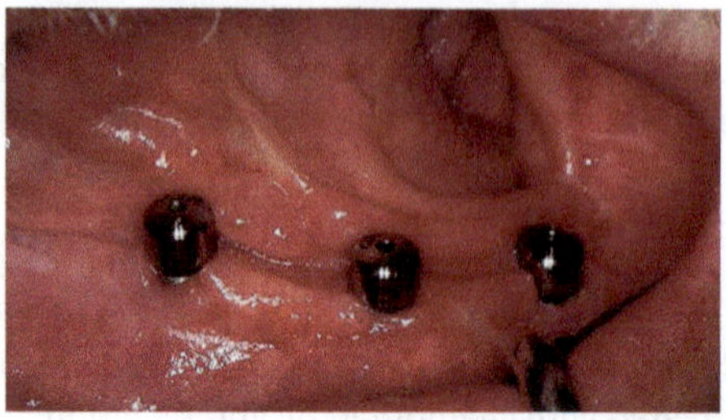

FIGURE 8: Placing gingival healing abutments.

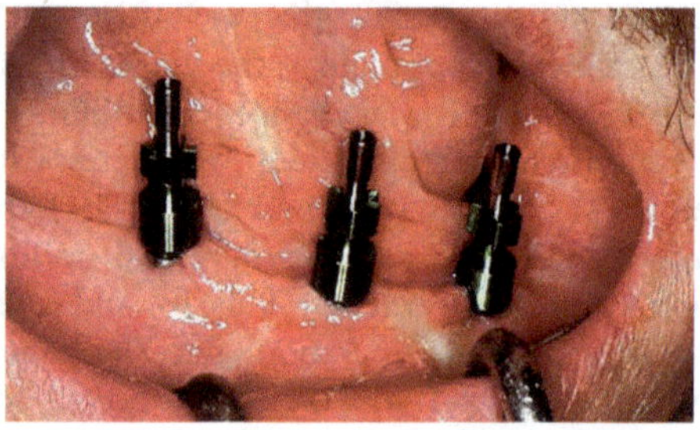

FIGURE 9: Transfers for open-tray impression.

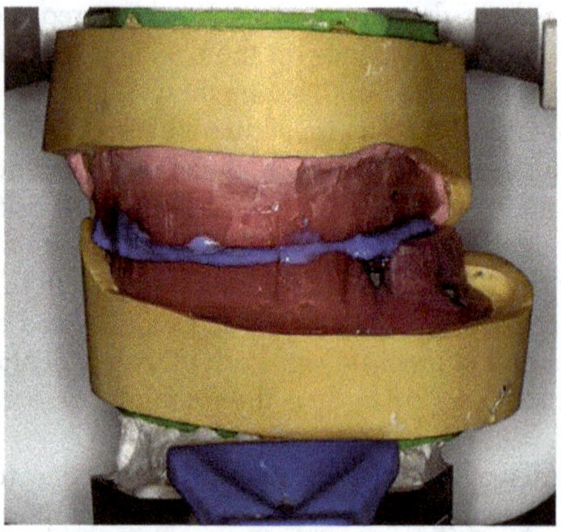

FIGURE 10: Maxillomandibular relationship.

bone should be allowed to recover from the radiation insult for some time before dental implant therapy, while Schepers et al. [23] reported that radiation therapy after dental implant placement did not affect osseointegration. A review by Nooh [24] found that postimplantation radiation therapy had a slightly better overall dental implant survival rate (92.2%) than preimplantation radiation therapy (88.9%), but these findings did not reach statistical significance. Although the

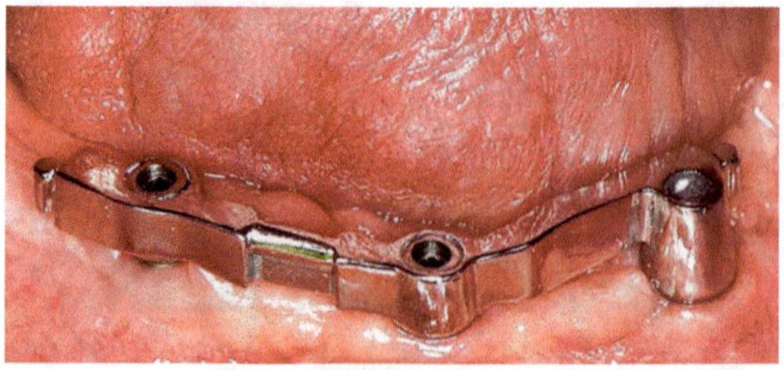

FIGURE 11: Individual milled bar for retaining mandibular overdenture.

mandible is more prone to ORN, it was reported that dental implants osseointegrate with greater success in the irradiated mandible in regard to its anatomy [25]. The anterior part of the mandible is usually exposed to a lower radiation dose and has a better remodelling capability due to the additional vascular supply from the facial artery [26]. In the presented case report, three dental implants were inserted into the anterior region of the mandible during the postimplantation period, and there were no signs of complications after 1-year follow-up (Figure 13).

Colella et al. [25] reported a correlation between implant failure and a radiation dose greater than 45 Gy. In the review by Nooh [24], radiation doses among individual studies ranged from 25 to 72 Gy; the uncommon incidence of low-dose radiation therapy was also 45 Gy, while a radiation dose above 55 Gy was associated with a significantly reduced survival rate of implants inserted during the postradiation period. The total dose of radiotherapy in the presented patient was 64 Gy because this is the dose prescribed for the treatment of squamous cell carcinoma of the head and neck, which is above marginal value range in which dental implant rehabilitation is recommended.

The recovery period after ionising radiation has a bipolar flow, consisting of a short positive phase lasting a few weeks and a long negative phase that lasts for years, characterised by hypovascularity, hypoxia, and hypocellularity [27]. In the study by Linsen et al. [28], the time between radiation therapy and dental implant placement varied from 6 weeks to 24 months, while other studies [24] reported intervals ranging from 4 to 228 months for the preimplantation period. In most studies, implant therapy was accomplished within a mean of 24 months after irradiation. Although the review by Nooh [24] found no statistical significance between time interval and dental implant survival rate, there was a higher overall implant survival rate after a mean of 30 months following the end of radiation. The recovery period in this case was 40 months after radiation therapy.

In the literature, there are no recent cases or studies involving TM implants in irradiated jaws. Joglekar et al. [29] found that tantalum trabecular metal acetabular components provided reliable reconstructions in patients following prior pelvic radiation. After a 5-year follow-up, they did not report any clinical or radiographic failures. In a study by Bencharit et al. [30], the authors mentioned that modern root-form endosseous titanium dental implants are commonly used due to their high success rate, but it is obvious

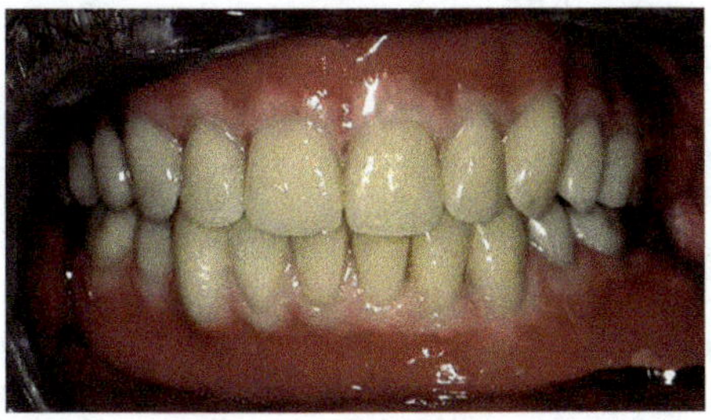

FIGURE 12: Upper partial denture and the bar-retained mandibular overdenture.

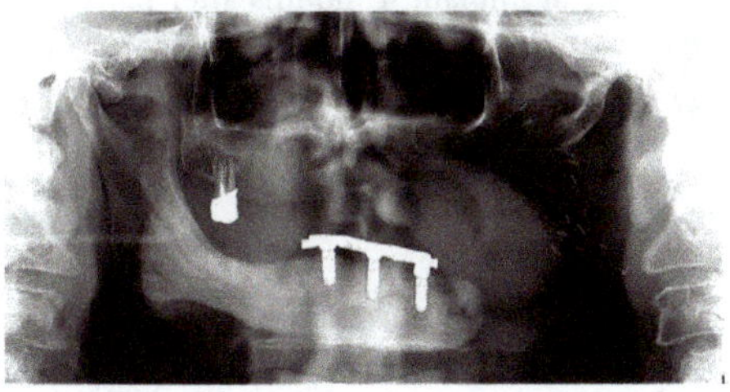

FIGURE 13: Panoramic image after 1-year follow-up.

that its osseointegration should be enhanced in patients with certain systemic medical conditions. In cases with poor tissue healing, such as patients with osteoporosis, diabetes mellitus, or irradiated bone, the findings related to TM implants suggest that there should be benefits from this type of implant. This case report demonstrated oral rehabilitation with TM dental implants with excellent ingrowth promotion for secondary implant stability, although further evidence is needed. During placement, implants were submerged 1 mm below the crestal bone, so from a theoretical point of view, there was no influence of the oral cavity or to bacteria. Spinato et al. [31] presented a case report of a healthy patient with a trabecular metal implant, in whom bone resorption was observed only in the coronal third of the implant, which was primarily composed of titanium. The greatest amount of bone was around the tantalum trabeculae compared to the apical part of the implant. The main reason for this result was bone remodelling following surgery and bone loss due to implant unloading. In many cases, bone disappearance from the coronal third can be related to bone remodelling after surgery and consequent erosion of the basal bone. The amount of bone around the middle trabecular part was greater because of the well-known properties of TM, in addition to the fact that the implant was unloaded. Spinato et al. [31] observed that the architecture of TM not only enhanced bone growth into the pores but also permitted more mechanical retention. Analysis of the orthopantomograph of our patient after 1-year follow-up showed consistent findings to those observed by Spinato et al. [31], who observed a small amount of bone loss around the implant in the coronal part, but without any clinical signs of peri-inflammation.

4. Conclusion

Implant prosthodontic rehabilitation of head and neck cancer patients is usually challenging in terms of achieving an improvement in its main aim, quality of life; however, today it is a safe and reliable therapy. Although radiation therapy may negatively affect the patient's oral condition and influence the short- and long-term success of the implant, the presented case report showed that the excellent properties of PTTM-enhanced dental implants may give great basis for future comparative researches of using these implants in the treatment of oncologic patients.

References

[1] J. Ferlay, I. Soerjomataram, R. Dikshit et al., "Cancer incidence and mortality worldwide: sources, methods and major patterns in GLOBOCAN 2012," *International Journal of Cancer*, vol. 136, no. 5, pp. E359–E386, 2015.

[2] C. Allen, S. Duffy, T. Teknos et al., "Nuclear factor-kappaB-related serum factors as longitudinal biomarkers of response and survival in advanced oropharyngeal carcinoma," *Clinical Cancer Research*, vol. 13, no. 11, pp. 3182–3190, 2007.

[3] M. S. Leibowitz, P. A. Andrade Filho, S. Ferrone, and R. L. Ferris, "Deficiency of activated STAT1 in head and neck cancer cells mediates TAP1-dependent escape from cytotoxic T lymphocytes," *Cancer Immunology, Immunotherapy*, vol. 60, no. 4, pp. 525–535, 2011.

[4] M. E. McLaughlin-Drubin and K. Munger, "Oncogenic activities of human papillomaviruses," *Virus Research*, vol. 143, no. 2, pp. 195–208, 2009.

[5] B. S. Ducatman, "The role of human papillomavirus in oropharyngeal squamous cell carcinoma," *Archives of Pathology & Laboratory Medicine*, vol. 142, no. 6, pp. 715–718, 2018.

[6] N. Munoz, X. Castellsagué, A. B. de González, and L. Gissmann, "Chapter 1: HPV in the etiology of human cancer," *Vaccine*, vol. 24, Suppl 3, pp. S1–S10, 2006.

[7] J. D. Combes and S. Franceschi, "Role of human papillomavirus in non-oropharyngeal head and neck cancers," *Oral Oncology*, vol. 50, no. 5, pp. 370–379, 2014.

[8] J. P. Shah, S. G. Patel, and B. Singh, *Jatin Shah's Head and Neck Surgery and Oncology*, Elsevier/Mosby, Philadelphia, 4th edition, 2012.

[9] S. Lavenus, G. Louarn, and P. Layrolle, "Nanotechnology and dental implants," *International Journal of Biomaterials*, vol. 2010, Article ID 915327, 9 pages, 2010.

[10] P. Trisi, C. Marcato, and M. Todisco, "Bone-to-implant apposition with machined and MTX microtextured implant surfaces in human sinus grafts," *The International Journal of Periodontics & Restorative Dentistry*, vol. 23, no. 5, pp. 427–437, 2003.

[11] M. Schlee, G. Pradies, W. U. Mehmke et al., "Prospective, multicenter evaluation of trabecular metal-enhanced titanium dental implants placed in routine dental practices: 1-year interim report from the development period (2010 to 2011)," *Clinical Implant Dentistry and Related Research*, vol. 17, no. 6, pp. 1141–1153, 2015.

[12] J. D. Bobyn, G. J. Stackpool, S. A. Hacking, M. Tanzer, and J. J. Krygier, "Characteristics of bone ingrowth and interface mechanics of a new porous tantalum biomaterial," *Journal of Bone and Joint Surgery. British Volume (London)*, vol. 81-B, no. 5, pp. 907–914, 1999.

[13] B. R. Levine, S. Sporer, R. A. Poggie, C. J. Della Valle, and J. J. Jacobs, "Experimental and clinical performance of porous tan-

talum in orthopedic surgery," *Biomaterials*, vol. 27, no. 27, pp. 4671–4681, 2006.

[14] R. Cohen, "A porous tantalum trabecular metal: basic science," *The American Journal of Orthopedics*, vol. 31, no. 4, pp. 216-217, 2002.

[15] D. J. Kim, S. S. Huja, B. C. Tee et al., "Bone ingrowth and initial stability of titanium and porous tantalum dental implants: a pilot canine study," *Implant Dentistry*, vol. 22, no. 4, pp. 399–405, 2013.

[16] A. Vissink, F. R. Burlage, F. K. Spijkervet, J. Jansma, and R. P. Coppes, "Prevention and treatment of the consequences of head and neck radiotherapy," *Critical Reviews in Oral Biology and Medicine*, vol. 14, no. 3, pp. 213–225, 2003.

[17] T. I. Tanaka, H. L. Chan, D. I. Tindle, M. Maceachern, and T. J. Oh, "Updated clinical considerations for dental implant therapy in irradiated head and neck cancer patients," *Journal of Prosthodontics*, vol. 22, no. 6, pp. 432–438, 2013.

[18] S. Nabil and N. Samman, "Risk factors for osteoradionecrosis after head and neck radiation: a systematic review," *Oral Surgery, Oral Medicine, Oral Pathology, Oral Radiology*, vol. 113, no. 1, pp. 54–69, 2012.

[19] S. Nabil and N. Samman, "Incidence and prevention of osteoradionecrosis after dental extraction in irradiated patients: a systematic review," *International Journal of Oral and Maxillofacial Surgery*, vol. 40, no. 3, pp. 229–243, 2011.

[20] L. Anderson, S. Meraw, K. Al-Hezaimi, and H. L. Wang, "The influence of radiation therapy on dental implantology," *Implant Dentistry*, vol. 22, no. 1, pp. 31–38, 2013.

[21] S. Ihde, K. Gundlach, and V. S. Konstantinovic, "Effects of radiation therapy on craniofacial and dental implants: a review of the literature," *Oral Surgery, Oral Medicine, Oral Pathology, Oral Radiology, and Endodontics*, vol. 107, no. 1, pp. 56–65, 2009.

[22] G. Granström, "Osseointegration in irradiated cancer patients: an analysis with respect to implant failures," *Journal of Oral and Maxillofacial Surgery*, vol. 63, no. 5, pp. 579–585, 2005.

[23] R. H. Schepers, A. P. Slagter, J. H. Kaanders, F. J. van den Hoogen, and M. A. Merkx, "Effect of postoperative radiotherapy on the functional result of implants placed during ablative surgery for oral cancer," *International Journal of Oral and Maxillofacial Surgery*, vol. 35, no. 9, pp. 803–808, 2006.

[24] N. Nooh, "Dental implant survival in irradiated oral cancer patients: a systematic review of the literature," *The International Journal of Oral & Maxillofacial Implants*, vol. 28, no. 5, pp. 1233–1242, 2013.

[25] G. Colella, R. Cannavale, M. Pentenero, and S. Gandolfo, "Oral implants in radiated patients: a systematic review," *The International Journal of Oral & Maxillofacial Implants*, vol. 22, no. 4, pp. 616–622, 2007.

[26] J. A. de Oliveira, A. L. do Amaral Escada, M. C. Alves Rezende, M. B. Mathor, and A. P. R. Alves Claro, "Analysis of the effects of irradiation in osseointegrated dental implants," *Clinical Oral Implants Research*, vol. 23, no. 4, pp. 511–514, 2012.

[27] L. L. Visch, M. A. van Waas, P. I. Schmitz, and P. C. Levendag, "A clinical evaluation of implants in irradiated oral cancer patients," *Journal of Dental Research*, vol. 81, no. 12, pp. 856–859, 2002.

[28] S. S. Linsen, M. Martini, and H. Stark, "Long-term results of endosteal implants following radical oral cancer surgery with and without adjuvant radiation therapy," *Clinical Implant Dentistry and Related Research*, vol. 14, no. 2, pp. 250–258, 2012.

[29] S. B. Joglekar, P. S. Rose, D. G. Lewallen, and F. H. Sim, "Tantalum acetabular cups provide secure fixation in THA after pelvic irradiation at minimum 5-year followup," *Clinical Orthopaedics and Related Research*, vol. 470, no. 11, pp. 3041–3047, 2012.

[30] S. Bencharit, W. C. Byrd, S. Altarawneh et al., "Development and applications of porous tantalum trabecular metal-enhanced titanium dental implants," *Clinical Implant Dentistry and Related Research*, vol. 16, no. 6, pp. 817–826, 2014.

[31] S. Spinato, D. Zaffe, P. Felice, L. Checchi, and H. L. Wang, "A trabecular metal implant 4 months after placement: clinical-histologic case report," *Implant Dentistry*, vol. 23, no. 1, pp. 3–7, 2014.

11

Rehabilitation of an Extremely Edentulous Atrophic Maxilla with a Pseudoskeletal Class III Relationship

Gregor-Georg Zafiropoulos,[1] Tae Ho Yoon,[2] and Moosa Abuzayda[2]

[1] *University of Sharjah, College of Dental Medicine, Sharjah, UAE*
[2] *Hamdan Bin Mohammed College of Dental Medicine, Mohammed Bin Rashid University, Dubai, UAE*

Correspondence should be addressed to Gregor-Georg Zafiropoulos; ggzafi@gmx.de

Academic Editor: Daniel Torrés-Lagares

The skeletal class III relationship presents complex dentoalveolar problems, requiring multidisciplinary treatment. In edentulous people, severe atrophy of the jawbone simulates the clinical appearance of a skeletal class III relationship (pseudoskeletal class III), which presents major problems for rehabilitation. This article describes the rehabilitation of a 67-year-old patient with a pseudoskeletal class III relationship. The mandible was restored with two implant-supported bar-retained overdentures using clips for retention. The extremely atrophic maxilla was restored with a combination of sinus augmentation, implant placement, and classic prosthodontic treatment using an electroformed mesostructured overdenture with swivel lock attachments on an implant-supported bar. By performing minimal augmentative and implant surgeries and using the possibilities and advantages of classic prosthetic dentistry, the clinical situation described here could be managed and the atrophic maxilla could be rehabilitated.

1. Introduction

The prosthetic rehabilitation of a fully edentulous and atrophic arch with implant-retained dentures requires thorough planning and should not only provide the correct vertical height and maxillary-mandibular relationship but also be esthetically acceptable [1–4]. The use of implant-supported overdentures is a treatment option for the restoration of fully edentulous jaws when conventional dentures have deficient retention due to advanced bone atrophy [1–4]. In older complete denture wearers, advanced jawbone atrophy simulates the clinical situation of a skeletal class III relationship combined with vertical alveolar bone loss; this condition is classified as pseudoskeletal class III. The true skeletal class III condition presents complex dentoalveolar problems, resulting from maxillary retrognathism and mandibular prognathism [5]. In such cases, rehabilitation presents a major challenge and multidisciplinary treatment is necessary. The application of regenerative techniques to the soft and hard tissues, sinus augmentation, implant placement, and/or Le Fort I osteotomy (e.g., orthognathic surgery) is often required, necessitating the involvement of periodontists, prosthodontists, and orthodontists, as well as oral and maxillofacial surgeons [5–10]. In pseudoskeletal class III cases in aged persons, resulting from multiple tooth extractions and severe or advanced atrophy of the jawbone over time, rehabilitation is also a major problem due not only to high levels of discomfort in the surgical and postsurgical phases but also the reduced regenerative capacity of the soft and hard tissues in this population. For this reason, less-invasive procedures for the implant-supported restoration of severely atrophic jaws, such as the placement of tilted or pterygoid implants, have been introduced [6–8].

There is debate of how many implant support will be sufficient for the retention of fully edentulous mandibular prosthesis. Recently, it has been concluded that two implant removable overdentures should become the first choice of the treatment for the mandible supporting the McGill and York consensus statement [11–13].

This article describes the rehabilitation of an elderly patient with a pseudoskeletal class III relationship. In this case, the mandible was restored with two implant-supported

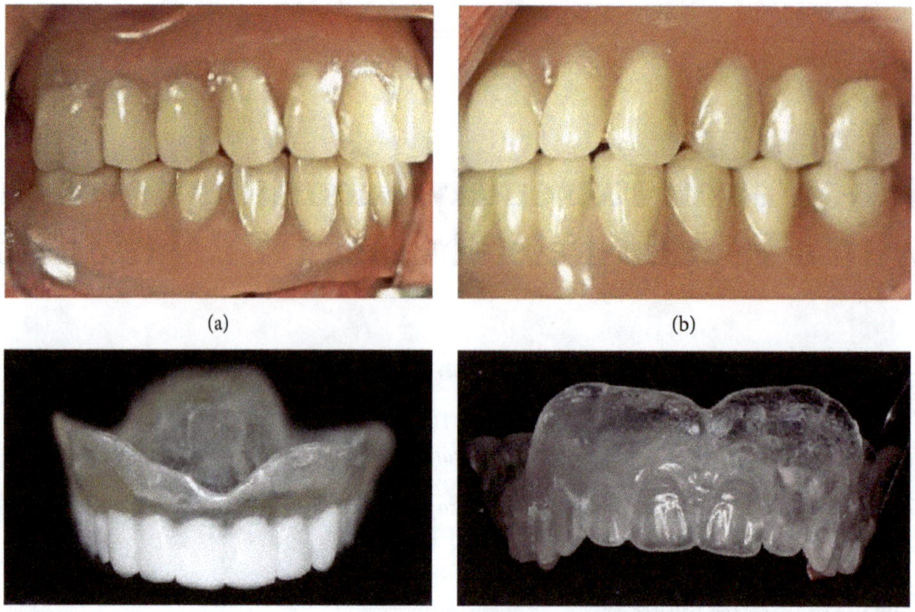

(a) (b) (c) (d)

FIGURE 1: Initial examination: (a) patient's dentures, right side; (b) patient's dentures, left side; (c) DentDu-Brm for the implant planning using barium sulfate resin for the teeth; (d) DentDu fabricated from clear resin.

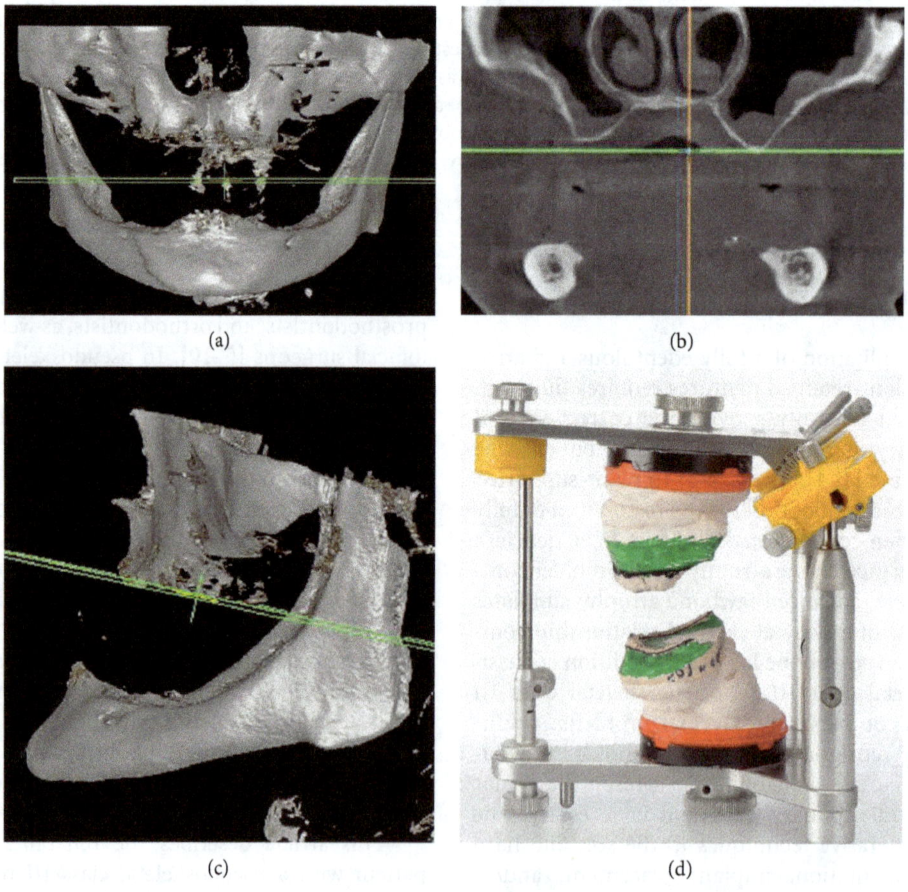

(a) (b) (c) (d)

FIGURE 2: CBCT bone masking showing generalized advanced atrophy of the maxilla and posterior mandibular atrophy: (a) front view; (b) sinuses in sagittal section; (c) side view; (d) articulated casts show patient's jaw relationship.

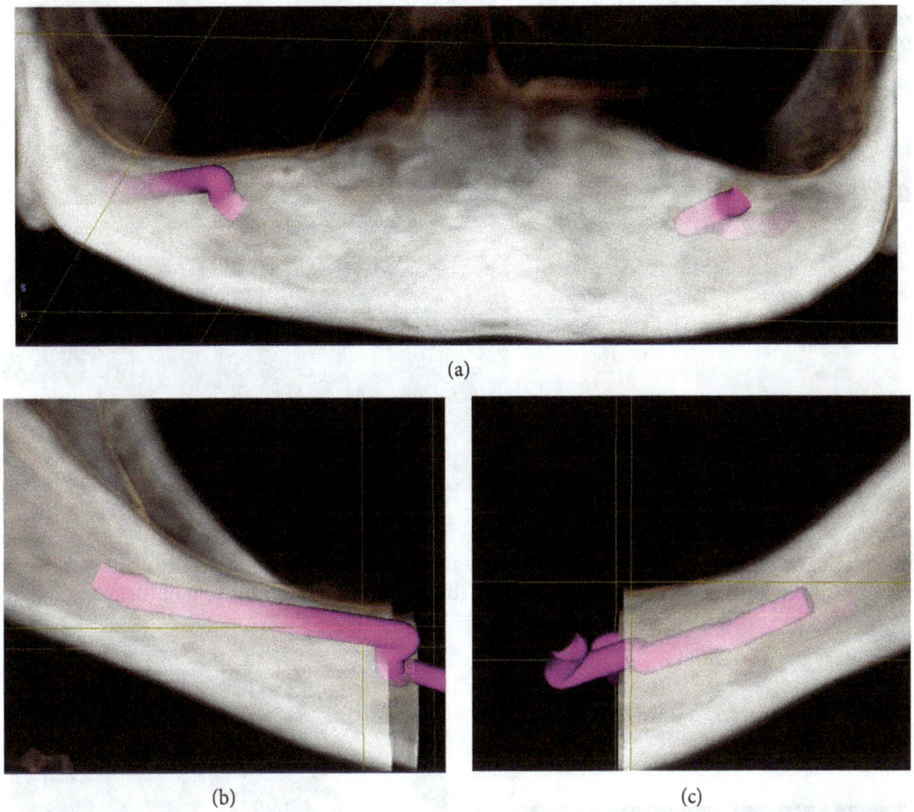

FIGURE 3: Tracking the path of inferior alveolar nerve and location of mental foramen for surgical implant placement: (a) frontal; (b) right side; (c) left side.

bar retained overdentures using clips for retention, and the extremely atrophic maxilla was restored with a combination of implant placement, sinus augmentation, and classic prosthodontic treatment using an electroformed mesostructured overdenture with swivel lock attachments on an implant-supported bar.

2. Case

A 67-year-old nonsmoker female patient in good general health was referred for implant placement and prosthetic rehabilitation in March 2012. She was completely edentulous and had worn full dentures in both arches for 17 years. The dentures at the time of presentation had been fabricated 3 months previously, and the patient was satisfied with the extraoral appearance of the lips and face and tolerated the vertical dimension (Figures 1(a) and 1(b)). Her main complaint was the loss of denture retention even though she used denture adhesive daily. The patient did not grant permission for extraoral photography.

Two (2) duplicates of patient's maxillary dentures were fabricated. One (DentDu-Brm) for the implant planning using clear resin (Paladur; Heraeus Kulzer, Hanau, Germany) for the base and barium sulfate resin (Acryline DVT, Anaxdent, Stuttgart, Germany) for the teeth (Figure 1(c)). The second one was using the same clear resin for the base and the teeth in order to serve as a transfer guide during restoration (DentDu) (Figure 1(d)). Duplicates were checked for intraoral fit before use.

Clinical examination and cone beam computed tomography (CBCT) revealed an extreme atrophy of the maxilla and mandible (Figures 2(a)–2(c)).

The patient's dentures were used for impressions with an alginate material (Alginat rosa; Omnident, Rodgau, Germany) and as guides for the articulation of the casts. Analysis of the articulated casts showed large vertical distances between the maxillary and mandibular alveolar crests (2.3–2.4 cm in the premolar/molar area, 1.9 cm in the anterior area) and a horizontal distance of 1.3 cm in the anterior area (Figure 2(d)). Therefore, rehabilitation with removable restorations was suggested. As the patient refused lateral and vertical augmentation, the decision was made to refabricate implant-retained removable dentures.

Both sinuses were grafted using a bovine xenograph (CompactBoneB; Dentegris, Duisburg, Germany), and the lateral windows were covered with porcine collagen membranes (BoneProtectGuide; Dentegris). In the same session, based on the CBCT, two implants were placed in positions #22 and #27 (SB line, 3.75 mm × 11 mm, Dentegris) and loaded immediately with a bar-retained overdenture using system-specific, prefabricated, angled, and tapered abutments (Figure 3). A bar was milled from type 3 cobalt-chromium-molybdenum alloy (CoCrMo; ZENOTEC NP; Wieland, Pforzheim, Germany), and a metal base (housing) was cast with CoCrMo (Ankatit, Anka Guss, Waldaschaff,

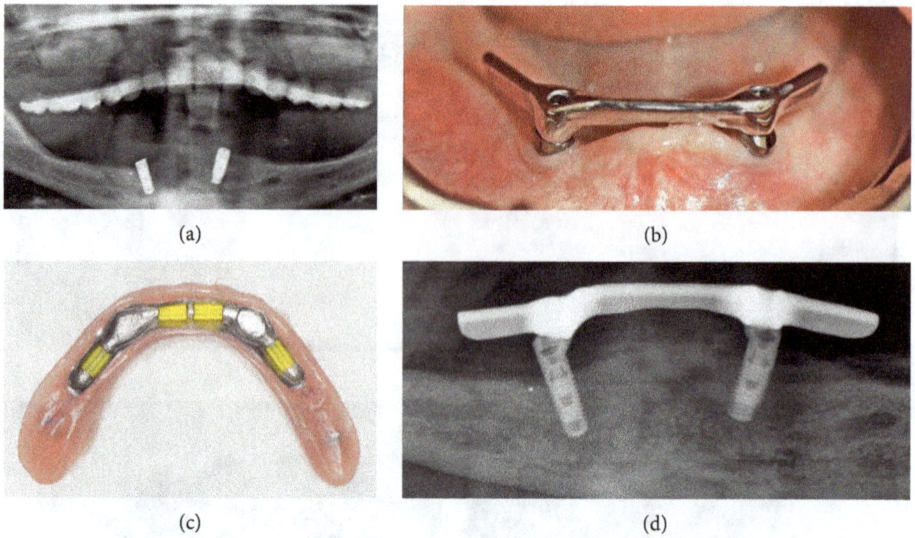

FIGURE 4: Sinus augmentation and mandibular restoration: (a) OPG after sinus augmentation and implant placement in the mandible; (b) implant-retained bar; (c) clips for retention of the base over the bar; (d) OPG section after loading of the mandibular implants.

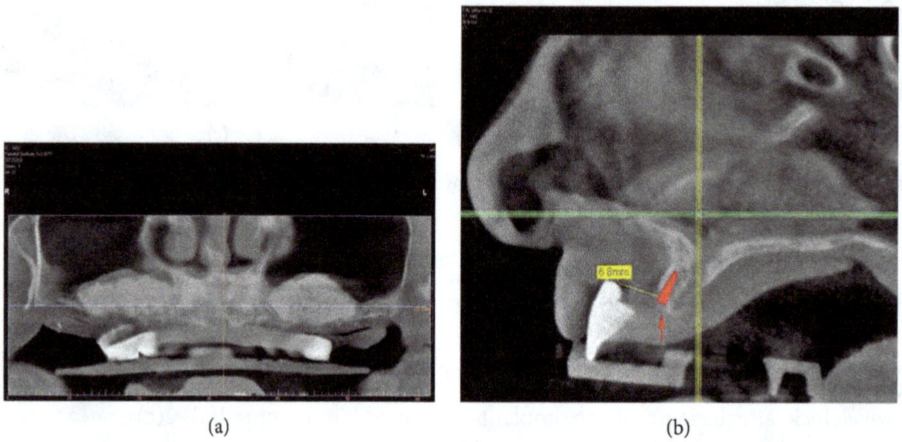

FIGURE 5: Implant planning. CBCT of the maxilla with DentDu-Brm *in situ* before implant placement: (a) sagittal section and (b) axial section.

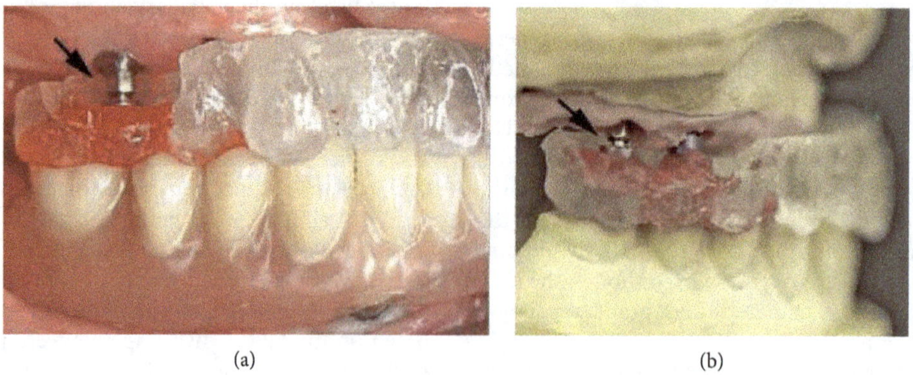

FIGURE 6: (a) DentDu retained on BATTs in occlusion and (b) articulated master cast with the BATTs and DentDu.

Germany). Elastic plastic clips (Preci Matrice; CEKA, Waregem, Belgium) were used to retain the base over the bar (Figure 4).

Five months after sinus augmentation, a total of six implants (#3, 4, 6, 11, and 13; SB line; Dentegris) were placed. CBCT planning software (Sicat Implant, Sicat GmbH, Bonn,

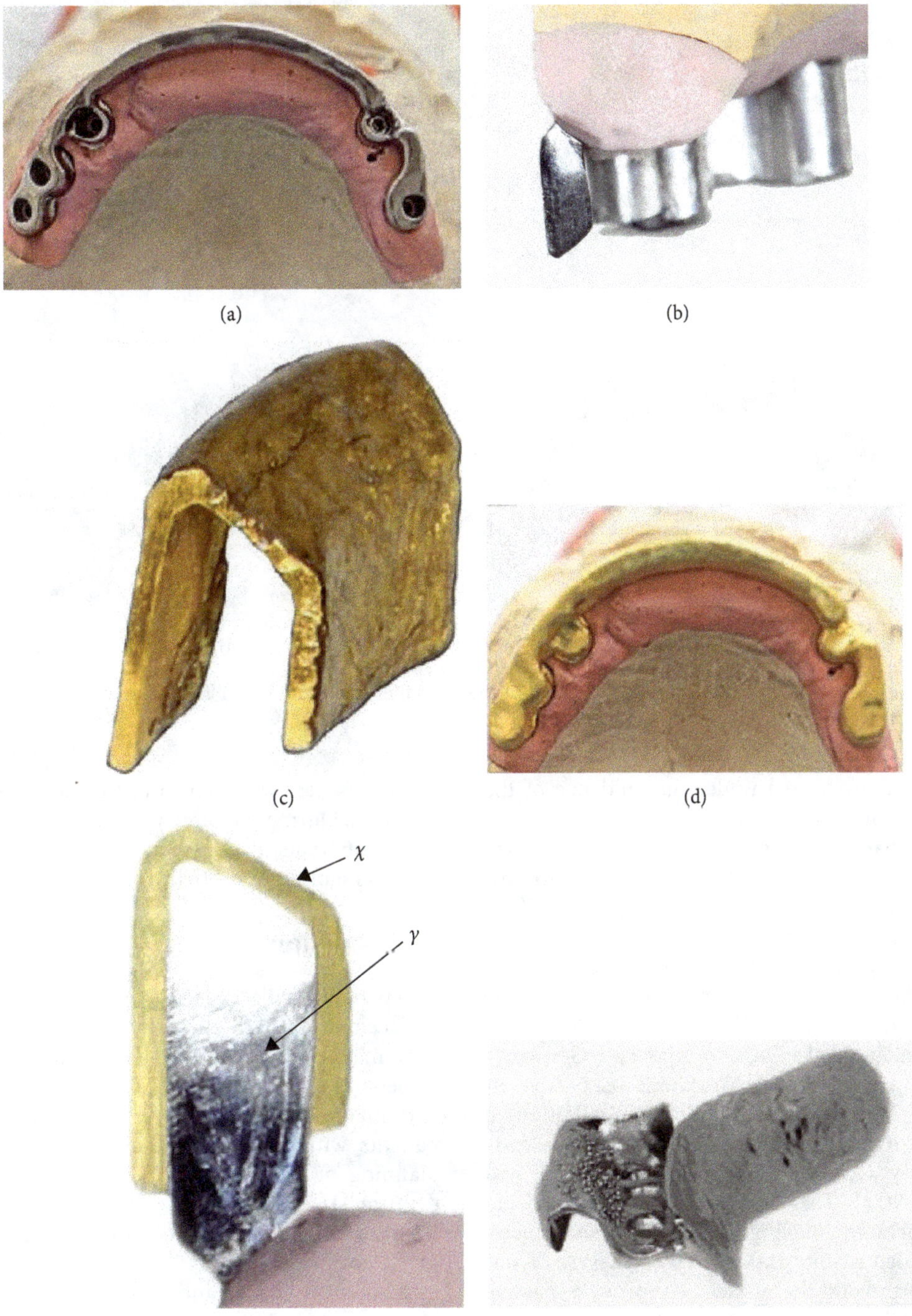

(a) (b) (c) (d) (e) (f)

FIGURE 7: (a) The fabricated maxillary bar; (b) cross section of the bar on a model; (c) ELMES; (d) ELMES conforming to the shape of the bar; (e) cross section on a model demonstrating the use of the ELMES (X) over the bar (Y); (f) casted metal framework (laboratory work shown on a demonstration cast).

Germany) showed that the ideal tooth position was 6.8 mm in front of the alveolar ridge (Figure 5). However, one implant (left sinus, #11) could not be stabilized, so treatment proceeded with the five remaining implants.

The maxillary implants were uncovered 6 months after placement, and impressions were made using an open-tray technique and a polyether impression material (Impregum Penta Soft; 3M ESPE, Neuss, Germany). System-specific ball attachments (BATTs) with their retention elements were mounted on three implants for laboratory transfer. Access windows were created on the buccal side of the DentDu in the areas of the BATTs, and the retention elements were fixed to the DentDu with self-curing modeling resin (Pattern Resin; GC, Alsip, IL, USA). Centric jaw relation was recorded using the same resin (Pattern Resin; GC America Inc., Alsip, IL, USA; Figure 6(a)). A master cast was fabricated, and the BATTs were mounted on the implant analogs. The DentDu with retention elements was then positioned on the master

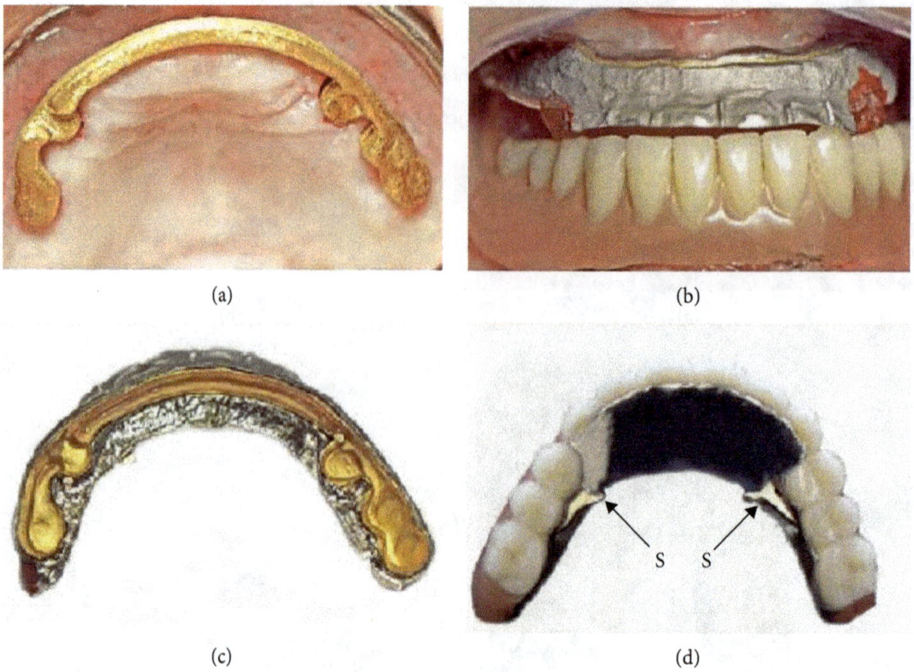

Figure 8: (a) ELMES try-in; (b) verification of the occlusal relationship with the framework in; (c) ELMES fixed in the framework; (d) external view of the metal framework (S: swivel-type lock attachments).

cast, and casts were articulated under the guidance of the DentDu and jaw record (Figure 6(b)).

The maxillary bar was designed using a superimposed DentDu and was positioned as far labial as possible to provide support for the denture base (Figures 7(a) and 7(b)). After verification of the bar's fit, an electroformed mesostructure (ELMES; Galvanogold, Wieland) with a thickness of 0.25 mm was fabricated to conform to the shape of the bar (Figures 7(c)–7(e)) [14, 15]. Framework was cast with CoCrMo alloy (Ankatit, Anka Guss, Waldaschaff, Germany) and tried in the patient's mouth to check its passive fit (Figure 7(f) and Figures 8(a) and 8(b)). In addition, a framework for an overdenture base was fabricated by casting CoCrMo alloy (Ankatit, Anka Guss; Figure 8 and Figures 9(a) and 9(b)). The U-shape framework covering the entire ridge including the lingual slope and partial palatal coverage provided rigidity and gains some degree of stability and support from the tissue. To provide passive retention and locking, two swivel-type lock attachments (swivel-type lock, Heraeus Kulzer, Hanau, Germany) were cast with a gold alloy (Hera; Heraeus Kulzer) (Figure 8(d) and Figures 9(c) and 9(d)) [16].

The fabricated maxillary bar was mounted on the implants, the ELMES was placed on the bar (Figure 8(b)), and the jaw relationship was verified with the framework in place (Figure 8(c)). Subsequently, the ELMES was fixed to the framework using a self-cure compomer (AGC Cem, Wieland; Figure 9(c)). Denture teeth (SR; Ivoclar Vivadent, Ellwangen, Germany) were set and tried in before the finishing process. The denture was finished with the use of an autopolymerizing acrylic resin base material (PalaXpress Ultra; Heraeus Kulzer; Germany) and delivered back to the office on the same day (Figures 10–12) [1–4, 17, 18].

The patient was then enrolled in a 6-month maintenance program. During the three years of observation period, at the follow-up visits, oral hygiene was reinforced together with debridement and prophylaxis.

3. Discussion

For patients with extensive residual ridge resorption, the replacement of hard and soft tissues with a removable denture may be a more suitable option than the use of a cemented (or fixed type) restoration [1–4]. The analysis and management of the restorative space in edentulous patients with implant overdentures are important for the planning of implant placement and for the design of the denture [16, 19, 20]. To retain dentures in patients who have lost large segments of alveolar ridge, the use of clips or electroformed copings on the bars, horizontal path bar attachment systems, and locking attachment systems has been reported [5, 6, 14–22].

In treatments involving removable dentures, decisions about tooth length and position are critical because they affect esthetics and function. In the case described here, the patient accepted the profile and appearance of the original denture, and a duplication of this denture was used as a guide for new denture fabrication in terms of tooth position and tissue and lip support, as well as for the CBCT-based implant placement plan and the design of overdenture substructures. As a general rule, OPGs are made at initial examination in order to assess the situation and after sinus augmentation. In the case presented here, we used a CBCT at the initial examination. The reason was the advanced atrophy on clinical examination; 3D imaging provided more accurate assessment of the sinuses and the existing bone.

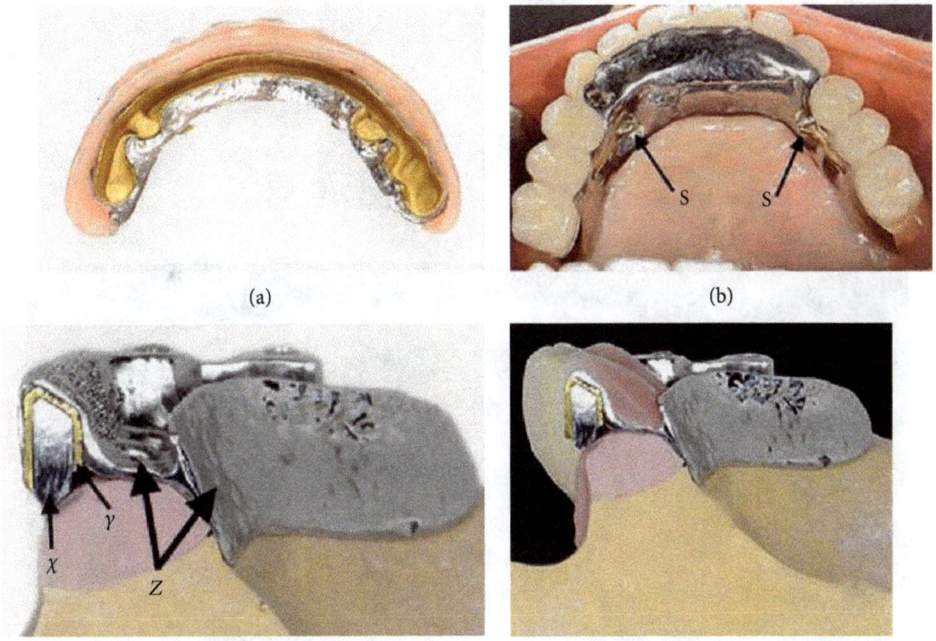

(a) (b) (c) (d)

FIGURE 9: (a) Finished maxillary restoration inner side; (b) maxillary restoration *in situ* (S: swivel-type lock attachments); (c) cross section of the construction on a model: bar (X), ELMES (Y), and metal framework (Z); (d) the veneered construction. (a, d) Laboratory work shown on a demonstration cast.

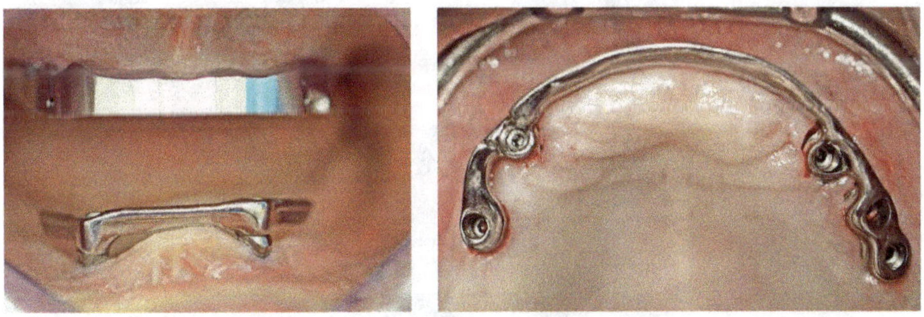

(a) (b)

FIGURE 10: Bars mounted onto the implants: (a) front view and (b) palatal view.

It is recommended to utilize the dental implants as a means for improving retention in cases of poor ridge support and its retention would be compromised. Only two implant placements were possible in this severely resorbed mandibular ridge, and their primary stability was good that additional augmentation to place more implants was not performed. The mandibular arch was restored with an implant-supported bar-retained overdenture using clips for retention, which is a treatment option for edentulous jaws because of the high implant/prosthesis survival rate and limited incidence of technical complications [23–28].

The quality and longevity of implant-supported removable dentures are affected by the passive fit of the superstructure. In the case presented here, ELMES used in the maxillary restoration allows for precise fitting of dental restorations and is particularly useful to achieve passive fit because it enables tension-free placement of the framework onto the abutments [5, 6, 17, 22, 29]. Furthermore, the palatal edge of the prosthesis remained in contact with the mucosa as the palate did not appear to resorb to any appreciable degree.

In the case described here, an implant-supported bar was placed buccally to the ridge crest to support the denture base and teeth, an ELMES was fabricated over it, and a U-shaped metal framework for the denture was designed to rest on the ridge crest and extend palatal to provide support and resistance with rigidity. This approach also strengthened the denture base and relieved the biting forces generated anteriorly by distributing stresses to the metal base. The swivel lock attachment provided rigid fixation on the implant-retained bar with minimal strain, preventing rocking movements of the denture during function. Therefore, this fixed-detachable denture with a swivel lock attachment system

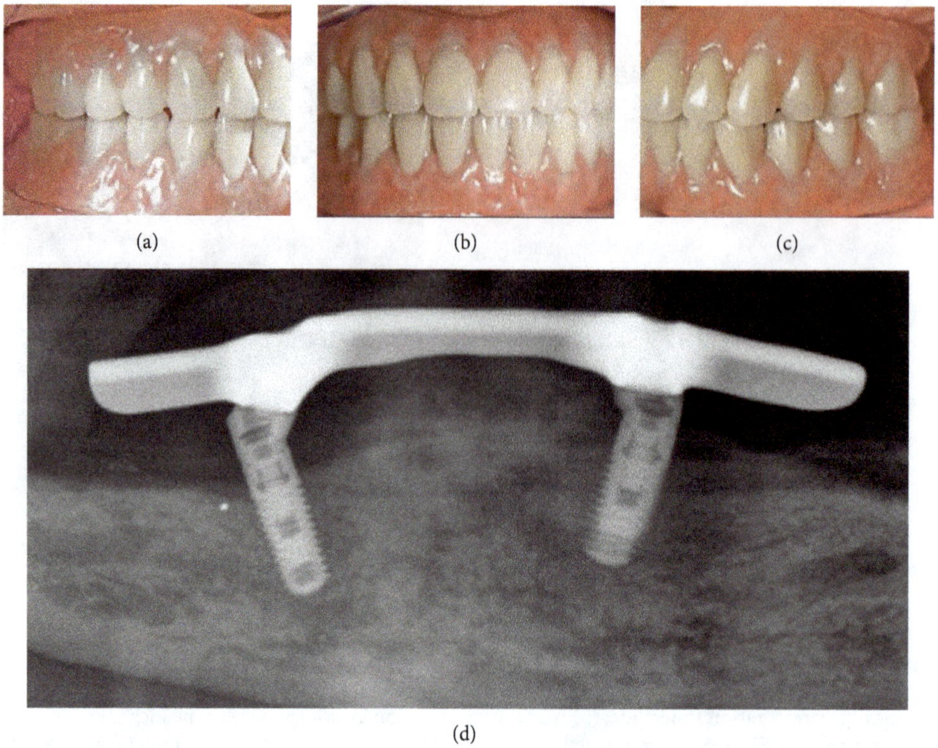

Figure 11: Final restorations in situ: (a) right; (b) front; (c) left; (d) OPG 3 years after treatment.

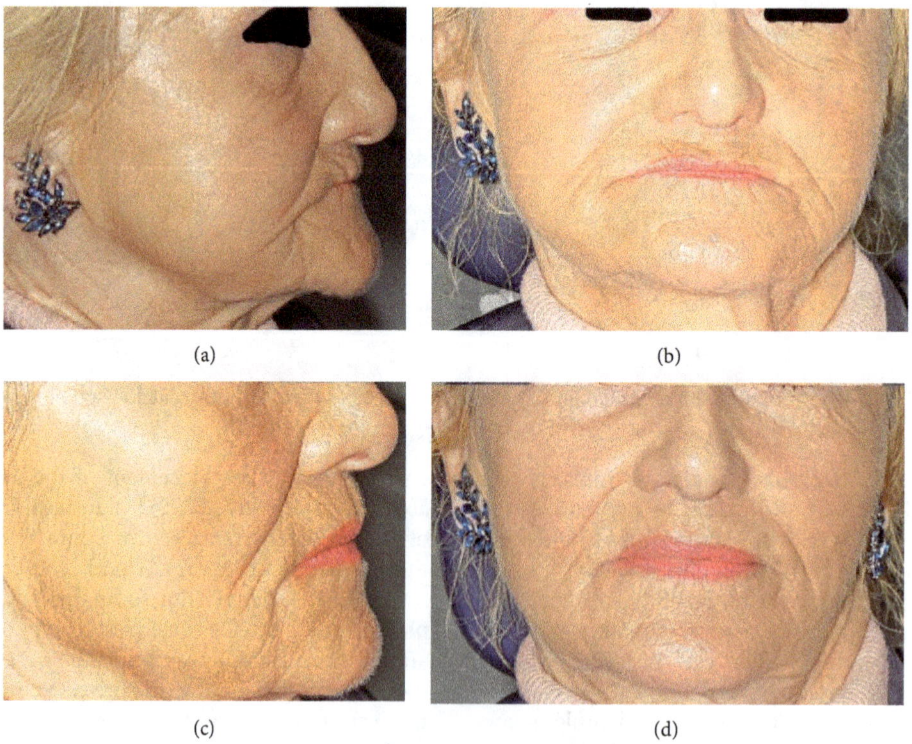

Figure 12: Final restoration delivered: (a) before treatment (lateral); (b) before treatment (frontal); (c) after treatment (lateral); (d) after treatment (frontal).

provided the comfort and assurance of a fixed implant-supported denture, as well as improved efficacy of masticatory function [16].

In the first three weeks following the delivery of the dentures, the patient learned to actuate the swivel lock attachment. It is reported from the systematic review that overdenture with two implants and with bar attachment has the least number of complications [30], and during the three years of follow-up period, no biological or prosthetic complications were observed.

Patient reported a high level of satisfaction with the dentures and an improved quality of life [31, 32].

A disadvantage of this approach is the initially higher laboratory cost due to the need for fabrication of multiple components. However, this cost may be offset by the need for fewer repairs and reduced patient discomfort. Furthermore, the application of the described technique, which combines surgical approaches with classic prosthetic treatment options, improves quality of life and avoids the need for more invasive surgery in elderly patients.

References

[1] J. Hobkirk and G. A. Zarb, "The edentulous state," in *Prosthodontic Treatment for Edentulous Patients: Complete Dentures and Implant-supported Prostheses*, G. A. Zarb, J. Hobkirk, S. Eckert, and R. Jacob, Eds., pp. 1–27, Mosby, St. Louis, 13th ed. edition, 2012.

[2] A. G. T. Payne and G. A. Zarb, "Implant overdentures," in *Prosthodontic Treatment for Edentulous Patients: Complete Dentures and Implant-supported Prostheses*, G. A. Zarb, J. Hobkirk, S. Eckert, and R. Jacob, Eds., pp. 330–340, Mosby, St. Louis, 13th ed. edition, 2012.

[3] C. R. Leles, D. R. Dias, T. E. Nogueira, G. McKenna, M. Schimmel, and L. M. R. Jordão, "Impact of patient characteristics on edentulous subjects' preferences for prosthodontic rehabilitation with implants," *Clinical Oral Implants Research*, vol. 30, no. 3, pp. 285–292, 2019.

[4] M. A. ELsyad, R. M. Emera, and T. M. Ashmawy, "Effect of different bar designs on axial and nonaxial retention forces of implant-retained maxillary overdentures: an in vitro study," *The International Journal of Oral & Maxillofacial Implants*, vol. 34, no. 1, pp. 31–38, 2019.

[5] S. Bencharit, D. J. Misiek, L. A. Simon, and A. Malone-Trahey, "Full mouth rehabilitation with dental implants for a patient with skeletal class III malocclusion: a case report," *Journal of Oral Implantology*, vol. 38, no. 1, pp. 63–70, 2012.

[6] M. A. Bassi, M. A. Lopez, C. Andrisani, Z. Ormanier, and M. Gargari, "Full arch rehabilitation in severe maxillary atrophy with palatal approach implant placement: a case report," *Oral & Implantology*, vol. 9, no. 3, pp. 115–122, 2016.

[7] X. Rodríguez, E. Lucas-Taulé, B. Elnayef et al., "Anatomical and radiological approach to pterygoid implants: a cross-sectional study of 202 cone beam computed tomography examinations," *International Journal of Oral and Maxillofacial Surgery*, vol. 45, no. 5, pp. 636–640, 2016.

[8] A. Lopes, P. Maló, M. de Araújo Nobre, E. Sánchez-Fernández, and I. Gravito, "The nobelguide®all-on-4®treatment concept for rehabilitation of edentulous jaws: a retrospective report on the 7-years clinical and 5-years radiographic outcomes," *Clinical Implant Dentistry and Related Research*, vol. 19, no. 2, pp. 233–244, 2017.

[9] Y. J. Seo, L. Lin, S. H. Kim, K. R. Chung, and G. Nelson, "Strategic camouflage treatment of skeletal class III malocclusion (mandibular prognathism) using bone-borne rapid maxillary expansion and mandibular anterior subapical osteotomy," *American Journal of Orthodontics and Dentofacial Orthopedics*, vol. 149, no. 1, pp. 114–126, 2016.

[10] M. Schlund, R. Nicot, L. Lauwers, G. Raoul, and J. Ferri, "Le Fort 1 osteotomy and calvarial bone grafting for severely resorbed maxillae," *Journal of Cranio-Maxillofacial Surgery*, vol. 44, no. 7, pp. 859–867, 2016.

[11] J. M. Thomason, S. A. M. Kelly, A. Bendkowski, and J. S. Ellis, "Two implant retained overdentures- a review of the literature supporting the McGill and York consensus statements," *Journal of Dentistry*, vol. 40, no. 1, pp. 22–34, 2012.

[12] J. S. Feine, G. E. Carlsson, M. A. Awad et al., "The McGill consensus statement on overdentures. Mandibular two-implant overdentures as first choice standard of care for edentulous patients. Montreal, Quebec, May 24-25, 2002," *International Journal of Oral & Maxillofacial Implants*, vol. 17, no. 4, pp. 601-602, 2002.

[13] J. M. Thomason, J. Feine, C. Exley et al., "Mandibular two implant-supported overdentures as the first choice standard of care for edentulous patients - the York Consensus Statement," *British Dental Journal*, vol. 207, no. 4, pp. 185-186, 2009.

[14] F. Behrend, "Gold electroforming system: GES restorations," *Journal of Dental Technology*, vol. 14, no. 2, pp. 31–37, 1997.

[15] Z. P. Biewer, "Development of the G.E.S. electroforming technique: biocompatible, corrosion-free production of telescopic crowns," *Journal of Dental Technology*, vol. 16, no. 6, pp. 24–29, 1999.

[16] L. W. Höhl, "Swing-lock as a holding and support element of the unilateral free-end prosthesis," *Die Quintessenz der Zahntechnik*, vol. 7, no. 1, pp. 15–17, 1981.

[17] T. Kimura, T. C. Yang, and Y. Maeda, "Influence of rigid bar and nonrigid double crown attachments on maxillary implant overdentures: an in vitro study with differential bone quality," *The International Journal of Oral & Maxillofacial Implants*, vol. 33, no. 4, pp. 764–769, 2018.

[18] A. G. T. Payne, N. H. M. Alsabeeha, M. A. Atieh et al., "Interventions for replacing missing teeth: attachment systems for implant overdentures in edentulous jaws," *Cochrane Database of Systematic Reviews*, vol. 10, 2018.

[19] M. Korbich and P. F. Ruskin, "Occlusal rests and stress equalizers incorporated into swing-lock partial denture design," *General Dentistry*, vol. 27, no. 1, pp. 24–28, 1979.

[20] S. Ahuja and D. R. Cagna, "Classification and management of restorative space in edentulous implant overdenture patients," *The Journal of Prosthetic Dentistry*, vol. 105, no. 5, pp. 332–337, 2011.

[21] W. Slot, G. M. Raghoebar, G. van Dijk, and H. J. A. Meijer, "Attachment of clips in a bar-retained maxillary implant overdenture: a clinical report," *The Journal of Prosthetic Dentistry*, vol. 107, no. 6, pp. 353–357, 2012.

[22] B. Greven, M. Luepke, and S. H. von Dorsche, "Telescoping implant prostheses with intraoral luted Galvano mesostructures to improve passive fit," *The Journal of Prosthetic Dentistry*, vol. 98, no. 3, pp. 239–244, 2007.

[23] M. F. Solá-Ruíz, R. Agustin-Panadero, A. Fons-Font, and C. Labaig-Rueda, "An implant-supported overdenture design with a horizontal path of insertion," *The Journal of Prosthetic Dentistry*, vol. 110, no. 4, pp. 239–242, 2013.

[24] R. Agustin-Panadero, D. Penarrocha-Oltra, S. Gomar-Vercher, A. Ferreiroa, and M. Penarrocha-Diago, "Implant-supported overdenture manufactured using CAD/CAM techniques to achieve horizontal path insertion between the primary and secondary structure: a clinical case report," *The Journal of Advanced Prosthodontics*, vol. 7, no. 3, pp. 264–270, 2015.

[25] E. D. de Avila, L. A. B. de Barros, M. A. del'Acqua, S. S. Nogueira, and F. de Assis Mollo Jr., "Eight-year follow-up of a fixed-detachable maxillary prosthesis utilizing an attachment system: clinical protocol for individuals with skeletal class III malocclusions," *Journal of Oral Implantology*, vol. 40, no. 3, pp. 307–312, 2014.

[26] R. Semsch and R. Muche, "Implant-supported bar-latch overdenture for the severely atrophied, edentulous jaw: a case report," *Quintessence International*, vol. 36, no. 7-8, pp. 565–576, 2005.

[27] S. Rinke, H. Rasing, N. Gersdorff, R. Buergers, and M. Roediger, "Implant-supported overdentures with different bar designs: a retrospective evaluation after 5-19 years of clinical function," *The Journal of Advanced Prosthodontics*, vol. 7, no. 4, pp. 338–343, 2015.

[28] O. Savabi, F. Nejatidanesh, and F. Yordshahian, "Retention of implant-supported overdenture with bar/clip and stud attachment designs," *Journal of Oral Implantology*, vol. 39, no. 2, pp. 140–147, 2013.

[29] J. Wirz and A. Hoffmann, *Electroforming in restorative dentistry: new dimensions in biologically based prostheses*, vol. 238-267, Quintessence, Chicago, 2000.

[30] E. Klemetti, "Is there a certain number of implants needed to retain an overdenture?," *Journal of Oral Rehabilitation*, vol. 35, Supplement 1, pp. 80–84, 2008.

[31] D. Beresford and I. Klineberg, "A within-subject comparison of patient satisfaction and quality of life between a two-implant overdenture and a three-implant-supported fixed dental prosthesis in the mandible," *The International Journal of Oral & Maxillofacial Implants*, vol. 33, no. 6, pp. 1374–1382, 2018.

[32] R. Sharka, H. Abed, and M. Hector, "Oral health-related quality of life and satisfaction of edentulous patients using conventional complete dentures and implant-retained overdentures: an umbrella systematic review," *Gerodontology*, 2019.

12

Oral Rehabilitation with Zygomatic Implants in a Patient with Cleft Palate

Guilherme José Pimentel Lopes de Oliveira[1] **Mariana Schaffer Brackmann,**[2] **Larissa Carvalho Trojan,**[3] **Paulo Domingos Ribeiro Júnior,**[4] **and Luis Eduardo Marques Padovan**[3]

[1]*Department of Periodontology/Implantology, Dental School, Federal University of Uberlândia-UFU, Uberlândia 38405-266, Brazil*
[2]*Department of Diagnosis and Surgery, Univ. Est. Paul.-UNESP, Araraquara 14801-903, Brazil*
[3]*Instituto Latino Americano de Ensino e Pesquisa Odontológico-ILAPEO, Curitiba 80710-150, Brazil*
[4]*Univ. Sagrado Coração, Bauru 17011-160, Brazil*

Correspondence should be addressed to Luis Eduardo Marques Padovan; padovan@iocp.com.br

Academic Editor: Jamil Awad Shibli

Edentulous patients with an atrophic maxilla associated with lip-palate fissures have unpredictable results after undergoing grafting procedures. In situations where the atrophic maxilla does not adequately allow reconstruction, the use of zygomatic implants has been indicated, and probably these implants can be indicated for the rehabilitation of patients with lip-palate fissures. This case report describes the oral rehabilitation treatment of a patient with a lip-palate cleft treated with zygomatic implants and implant-supported fixed prosthesis with two years of follow-up. A 65-year-old female patient had a lip-palate cleft and previously underwent surgery to close the cleft. The patient had a severely atrophic maxilla and had difficulty adapting to a removable total prosthesis. Due to the small amount of bone remaining and extensive fibrous tissue in the palate region, a rehabilitation with conventional implants associated with zygomatic implants was chosen. Two zygomatic implants and a conventional implant were placed on the right side, and a zygomatic implant and conventional implant were placed on the left side; these implants were later activated by a protocol-type prosthesis. The zygomatic implants provided an adequate aesthetic and functional outcome of the prosthesis in a patient with cleft palate.

1. Introduction

The use of implant-supported prostheses has been shown to be a predictable treatment with a high success rate for the treatment of any type of edentulism [1, 2]. However, in some clinical situations, it is not possible to place implants in a good position due to the limited availability of the bone tissue [3, 4]. In these situations, the rehabilitation of the atrophic maxilla may represent the greatest challenge because it is a bone with low biological quality compared to the mandible and contains a sinus cavity that tends to increase its degree of pneumatization after tooth loss [3, 5].

To address this problem, bone substitute biomaterials associated with maxillary sinus floor elevation techniques [6], guided bone regeneration [5], osteogenic distraction [4], and the use of block grafts [7] have previously been proposed to treat the atrophic maxilla before implant placement. However, in some cases, maxillary atrophy may be of a high degree of severity that renders bone reconstruction procedures unpredictable.

Edentulous patients with an atrophic maxilla associated with lip-palate fissures have unpredictable results after undergoing grafting because they have a compromised local vascularization, low tissue elasticity, and impaired psychological aspects. In addition, the limitation of the openness of the mouth makes it difficult to place implants correctly [8]. In situations where the atrophic maxilla does not adequately allow reconstruction, the use of zygomatic implants has been indicated. These implants were originally designed for the treatment of maxillectomized patients who were tumour or trauma victims [9, 10] and may be an excellent alternative in the rehabilitative treatment of patients with lip-palate fissures [11].

This case report is aimed at describing and presenting the outcomes of the oral rehabilitation treatment of a patient with a lip-palate cleft who was treated with zygomatic implants and implant-supported fixed prosthesis after two years of follow-up.

2. Case Presentation

A 65-year-old female patient who presented with a lip-palate cleft previously underwent a surgical procedure to close the lip-palate cleft. However, even after this procedure, the patient had a clearly atrophic maxilla (class V of Cawood and Howell) and had difficulty adapting to a total removable of prosthesis. Due to the small amount of bone remaining and extensive fibrous tissue in the palate region, rehabilitation with conventional implants associated with zygomatic implants was chosen instead of subjecting the patient to a reconstruction with large bone grafts (Figure 1(a)). For the preoperative evaluation, panoramic radiography and cone-beam computed tomography of the maxilla and zygomas were requested, which confirmed the low bone availability in this case (Figures 1(b) and 1(c)). Two zygomatic implants and a conventional implant were placed in the right side, and one zygomatic implant and one conventional implant were placed in the left side under general anaesthesia and nasotracheal intubation. Zygomatic implants with the Cone Morse platform (Neodent®, Curitiba, Brazil) and conventional implants with the Cone Morse platform and a hydrophilic surface (Acqua surface, Neodent®, Curitiba, Brazil) were used. Of these implants, a zygomatic implant with 4.4 × 52.5 mm was installed in the region of tooth 12, a 4.4 × 40 mm zygomatic implant was installed in the region of tooth 16, a zygomatic implant with 4.4 × 52.5 mm was installed in the region of tooth 26, and two conventional conical implants with 3.5 × 11.5 mm were placed in the region of teeth 14 and 23. Furthermore, more than 60 N·cm of insertion torque was obtained during the placement of all the implants.

During the milling of the surgical site, the following sequence of drills was used: spherical drill zygomatic plus 2, spiral drill 2.7 zygomatic plus, pilot spiral drill zygomatic plus 2.7/3.3, spiral drill zygomatic plus 3.3, pilot spiral drill zygomatic plus 3.3/3.7, and countersink drill for Cone Morse zygomatic implant placement, and then the implant installation was performed. A surgical guide was used during the implant surgical site preparation. An antibiotic (amoxicillin) was given intraoperatively and maintained for seven days. Miniabutments were selected and installed at the time of surgery. After 24 hours, the castings were performed, and 48 hours after surgery, a screwed fixed-implant protocol prosthesis with CrCo infrastructure and acrylic teeth was installed on the implants. During the postoperative period, radiographic and clinical examinations showed that there were no complications (Figures 2(a) and 2(b)). The patient underwent follow-up after 15, 30, and 90 days and then every six months thereafter. Currently, the patient has been followed up for two years without any complaint and with a functional prosthesis (Figures 3(a)–3(c)). Furthermore, the patient expressed satisfaction with the obtained aesthetic and functional outcome. The patient gave the researchers a signed consent for the publication of this case.

3. Discussion

In general, it was verified in this case report that the use of zygomatic implants was effective for providing a basis for the rehabilitative treatment of a patient who presented with a lip-palate cleft. As the patient had already undergone grafting procedures and because she was not of ideal age to undergo other grafting procedures to reduce the fibrous tissue present on the palate, the grafting technique was contraindicated for the use of zygomatic implants.

Lip-palate clefts are the most frequent craniofacial malformations. These deformities were considered by the World Health Organization to be a public health problem. In 2002, this type of malformation accounted for 1 in 650 babies born worldwide [12]. The fissures present a multifactorial aetiology, with the involvement of genetic and environmental factors. Treatment of patients affected by these malformations should begin soon after birth and extend into adulthood [13]. As the patient of the present case report did not undergo treatment in the early stage, there was a reduced chance of success with the grafting procedures.

Zygomatic implants were initially designed to be used to treat atrophic maxilla to avoid graft procedures; these implants reduce the degree of morbidity of the surgical procedure and costs and accelerate prosthetic rehabilitative treatment [14]. However, it has been reported that the success of installing zygomatic implants is related to the degree of experience and skill of the surgeon and that some complications, such as haemorrhages during the procedure or the occurrence of sinusitis after the procedure, are not uncommon [15]. On the other hand, some studies have shown that zygomatic implants have high success and survival rates [10, 14, 16], which shows that rehabilitation treatment with this type of implant is safe, as confirmed in the case report described. In this case report, the indication of the use of the zygomatic implant was due to the lacking of enough bone tissue which enables the placement of an adequate number of implants of conventional size suitable for the installation of a fixed-implant protocol prosthesis due to atrophy of the maxilla associated with the presence of the cleft palate.

It has been a tendency in medical areas to indicate less invasive surgical procedures that are associated with lower morbidity for patients [17, 18]. Less invasive procedures accelerate the healing process and generate a high degree of satisfaction of patients, and whenever possible, less invasive surgical procedures should be indicated. Although grafting procedures are related to high rates of clinical success, this additional surgical step requires more time due to implant placement in most cases [14, 16]. In addition, in cases of severe atrophy, the use of an autogenous bone graft isolated or associated with other bone substitutes is more appropriate because it is necessary that the graft presents good biological

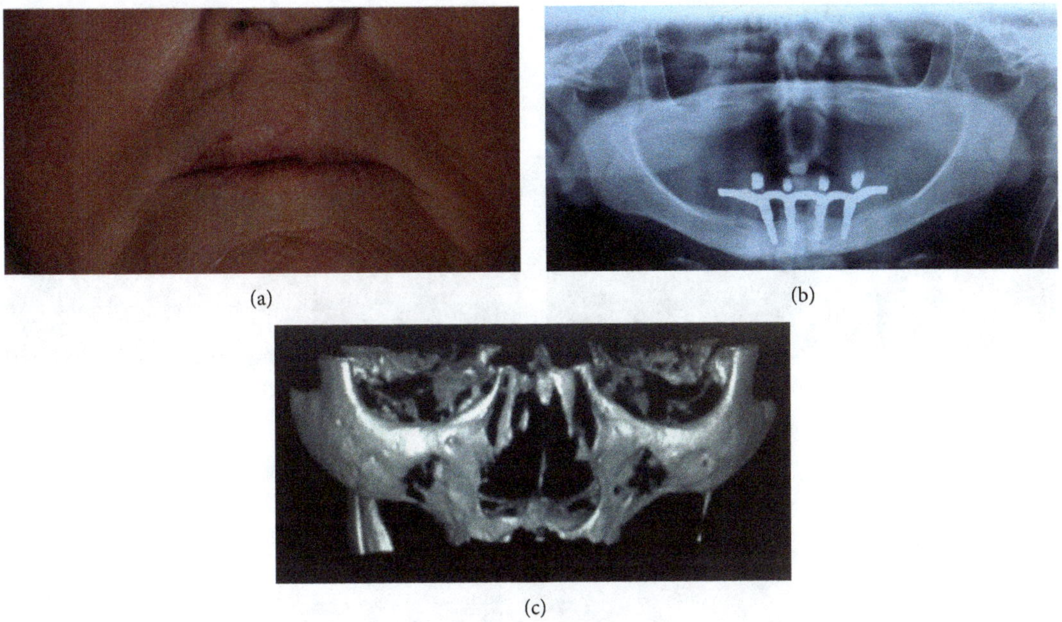

FIGURE 1: (a) Preoperative clinical condition of the patient, (b) preoperative panoramic radiography, and (c) preoperative cone beam computed tomography. Note the large degree of maxilla atrophy presented by the patient before the surgical procedure.

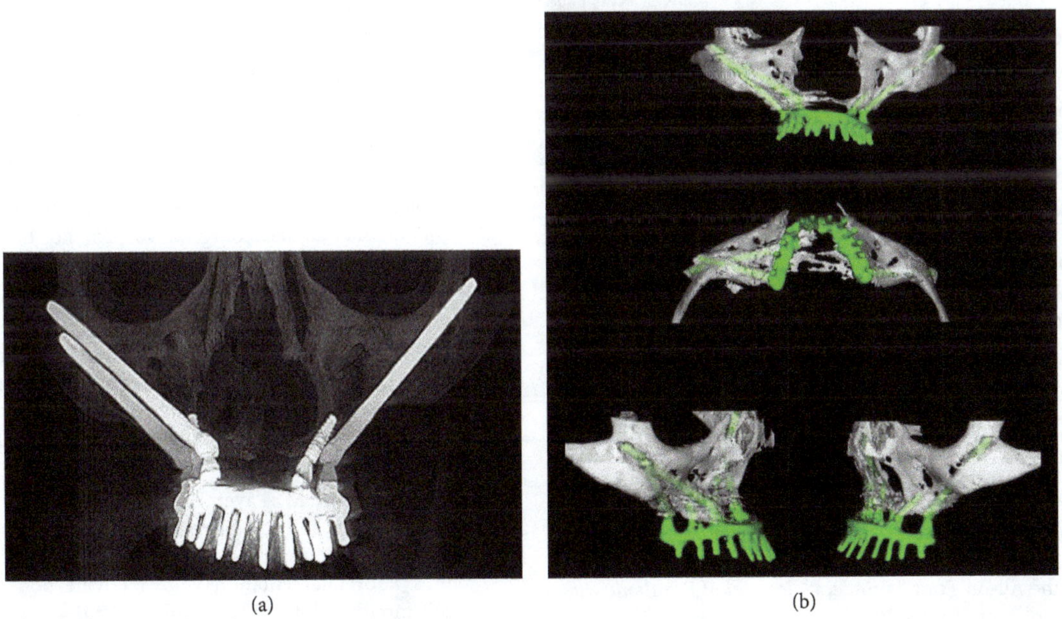

FIGURE 2: (a) Panoramic tomography and (b) tomographic image of the patient after 2 years of follow-up. Note the good position of the implants placed and the absence of complications.

properties to integrate into the surgical beds of the native bone with little thickness [5]. In these cases, morbidity in the donor sites generates a great discomfort to patients [19]. In fact, the option to install zygomatic implants in this case promoted the application of a more conservative surgical technique with a smaller possibility of causing morbidity to the patient and promoted acceleration of prosthetic rehabilitation, thus promoting a greater patient satisfaction with the surgical procedure performed.

Another possibility for rehabilitation of this case would be the use of overdenture-type prosthesis that has been shown to be a conservative treatment with high rates of success and patient satisfaction [20]. However, in this specific case, the patient's previous positive experience with the protocol-fixed prostheses used to rehabilitate the inferior jaw was taken into account. In addition, there was no communication of the nasal with the buccal cavity due to the grafting attempt that sealed this communication.

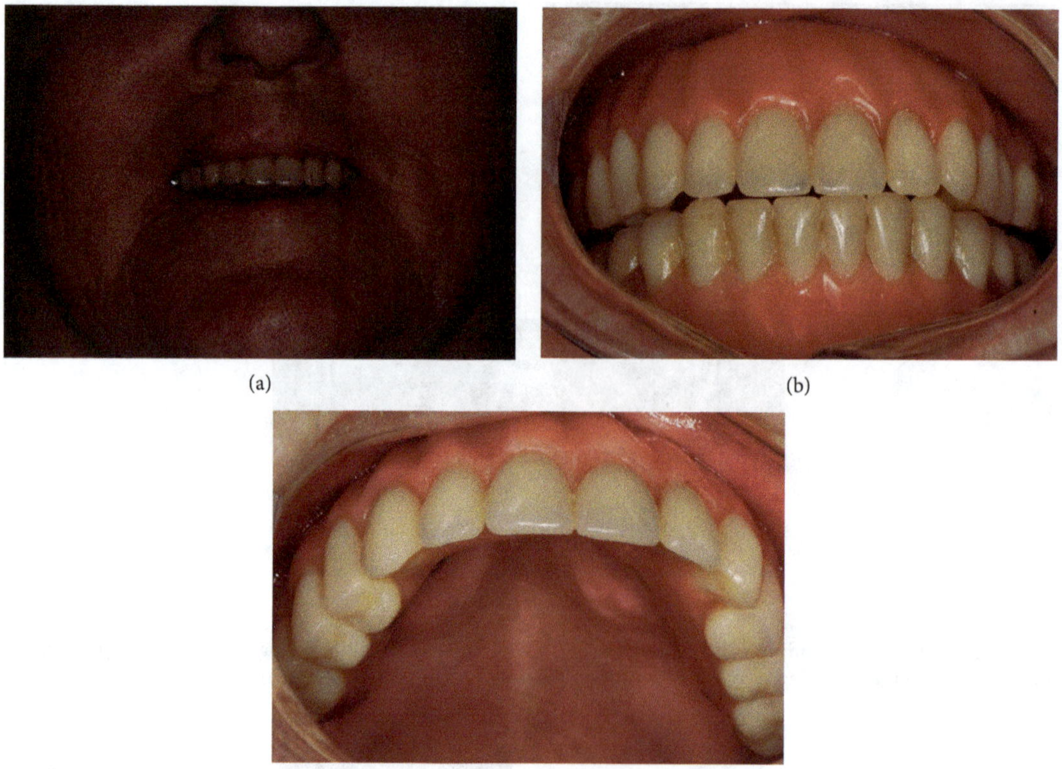

(a) (b) (c)

Figure 3: (a) Postoperative clinical condition of the patient with the upper protocol-type prosthesis in function, (b) postoperative condition of the prosthesis, and (c) postoperative condition of the palate. Note the good clinical outcome of the upper protocol-type prosthesis after 2 years of follow-up. Furthermore, a good condition of the palate with the communication of the nasal and oral cavities is showed.

4. Conclusion

This case report showed that the use of zygomatic implants in a severely atrophic maxilla provides a sufficiently stable support for the installation of a total-fixed prosthesis in the atrophic maxilla of a lip-palate cleft patient with good clinical outcomes after two years of follow-up.

References

[1] T. J. Balshi, G. J. Wolfinger, R. W. Slauch, and S. F. Balshi, "A retrospective analysis of 800 Brånemark System implants following the All-on-Four™ protocol," *Journal of Prosthodontics* vol. 23, no. 2, pp. 83–88, 2014.

[2] P. Maló, M. de Araújo Nobre, A. Lopes, A. Ferro, and I. Gravito, "Single-tooth rehabilitations supported by dental implants used in an immediate-provisionalization protocol: report on long-term outcome with retrospective follow-up," *Clinical Implant Dentistry and Related Research*, vol. 17, Supplement 2, pp. e511–e519, 2015.

[3] C. Aparicio, W. Ouazzani, R. Garcia, X. Arevalo, R. Muela, and V. Fortes, "A prospective clinical study on titanium implants in the zygomatic arch for prosthetic rehabilitation of the atrophic edentulous maxilla with a follow-up of 6 months to 5 years," *Clinical Implant Dentistry and Related Research*, vol. 8, no. 3, pp. 114–122, 2006.

[4] T. Binger, M. Rücker, and W. J. Spitzer, "Dentofacial rehabilitation by osteodistraction, augmentation and implantation despite osteogenesis imperfecta," *International Journal of Oral & Maxillofacial Surgery*, vol. 35, no. 6, pp. 559–562, 2006.

[5] I. A. Urban, A. Monje, J. L. Lozada, and H. L. Wang, "Long-term evaluation of peri-implant bone level after reconstruction of severely atrophic edentulous maxilla via vertical and horizontal guided bone regeneration in combination with sinus augmentation: a case series with 1 to 15 years of loading," *Clinical Implant Dentistry and Related Research*, vol. 19, no. 1, pp. 46–55, 2017.

[6] A. Wildburger, M. Payer, N. Jakse, D. Strunk, N. Etchard-Liechtenstein, and S. Sauerbier, "Impact of autogenous concentrated bone marrow aspirate on bone regeneration after sinus floor augmentation with a bovine bone substitute–a split-mouth pilot study," *Clinical Oral Implants Research*, vol. 25, no. 10, pp. 1175–1181, 2014.

[7] B. A. Gultekin, E. Cansiz, and M. O. Borahan, "Clinical and 3-dimensional radiographic evaluation of autogenous iliac block bone grafting and guided bone regeneration in patients with atrophic maxilla," *Journal of Oral and Maxillofacial Surgery*, vol. 75, no. 4, pp. 709–722, 2017.

[8] K. Wermker, S. Jung, U. Joos, and J. Kleinheinz, "Dental implants in cleft lip, alveolus, and palate patients: a systematic review," *The International Journal of Oral & Maxillofacial Implants*, vol. 29, no. 2, pp. 384–390, 2014.

[9] A. V. Pham, M. Abarca, A. de Mey, and C. Malevez, "Rehabilitation of a patient with cleft lip and palate with an extremely edentulous atrophied posterior maxilla using zygomatic

implants: case report," *The Cleft Palate-Craniofacial Journal*, vol. 41, no. 5, pp. 571–574, 2017.

[10] E. M. Sartori, L. E. M. Padovan, I. A. de Mattias Sartori, P. D. Ribeiro Jr, A. C. Gomes de Souza Carvalho, and M. C. Goiato, "Evaluation of satisfaction of patients rehabilitated with zygomatic fixtures," *Journal of Oral and Maxillofacial Surgery*, vol. 70, no. 2, pp. 314–319, 2012.

[11] C. Aparicio, C. Manresa, K. Francisco et al., "The long-term use of zygomatic implants: a 10-year clinical and radiographic report," *Clinical Implant Dentistry and Related Research*, vol. 16, no. 3, pp. 447–459, 2014.

[12] W. Shaw, "Global strategies to reduce the health care burden of craniofacial anomalies: report of WHO meetings on international collaborative research on craniofacial anomalies," *The Cleft Palate-Craniofacial Journal*, vol. 41, no. 3, pp. 238–243, 2004.

[13] W. A. Pena, K. Vargervik, A. Sharma, and S. Oberoi, "The role of endosseous implants in the management of alveolar clefts," *Pediatric Dentistry*, vol. 31, no. 4, pp. 329–333, 2009.

[14] R. Davó, P. Felice, R. Pistilli et al., "Immediately loaded zygomatic implants vs conventional dental implants in augmented atrophic maxillae: 1-year post-loading results from a multicentre randomised controlled trial," *European Journal of Oral Implantology*, vol. 11, no. 2, pp. 145–161, 2018.

[15] B. R. Chrcanovic and M. H. N. G. Abreu, "Survival and complications of zygomatic implants: a systematic review," *Oral and Maxillofacial Surgery*, vol. 17, no. 2, pp. 81–93, 2013.

[16] M. Esposito, R. Davó, C. Marti-Pages et al., "Immediately loaded zygomatic implants vs conventional dental implants in augmented atrophic maxillae: 4 months post-loading results from a multicentre randomised controlled trial," *European Journal of Oral Implantology*, vol. 11, no. 1, pp. 11–28, 2018.

[17] M. Motta, R. Monsano, G. R. Velloso et al., "Guided surgery in esthetic region," *Journal of Craniofacial Surgery*, vol. 27, no. 3, pp. e262–e265, 2016.

[18] Y. N. R. Gallardo, I. R. T. da Silva-Olivio, E. Mukai, S. Morimoto, N. Sesma, and L. Cordaro, "Accuracy comparison of guided surgery for dental implants according to the tissue of support: a systematic review and meta-analysis," *Clinical Oral Implants Research*, vol. 28, no. 5, pp. 602–612, 2017.

[19] E. Nkenke and F. W. Neukam, "Autogenous bone harvesting and grafting in advanced jaw resorption: morbidity, resorption and implant survival," *European Journal of Oral Implantology*, vol. 7, Supplement 2, pp. S203–S217, 2014.

[20] M. Sánchez-Siles, J. F. Ballester-Ferrandis, N. Salazar-Sánchez, F. J. Gómez-García, R. Moraleja-Ruiz, and F. Camacho-Alonso, "Long-term evaluation of quality of life and satisfaction between implant bar overdentures and conventional complete dentures: a 23 years retrospective study," *Clinical Implant Dentistry and Related Research*, vol. 20, no. 2, pp. 208–214, 2018.

13

Horizontal Ridge Augmentation and Contextual Implant Placement with a Resorbable Membrane and Particulated Anorganic Bovine Bone-Derived Mineral

Ferdinando Attanasio,[1] Andrea Pacifici,[2] Amerigo Giudice,[1] Antonella Polimeni,[2] and Luciano Pacifici[2]

[1]*Department of Health Sciences, Magna Graecia, University of Catanzaro, Catanzaro, Italy*
[2]*Department of Oral and Maxillo-Facial Science, Sapienza University of Rome, Rome 00100, Italy*

Correspondence should be addressed to Andrea Pacifici; andrea.pacifici@uniroma1.it

Academic Editor: Giuseppe Alessandro Scardina

Alveolar ridge deficiency is considered a major limitation for successful implant placement. Various approaches have been developed to horizontal augmentation of bone volume. This case report presents the medium-term results of one-stage guided bone augmentation using an anorganic bovine bone (70%) and autologous bone (30%), placed in layers, in association with resorbable collagen membrane for a subsequent implant placement. The patient presented with a localized horizontal ridge defect in the posterior zone of the jaw. The clinical and radiographic presentations, as well as relevant literature, are presented.

1. Introduction

Over the years, prosthetic rehabilitations supported by osteointegrated implant has become a common treatment modality in daily dental practice. After the development of the principles of osseointegration and their application to the most complex conditions, new methodologies have evolved with the aim of predicting the integration in the bone tissue [1]. With the improvement of surgical techniques, materials, and knowledge, implant therapy went from an anatomically guided procedure to a prosthetically guided procedure. In the past, surgeons used to decide to place implants where there was a sufficient amount of bone in order to ensure long-term success of osteointegrated implants. However, this procedure could lead to two types of problems: an aesthetic and a mechanical one. From a mechanical point of view, the positioning of an implant should ideally take place along the direction of the load force of the tooth or of the group of teeth to be rehabilitated in order to avoid overloading and peri-implant bone resorption's risks [2]. Thanks to the surgical techniques and the biomaterials available today, it is possible to reconstruct three-dimensional atrophic edentulous areas of the jaws thus allowing the clinician to correctly position the implants and protect themselves from failures and mechanical/prosthetic failures. GBR has been used for horizontal and vertical ridge augmentations and has demonstrated reproducible outcomes with high implant survival rates and low complication rates. Both resorbable and nonresorbable barrier membranes have proven clinical effectiveness [3–5]. Nevertheless, guided bone regeneration by means of titanium-reinforced expanded polytetrauoroethylene membrane (e-PTFE) has proven to be a successful and predictable technique for vertical and horizontal ridge augmentation both in short- and long-term studies [6–8]. However, the use of a barrier membrane is a technique-sensitive procedure, and it is not lacking in complications [9]. The most frequently reported problems involve the soft tissue; very often, the exposure of the membrane forces the operator to remove it with the possible compromise of the entire area subject to regeneration [10]. This clinical case report details the successful use of an

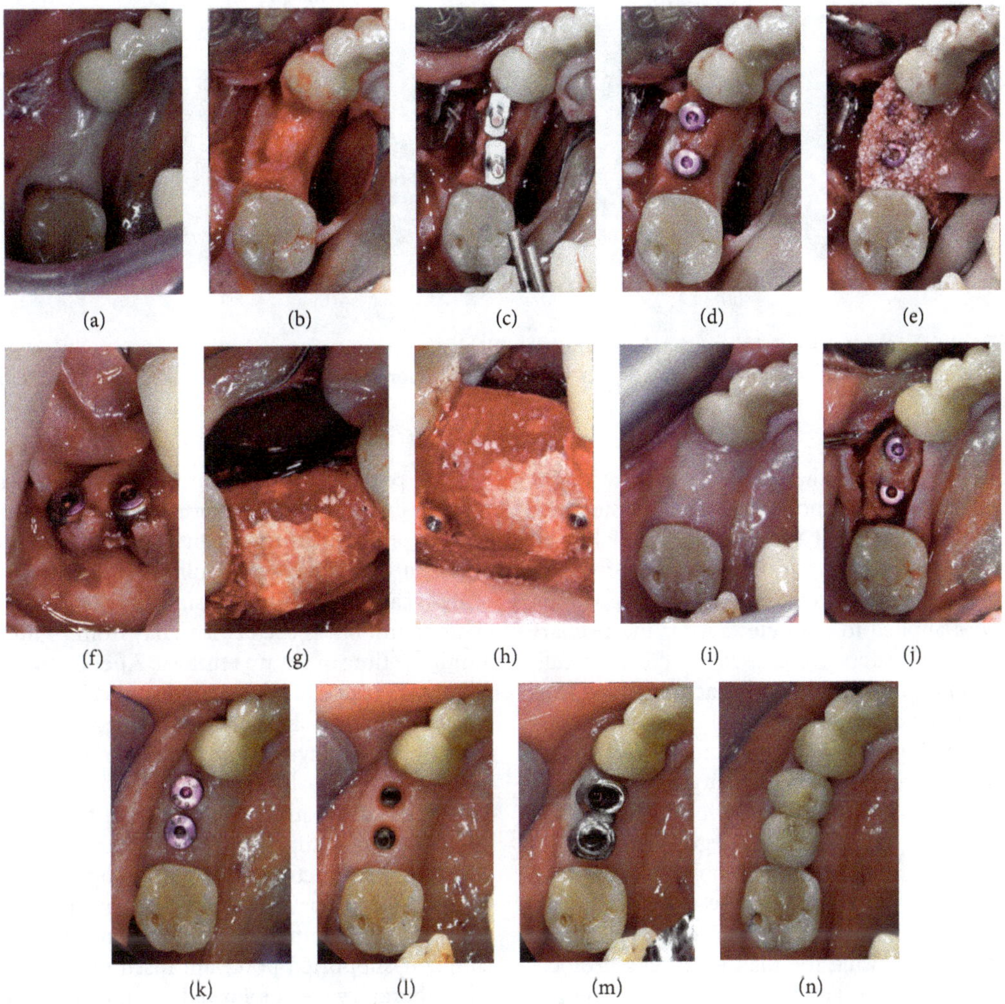

FIGURE 1: Occlusal views (a, b) of the posterior mandibular area show the thin bone crest. Occlusal view (c, d) of the two implant osteotomies and implant in place. (e) Autogenous particulate bone mixed with inorganic bovine bone-derived mineral (ABBM) in place. Buccal (f, h) and occlusal (g) views of the membrane fixed with titanium pins. Occlusal view (i) of the posterior mandibular area 6-months postsurgery. Occlusal view (j) of the regenerated bone. Second surgery performed by a lingual approach with roll flap technique that allows to increase the vestibular volume of soft tissues. (k) Healing screw in place. (l) Removal of healing screws and taking impressions. (m, n) Placement of the definitive crown (screw-retained).

inorganic bovine-derived bone mineral and a resorbable barrier membrane to reconstruct a severe alveolar posterior mandibulary bone defect.

2. Materials and Methods

A healthy 50-year-old woman presented for an evaluation of her posterior right mandibular and tooth loss in the premolar region. She reported that teeth were extracted several years previously due to a history of dentoalveolar infections. The patient was overall a healthy nonsmoker with good oral hygiene habits. Several years postextraction, the patient wanted implant therapy. As foreseen, there was a severe horizontal ridge defect, which meant the site was seriously compromised for implant reconstruction. Radio graphic examination showed that the bone width in this area was not sufficient for standard implant placement. Since the patient wanted a fixed prosthesis rehabilitation with implants, the treatment plan included regeneration of the alveolar defect to ideally restore form, function, and esthetics with the immediate placement of two fixtures (Figure 1).

2.1. Surgical Procedure. The surgical technique selection was made in accordance to the protocol established by Urban et al. [11]. The patient was premedicated with amoxicillin+clavulanic acid (2 g) 1 hour before surgery, and then, 875 mg of amoxicillin+125 mg of clavulanic acid was administered twice a day for 1 week following surgery. The patient rinsed with a 0.20% chlorhexidine gluconate solution (Curasept, Curaden HealthCare, Italy) for 1 minute, then the skin surrounding the surgical site was disinfected. The patient presented with a thick biotype. Under local anesthesia (2% lidocaine with 1 : 80,000 epinephrine), the flap was designed to provide a clear view of the surgical area and to ensure primary tension-free closure. A full-thickness, mid-crestal incision was made in the keratinized gingiva on the alveolar crest. For adequate surgical access, a divergent

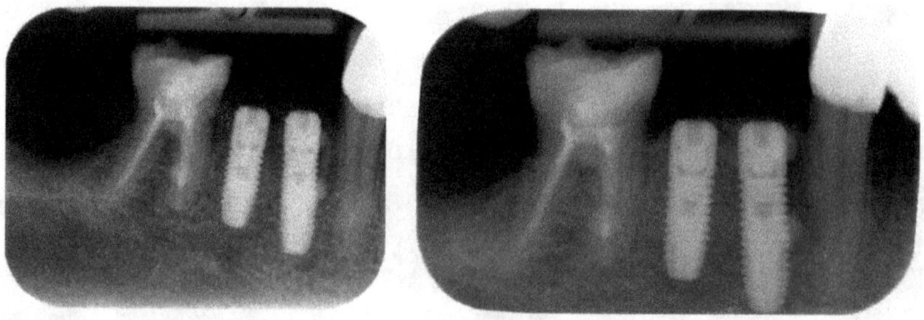

(a) (b)

FIGURE 2: Radiographic exams. (a) Rx right after implant surgery: it highlights the correct implant axis, the connection with the proximal roots, and the implant's fitness under the bone crest. (b) Rx control after 6 months: it shows the physiological bone remodeling around the implant's head.

vertical incision was made at the mesial line angle of the mandibular right canine and another vertical incision was made at the distal line angle of the mandibular right first molar. The flap design meant that primary tension-free closure would have to be achieved over a larger dimension after the bone graft was applied to the defect. After the primary incisions, periosteal elevators were used to create a full-thickness flap beyond the mucogingival junction and at least 5 mm beyond the bone defect [12].

A periosteal releasing incision connecting the two vertical incisions was performed to achieve elasticity of the flap; the crestal cut continued 5 mm distally from it; to preserve the lingual nerve, the blade was inclined 45 degrees with the tip in the buccal direction and the external oblique ridge [13]. One implant 3,6 Ø × 11 mm long and one implant 3,6 Ø × 9 mm long OsseoSpeed EV (Astra Tech, Dentsply, Molndal, Sweden) were placed following the manufacturer's protocol in the 4.4 and 4.5 tooth site. The implants were submerged in a two-stage procedure. Given that, as planned, the procedure led to an incomplete implant incorporation into the mandibular bone matrix and proceeded to a horizontal regeneration of the defect. Autogenous bone was then harvested by the use of a manual scraper from the bone adjacent to the area to be regenerated and mixed with anorganic bovine bone-derived mineral (ABBM) (Creos Xenogain, Nobel Biocare, Goteborg, Sweden) to form a composite bone graft. Multiple decortical holes were made in the bony bed using a small round burr in order to reveal the medullary space. The correct size of a collagen membrane (T-BARRIER, B&B Dental Implant Company, Bologna, Italy) was trimmed allowing for graft volume. The membrane was positioned on the lingual side using a titanium pin. The composite bone graft was put into the defect, and the membrane was folded over and positioned using the other two titanium pins on the vestibular side. Using an expanded polyester suture (Ethibond, Ethicon, Somerville, NJ), the flap was then stitched in two layers. Horizontal mattress stitches were made 4 mm from the incision line followed by single interrupted stitches to close the edges of the flap allowing a minimum of a 4 mm deep connective tissue layer between the membrane and the oral epithelium. Using single interrupted stitches, the vertical incisions were closed. These single stitches were removed 10 to 14 days after surgery while the mattress stitches were taken out after 3 weeks. In addition to the pre- and postoperative antibiotics described above, an anti-inflammatory medication (ibuprofen 600 mg) immediately after the surgical intervention and thereafter three times a day for 1 week following surgery was prescribed. Chemical plaque control using a 0.20% chlorhexidine gluconate solution was used twice a day from 24 hours postsurgery until the time of suture removal. After 6 months, an envelope flap was created for the second surgical stage which consisted in a paracrestal incision 3 mm lingual from the crest. The keratinized gingiva was positioned and stitched on the buccal aspect of the healing abutments. This uncovery procedure ensured good quality keratinized tissue all around the implants, thus improving not only the aesthetics of the area but also the function, preventing unpleasant accumulations of food for the patient in that area given by the concavity of the site. The implants were restored with screw-retained implant-supported porcelain fused-to-metal crowns, and all the laboratory steps followed a completely digital workflow.

3. Results and Discussion

The implants remained in function, and the patient did not complain of foreign body sensation, pain, or dysesthesia. Intraoral examinations showed healthy peri-implant mucosa without suppuration, swelling, or redness at any implant site. Radiologic examination showed the first bone-implant contact was located near the first implant thread (Figure 2).

Guided bone regeneration is still a daunting element in the dental implant treatment protocol.

In order to arrive at a good long-term scenario for osteointegrated implants, there has to be enough bone volume at the implantation sites. To replace the lost bone and to permit the complete implant's integration and maintained during functional loading [14–16], diverse approaches, such as bone-grafting techniques, alveolar distraction, and guided bone regeneration, have been practiced. Guided bone regeneration is thought to be the most commonly used alveolar bone's reconstructing method, also used to treat peri-implant bone deficiencies [17–20]. Research indicates that survival rates of implants positioned in the sites enlarged by GBR are comparable to those found for implants in pristine sites [16, 21–23]. In particular, the implant survival rate in the sites that have received GBR procedures through the use of xenogenic materials is greater compared to the sites that have received GBR procedures through the insertion of autogenous bone blocks; in a prospective study by Meloni et al. (2019), data confirm the 1-year results allowing for the use of collagen resorbable membrane in GBR procedures for horizontal ridge augmentation; although the two-stage approach needs a longer time before prosthesis delivery, this technique seems to be safe and predictable for large reconstruction and can be applied in daily practice [24].

The survival rate of implants positioned in enlarged sites oscillated between 79 and 100%, and the bulk of research showed a survival rate of over 90% after at least one year of utility [25]. An essential element in the treatment is the membrane and its various materials and adaptations used for GBR. The membrane used for GBR therapy should have biocompatibility, cell-occlusion properties, integration by the host tissues, clinical manageability, the ability to make space, and adequate mechanical and physical properties.

Nonresorbable membranes, for the most part polytetrafluoroethylene (PTFE) in its expanded form (e-PTFE), made up the first generation of barrier membranes. These membrane types generally showed biocompatibility and space-making capability [26], but nonresorbable membranes require another surgical operation to remove the membrane. Later, a second generation of resorbable membranes was developed, and their use became widespread in diverse clinical situations. Of late, work has been carried out to develop a further generation of membranes by using naturally derived membranes or employing principles of tissue engineering during the preparation of the membrane [27, 28]. In addition, the use of membranes in the defect, along with bone grafts and substitute materials, is regularly employed to give a structural support to the defect site and to advocate the intrinsic regenerative potential of the host tissue. Horizontal ridge augmentation has been illustrated using a variety of different techniques and materials [29]. In the case in question, we used a resorbable collagen membrane so as to avoid some of the drawbacks when using nonresorbable membranes, like the necessity for a second surgical procedure to remove the membrane combined with the risk of losing more of the regenerated bone due to flap reflection [30]. Moreover, the conclusion of an in vitro study which compared resorbable and nonresorbable membranes was that bioabsorbable membranes, particularly collagen and hyaluronic acid, may promote bone regeneration through their activity on osteoblasts which suggests that bioabsorbable membranes could be more apt than nonresorbable membranes because they encourage the regeneration and repair of bones [31].

Since they are not rigid, most bioabsorbable membranes have to be combined with a graft material to ensure space maintenance when used for bone augmentation; otherwise, barrier membranes could get compressed into the space of a bony defect by the overlying soft tissue during the healing process [29]. Thus, a blend of particulate of autogenous and xenogeneic grafts was used together with the membrane. Autograft is deemed the gold standard for the majority of craniofacial bone grafting as well as for the treatment of various dental implant-related defects. On the other hand, autografts have known weaknesses which include donor site morbidity, potential resorption, size mismatch, and insufficient quantity of graft material.

The most important complication with the autologous bone is certainly the comorbidity associated with the presence of a donor site which needs a second surgical site. The complications described in the literature with this type of material appear to be chronic pain in a range of 2.5% from 8% of cases, dysesthesia in 6% of cases, or infection in 2% of cases. An alternative to autologous bone is the use of allogenic, but some risk of disease transmission can exists. Moreover, the high cost of such materials should be considered. Another alternative to autograft could be the use of xenogenic bone [32]. In our case, none of these potential complications came up and healing was uneventful during the follow-up period. We were able to overcome the lack of titanium reinforcement for the resorbable membrane by securely fixing the membrane on both the lingual/palatal and the vestibular side. In this way, the graft material is immobilized permitting the formation of the required quantity of bone.

4. Conclusions

Within the confines of this case report, we can consider the GBR technique to be successful in the preprosthetic surgical treatment of horizontally deficient alveolar ridges, allowing in these cases the execution of prosthetically guided implant-supported oral rehabilitations. Anyway, the use of a barrier membrane is a technique-sensitive procedure and it is not lacking in complications. The GBR technique using autogenous bone, with ABBM, and a resorbable barrier membrane fixed with titanium pins, allows the patient to save further surgery and therefore reduces the comorbidity of the procedure and the risk of complications such as the loss of regenerated tissue. The regenerated bone showed to provide good osteointegration of the dental implants. We would stress that the study in question is a case report and so conclusions cannot be generalized. Further-reaching, long-term studies will be necessary to back up this premise so as to apply this technique for other clinical cases.

References

[1] T. L. Aghaloo and P. K. Moy, "Which hard tissue augmentation techniques are the most successful in furnishing bony support for implant placement?," *The International Journal of Oral & Maxillofacial Implants*, vol. 23, no. 1, p. 56, 2008.

[2] L. Ramaglia, P. Toti, C. Sbordone, F. Guidetti, R. Martuscelli, and L. Sbordone, "Implant angulation: 2-year retrospective analysis on the influence of dental implant angle insertion on marginal bone resorption in maxillary and mandibular osseous onlay grafts," *Clinical Oral Investigations*, vol. 19, no. 4, pp. 769–779, 2015.

[3] D. Buser, S. Ingimarsson, K. Dula, A. Lussi, H. P. Hirt, and U. C. Belser, "Long-term stability of osseointegrated implants in augmented bone: a 5-year prospective study in partially edentulous patients," *The International Journal of Periodontics & Restorative Dentistry*, vol. 22, no. 2, pp. 109–117, 2002.

[4] M. Simion, S. A. Jovanovic, C. Tinti, and S. P. Benfenati, "Long-term evaluation of osseo-integrated implants inserted at the time or after vertical ridge augmentation. A retrospective study on 123 implants with 1-5 year follow-up," *Clinical Oral Implants Research*, vol. 12, no. 1, pp. 35–45, 2001.

[5] I. A. Urban, S. A. Jovanovic, and J. L. Lozada, "Vertical ridge augmentation using guided bone regeneration (GBR) in three clinical scenarios prior to implant placement: a retrospective study of 35 patients 12 to 72 months after loading," *The International Journal of Oral & Maxillofacial Implants*, vol. 24, no. 3, pp. 502–510, 2009.

[6] I. Rocchietta, F. Fontana, and M. Simion, "Clinical outcomes of vertical bone augmentation to enable dental implant placement: a systematic review," *Journal of Clinical Periodontology*, vol. 35, Supplement 8, pp. 203–215, 2008.

[7] M. Esposito, M. G. Grusovin, S. Kwan, H. V. Worthington, and P. Coulthard, "Interventions for replacing missing teeth: bone augmentation techniques for dental implant treatment," *Cochrane Database of Systematic Reviews*, no. 3, article CD003607, 2008.

[8] F. Fontana, F. Santoro, C. Maiorana, G. Iezzi, A. Piattelli, and M. Simion, "Clinical and histologic evaluation of allogeneic bone matrix versus autogenous bone chips associated with titanium-reinforced E-PTFE membrane for vertical ridge augmentation: a prospective pilot study," *The International Journal of Oral & Maxillofacial Implants*, vol. 23, no. 6, pp. 1003–1012, 2008.

[9] F. Fontana, E. Maschera, I. Rocchietta, and M. Simion, "Clinical classification of complications in guided bone regeneration procedures by means of a nonresorbable membrane," *The International Journal of Periodontics & Restorative Dentistry*, vol. 31, no. 3, pp. 265–273, 2011.

[10] F. Briguglio, D. Falcomatà, S. Marconcini, L. Fiorillo, R. Briguglio, and D. Farronato, "The use of titanium mesh in guided bone regeneration: a systematic review," *International Journal of Dentistry*, vol. 2019, Article ID 9065423, 8 pages, 2019.

[11] I. A. Urban, H. Nagursky, and J. L. Lozada, "Horizontal ridge augmentation with a resorbable membrane and particulated autogenous bone with or without anorganic bovine bone-derived mineral: a prospective case series in 22 patients," *The International Journal of Oral & Maxillofacial Implants*, vol. 26, no. 2, pp. 404–414, 2011.

[12] I. A. Urban, J. L. Lozada, S. A. Jovanovic, and K. Nagy, "Horizontal guided bone regeneration in the posterior maxilla using recombinant human platelet- derived growth factor: a case report," *The International Journal of Periodontics and Restorative Dentistry*, vol. 33, no. 4, pp. 421–425, 2013.

[13] M. Ronda and C. Stacchi, "A novel approach for the coronal advancement of the buccal flap," *The International Journal of Periodontics & Restorative Dentistry*, vol. 35, no. 6, pp. 795–801, 2015.

[14] M. Chiapasco, M. Zaniboni, and M. Boisco, "Augmentation procedures for the rehabilitation of deficient edentulous ridges with oral implants," *Clinical Oral Implants Research*, vol. 17, Supplement 2, pp. 136–159, 2006.

[15] S. Bernstein, J. Cooke, P. Fotek, and H. L. Wang, "Vertical bone augmentation: where are we now?," *Implant Dentistry*, vol. 15, no. 3, pp. 219–228, 2006.

[16] N. Donos, N. Mardas, and V. Chadha, "Clinical outcomes of implants following lateral bone augmentation: systematic assessment of available options (barrier membranes, bone grafts, split osteotomy)," *Journal of Clinical Periodontology*, vol. 35, Supplement 8, pp. 173–202, 2008.

[17] C. H. Hammerle and R. E. Jung, "Bone augmentation by means of barrier membranes," *Periodontology 2000*, vol. 33, no. 1, pp. 36–53, 2003.

[18] Y. D. Rakhmatia, Y. Ayukawa, A. Furuhashi, and K. Koyano, "Current barrier membranes: titanium mesh and other membranes for guided bone regeneration in dental applications," *Journal of Prosthodontic Research*, vol. 57, no. 1, pp. 3–14, 2013.

[19] M. Chiapasco and M. Zaniboni, "Clinical outcomes of GBR procedures to correct peri-implant dehiscences and fenestrations: a systematic review," *Clinical Oral Implants Research*, vol. 20, Supplement 4, pp. 113–123, 2009.

[20] G. I. Benic, M. Bernasconi, R. E. Jung, and C. H. F. Hämmerle, "Clinical and radiographic intra-subject comparison of implants placed with or without guided bone regeneration: 15-year results," *Journal of Clinical Periodontology*, vol. 44, no. 3, pp. 315–325, 2017.

[21] S. M. Meloni, S. A. Jovanovic, I. Urban, E. Baldoni, M. Pisano, and M. Tallarico, "Horizontal ridge augmentation using GBR with a native collagen membrane and 1:1 ratio of particulate xenograft and autologous bone: a 3-year after final loading prospective clinical study," *Clinical Implant Dentistry and Related Research*, vol. 21, no. 4, pp. 669–677, 2019.

[22] G. I. Benic and C. H. Hämmerle, "Horizontal bone augmentation by means of guided bone regeneration," *Periodontology 2000*, vol. 66, no. 1, pp. 13–40, 2014.

[23] M. Clementini, A. Morlupi, L. Canullo, C. Agrestini, and A. Barlattani, "Success rate of dental implants inserted in horizontal and vertical guided bone regenerated areas: a systematic review," *International Journal of Oral and Maxillofacial Surgery*, vol. 41, no. 7, pp. 847–852, 2012.

[24] S. S. Jensen and H. Terheyden, "Bone augmentation procedures in localized defects in the alveolar ridge: clinical results with different bone grafts and bone-substitute materials," *The International Journal of Oral & Maxillofacial Implants*, vol. 24, pp. 218–236, 2009.

[25] C. H. Hämmerle, R. E. Jung, and A. Feloutzis, "A systematic review of the survival of implants in bone sites augmented with barrier membranes (guided bone regeneration) in partially edentulous patients," *Journal of Clinical Periodontology*, vol. 29, no. s3, pp. 226–231, 2002.

[26] J. Liu and D. G. Kerns, "Mechanisms of guided bone regeneration: a review," *The Open Dentistry Journal*, vol. 8, no. 1, pp. 56–65, 2014.

[27] M. C. Bottino, V. Thomas, G. Schmidt et al., "Recent advances in the development of GTR/GBR membranes for periodontal regeneration–a materials perspective," *Dental Materials*, vol. 28, no. 7, pp. 703–721, 2012.

[28] G. Sam and B. R. Pillai, "Evolution of barrier membranes in periodontal regeneration-"are the third generation membranes really here?"," *Journal of Clinical and Diagnostic Research*, vol. 8, no. 12, pp. ZE14–ZE17, 2014.

[29] B. S. McAllister and K. Haghighat, "Bone augmentation techniques," *Journal of Periodontology*, vol. 78, no. 3, pp. 377–396, 2007.

[30] L. Ramaglia, F. di Spirito, M. Sirignano, M. la Rocca, U. Esposito, and L. Sbordone, "A 5-year longitudinal cohort

study on crown to implant ratio effect on marginal bone level in single implants," *Clinical Implant Dentistry and Related Research*, pp. 1–7, 2019.

[31] L. Marinucci, C. Lilli, T. Baroni et al., "In vitro comparison of bioabsorbable and non-resorbable membranes in bone regeneration," *Journal of Periodontology*, vol. 72, no. 6, pp. 753–759, 2001.

[32] G. F. Grado, L. Keller, Y. Idoux-Gillet et al., "Bone substitutes: a review of their characteristics, clinical use, and perspectives for large bone defects management," *Journal of Tissue Engineering*, vol. 9, 2018.

14

Horizontal Ridge Augmentation using a Xenograft Bone Substitute for Implant-Supported Fixed Rehabilitation: A Case Report with Four Years of Follow-Up

Bruno Freitas Mello,[1] Márcio de Carvalho Formiga,[1] Luiz Fernando de Souza da Silva,[2] Gustavo dos Santos Coura,[2] and Jamil Awad Shibli[1]

[1]*Department of Periodontology and Oral Implantology, Dental Research Division, University of Guarulhos, Sao Paulo, Brazil*
[2]*Department of Implantology, Unisociesc, Florianópolis, Brazil*

Correspondence should be addressed to Márcio de Carvalho Formiga; marciocformiga@gmail.com

Academic Editor: Mine D ndar

The guided bone regeneration (GBR) technique has been used to achieve optimal bone volume augmentation and allow dental implant placement in atrophic maxilla and mandible, with predictable results and high survival rates. The use of bone substitutes has reduced the necessity of autogenous bone grafts, reducing the morbidity at the donor areas and thus improving the patients' satisfaction and comfort. This clinical case report shows a clinical and histological evaluation of the bone tissue behavior, in a case that required the horizontal augmentation of the alveolar ridge, with the use of xenograft biomaterial and further dental implant placement. After six months of healing time, six implants were placed, and a bone biopsy was done. The histological analysis depicted some fragments of the xenograft bone graft, integrated with the new-formed bone tissue.

1. Introduction

The rehabilitation of totally, partially, and single-unit edentulous patients with the use of dental implants is an established treatment with high success rates [1, 2]. However, there are several unfavorable clinical situations for the placement of implants, where there is not sufficient bone height and/or width in the alveolar bone ridge. Augmentation of the alveolar ridge using guided bone regeneration (GBR) became a treatment option to obtain bone support for osseointegrated dental implants [3]. The procedures for bone augmentation of the alveolar ridge through GBR present successful, long-term follow-up results [4–6].

Autogenous bone grafts are often used in GBR procedures and are considered as the gold standard because it is the only biomaterial that combines properties of osteogenesis, osteoinduction, and osteoconduction [7, 8]. However, disadvantages such as morbidity at the donor site, limited availability, tooth sensitivity, and risk of dehiscence of the wounds [1, 7, 9–11] have led to investigations on the development and application of bone substitutes for the regeneration of the alveolar bone ridge [11–13].

Xenografts have shown to have excellent properties for GBR, like its biocompatibility, formation of a scaffold (osteoconduction), slow resorption rates, and the ability to define and maintain the volume for bone gain [12–14]. The graft maturation period could be longer than that of autogenous bone grafts, taking from nine to twelve months [10, 12–14], and demand the need of collagen membranes for guided bone regeneration procedures, which must provide cell occlusion and a better biocompatibility with the soft tissue, reducing the risk of complications such as wound dehiscence [11, 14].

Therefore, the aim of this case report is to describe a GBR with xenograft and collagen membrane for horizontal augmentation for an implant-supported fixed rehabilitation and the four years of follow-up.

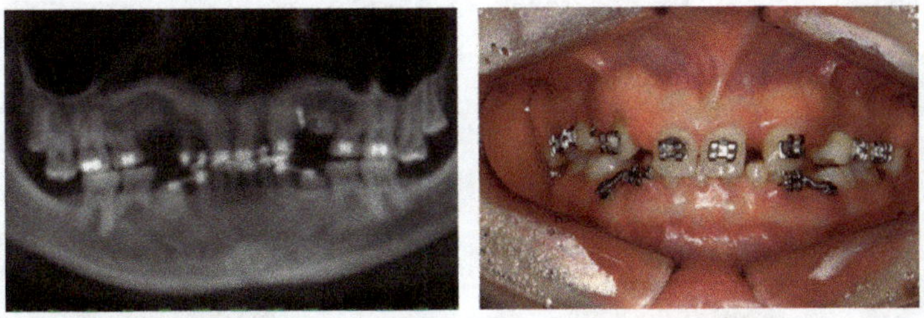

Figure 1: Panoramic radiograph (a) and intraoral buccal view, showing permanent tooth absences and presence of several deciduous teeth.

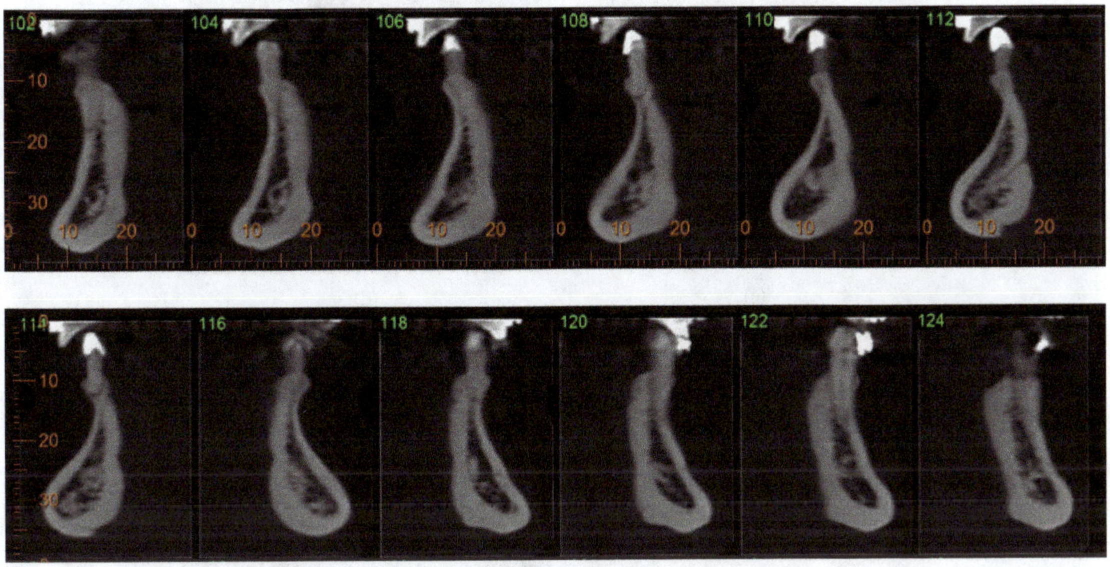

Figure 2: Preoperatory tomography of the anterior mandible region.

2. Case Report

An 18-year-old female patient attended a clinic/school seeking to solve aesthetic and functional problems. After an initial evaluation, several dental losses and the presence of some deciduous teeth were observed, revealing a multiple agenesis condition. Clinical examination and CT scans were performed. In the mandible, the patient presented all the deciduous teeth, and only permanent teeth present were #36 and #46 (Figure 1).

Analyzing the mandible CT scan, it was observed a sizeable horizontal deficiency of the alveolar ridge in the crestal symphysis region. This situation made impossible the placement of implants in the ideal three-dimensional position, requiring previous bone reconstruction (Figure 2).

It was decided to perform horizontal bone augmentation by guided bone regeneration with only a bovine bone substitute (Bio-Oss® Geistlich), because it presents reproducible results with acceptable success rates and low rate of complications, besides providing lower morbidity for the patient. The marginal gingiva was healthy and presented a good width of keratinized tissue. Amoxicillin 500 mg 1 every 8 hours for 7 days and 0.12% chlorhexidine gluconate rinse 3 times a day for 14 days were prescribed, initiating 2 days before surgery. Infiltration anesthesia was performed with 4% articaine anesthetic in the mental nerve plexus, bilaterally. The incision was intrasulcular in the region from 75 to 85, with small vertical releases at the distal of this incision. A mucoperiosteal flap was raised. At the recipient site, soft tissue debridement and small perforations with 1.3 drills were performed in the cortical bone with the purpose of providing irrigation and blood supply to the bone substitute. At this moment, 1.0 cc of bone substitute (Bio-Oss® Geistlich, large granules) was prepared to be placed at the recipient site and covered with double layer collagen resorbable membrane (Bio-Gide® Geistlich, 25 mm × 25 mm). Both bone substitute and collagen membrane were displaced on different recipients, with saline for 10 minutes of hydration prior use. The buccal flap was repositioned, covering all the membrane and avoiding displacement. The suture was performed with simple interrupted and sling sutures using the deciduous teeth as support, with silk 4.0 (Ethicon). After the surgical procedure, a bandage (Micropore®) was performed to compress the surgical area to diminish possible edema (Figure 3).

Nimesulide 100 mg twice a day for 3 days, paracetamol 750 mg 3 times a day (if necessary for pain control), and continuation of the preoperative antibiotic and antiseptic mouthwash protocols were prescribed. The patient was instructed to eat only soft foods, put ice bags on the surgical area for 48 hours, and avoid exercises for 7 days. The sutures were removed after 7 days.

After 12 months, the area of the horizontal bone augmentation was clinically evaluated and through cone-beam CT. After the analysis of the tomography radiograph and initial

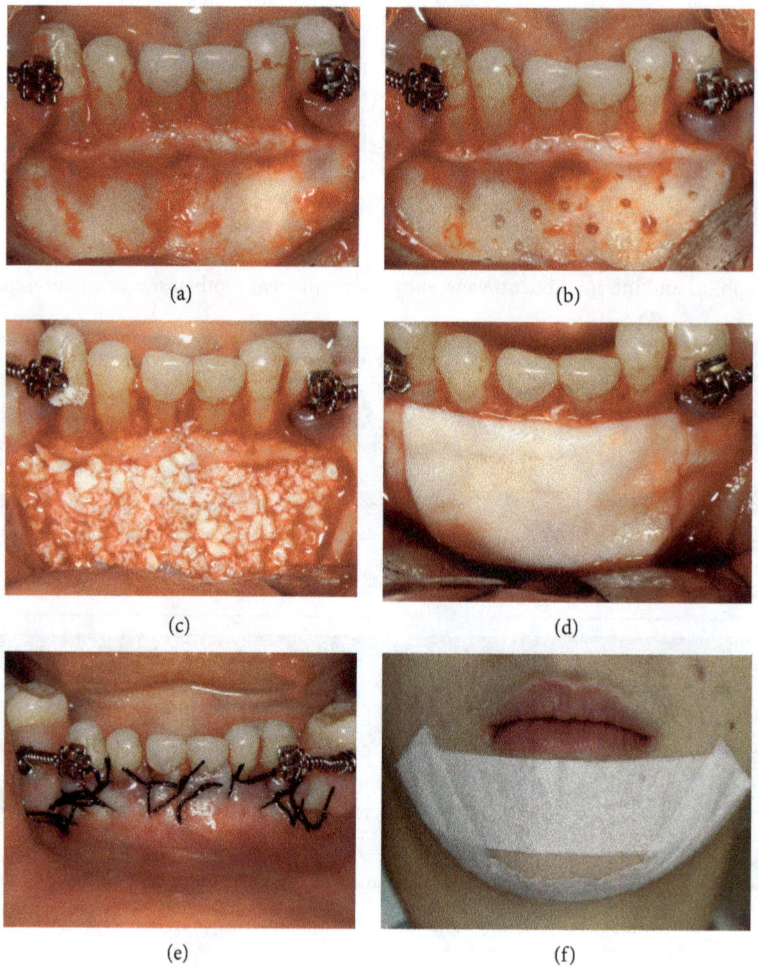

FIGURE 3: Intraoral view of the surgery steps: (a) incision and total flap detachment, (b) cortical perforations, (c) bone substitute accommodation, (d) double layer collagen membrane, (e) single sutures, and (f) bandage (Micropore®).

and final prototypes, the gain in bone thickness was approximately 5 mm. Clinically, the success of the procedure was confirmed, as well as the presence of good health of the gingival tissue (Figures 4 and 5).

The surgery to install 6 dental implants (Ankylos®, Dentsply) was performed 12 months following the horizontal bone augmentation, according to the reverse planning and surgical guide, between the region of #34 and #44. All implants presented initial stability above 35 N/cm. The deciduous teeth 74, 73, 72, 71, 81, 82, 83, and 84 were removed at this time. After detachment of the mucoperiosteal flap, we found new bone tissue with excellent quality with the native bone appearance and without the presence of loose particles of a bone substitute and surrounded by fibrous tissue. At this moment, a bone fragment of approximately 3 mm was removed using a 2.0 mm trephine drill in a buccolingual direction for histological analysis of the grafted area (Figure 6).

In the histological analysis, it was observed the formation of cortical bone with the presence of osteocytes found in several sizes and homogeneously distributed. Bone substitute particles were present in a graft/cortical bone interface. However, it could be confirmed on the clinical observation that the regenerated bone was similar to the natural bone (Figure 7).

Immediately after implant surgery, standard prosthetic abutments (A4) were installed (Ankylos®). After suturing, with 5.0 polypropylene (Atramat), because of its fewer biofilm accumulation, the impression-taking of the abutments and occlusal registration were accomplished. A temporary acrylic resin fixed prosthesis was installed immediately to the surgical procedure, within 24 hours (Figure 8). Pre- and postoperative recommendations and medication protocols were identic to the first surgery, but without the need for bandages.

Four years after bone augmentation of the alveolar ridge, a tomographic examination was requested to evaluate the bone tissue, as well as the implants, where bone normality and stability around the implants were seen, to confirm our clinical evaluation (Figures 9 and 10).

3. Discussion

Guided bone regeneration (GBR) performed within the concepts of the technique can be indicated to increase the width of alveolar bone ridges when associated with the use of collagen membranes and bovine bone substitute, with high survival rates of implants placed in sites with large bone volume deficiencies [6, 10, 15].

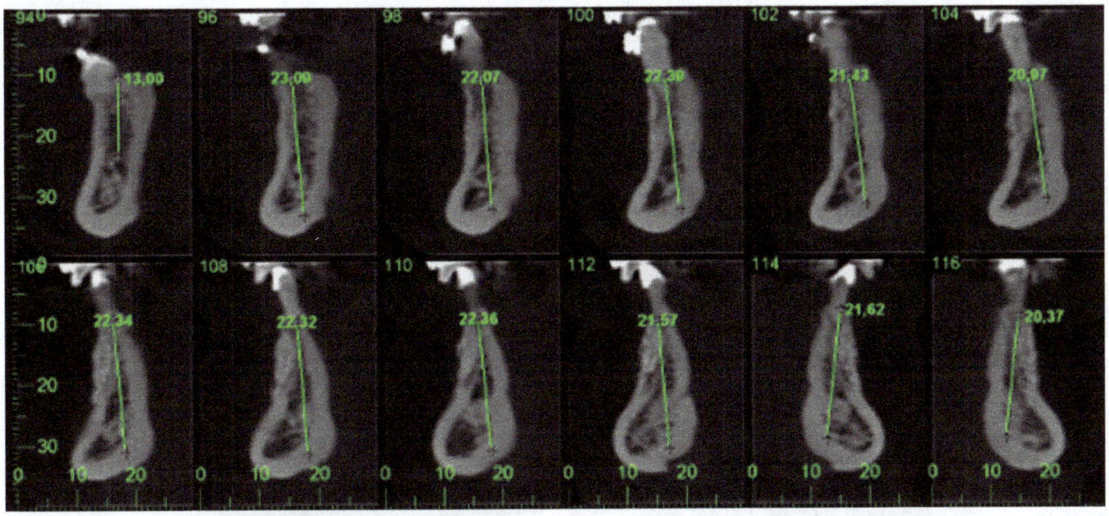

FIGURE 4: Postoperatory tomography radiograph 12 months after the horizontal bone augmentation, showing new bone formation, allowing the correct three-dimensional placement of dental implants.

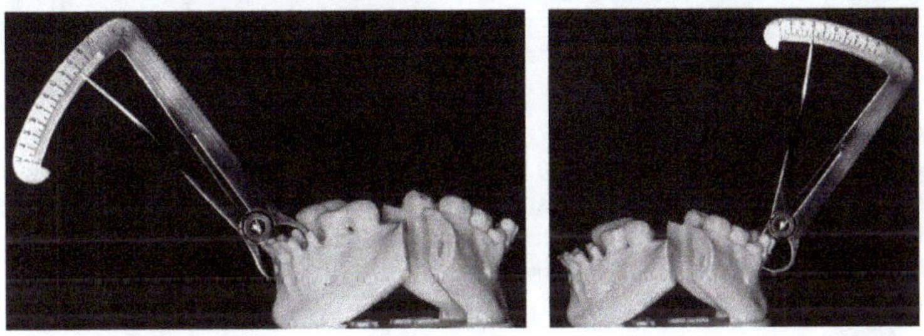

(a) (b)

FIGURE 5: 3D resin prototype of the appearance of the ridge before (a) and after (b) the volume increase of the alveolar ridge. There was a 5 mm gain in bone thickness.

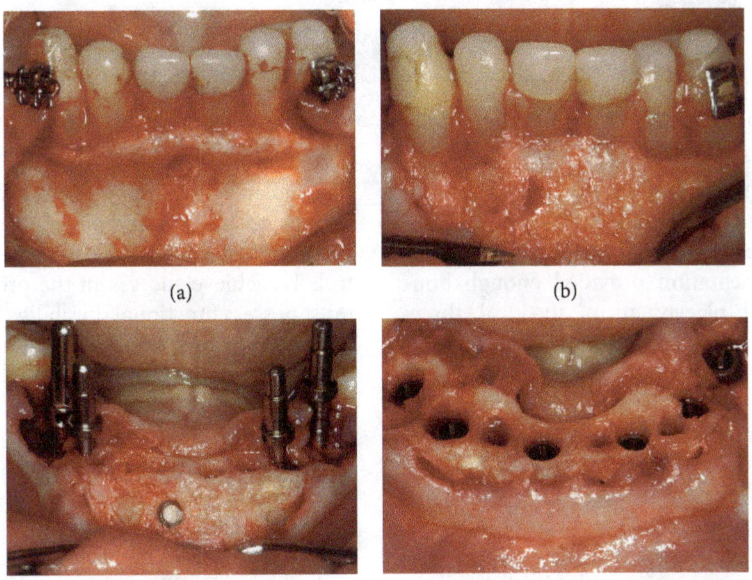

(a) (b) (c) (d)

FIGURE 6: Intraoral view of the alveolar ridge before (a) and after (b) augmentation. Removal of bone fragment using a 2.0 mm trephine for histological analysis of the grafted area (c). Six implants in place with initial torque of 35 N/cm (d).

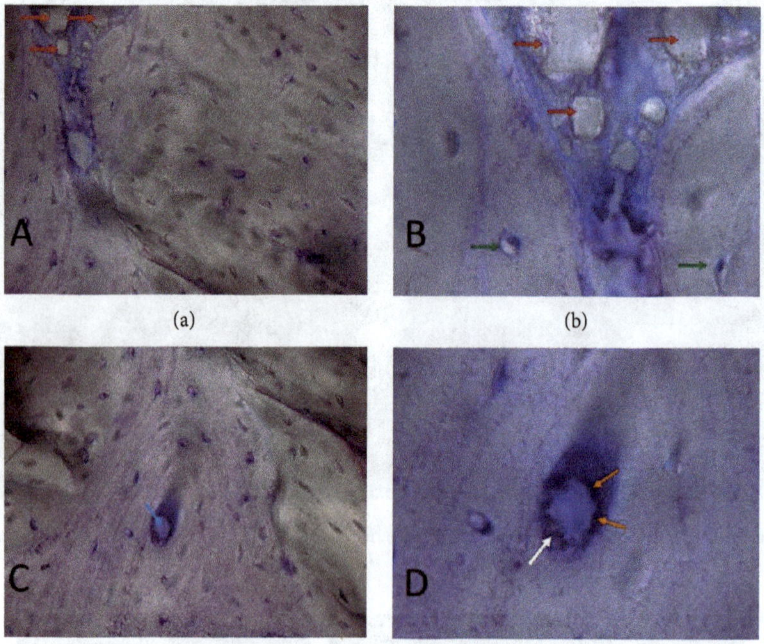

(a) (b) (c) (d)

FIGURE 7: (a) Image of a grafted material interface (red arrow) and cortical bone. It is clearly shown the formation of cortical bone with osteocytes; (b) enlarged image of (a). Grafted material (red arrow). Osteocytes present in the gaps (green arrow); (c) well-formed Haversian system: note the arrangement of concentric lamellae, with the central channel of Havers (blue arrow). Osteocytes homogeneously distributed, demonstrating the usual architecture of cortical bone; (c) enlarged image of (d). In detail, the Havers channel, with endosteum (orange arrow) and red blood cells (white arrow).

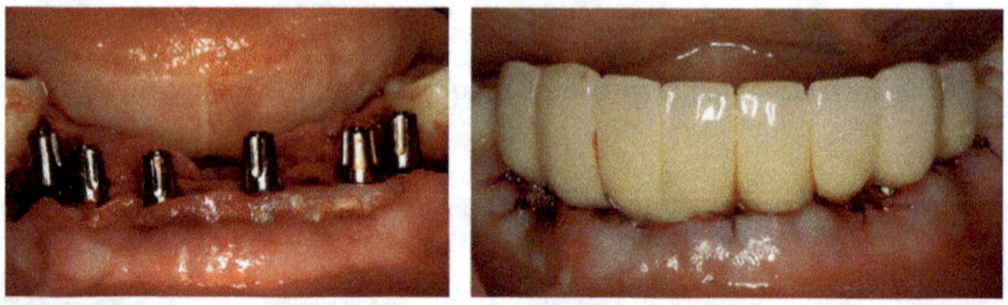

FIGURE 8: Installation of the definitive prosthetic abutments and delivery of the temporary cemented restoration with immediate load.

The horizontal bone gain of about 5 mm after 12 months observed in this clinical case is within the mean gain obtained by other clinical reports of GBR approach in the literature [11, 12]. This bone augmentation provided enough bone width for dental implant placement in an ideal three-dimensional position.

Soft tissue healing was excellent, with no intercurrences, such as membrane exposure or infections. This corroborated further studies on the compatibility of collagen membranes with soft tissue [9–12]. Studies reported that second intention healing occurred in all membrane exposures, with spontaneous reepithelialization, with no major complications [9].

The collagen absorbable membranes, due to its hydrophilic property and excellent interaction with blood clot fibrin in the surgical wound, facilitate the suture procedure [16] and have less tendency to soft tissue dehiscence [14]. In this case, we used silk suture on the GBR procedure because it was more comfortable for the patient, and the patient had excellent biofilm control. We realize it was not the best suture biomaterial, but the patient was very cooperative during all treatment. On the implant surgery, we preferred the use of polypropylene sutures because it remained above the temporary fixed prosthesis, and this material would provide a better biofilm control. To achieve success in the procedures, GBR membranes must possess functional durability, be resistant to degradation, and have biocompatibility with the soft tissue, providing tissue integration and avoiding spaces that may predispose to tissue dehiscence and infections [15]. The disadvantages of the collagen membrane are the resorption period between 4 and 8 weeks and lack of rigidity, leading to the need for filling material under the membrane thus providing the contour for bone augmentation [16].

Nonabsorbable membranes have greater stability in GBR and are more predictable regarding the time of permanence and maintenance of the scaffold in the alveolar ridge, with excellent results for bone augmentation [11, 16]. However, some reports have shown that nonresorbable membranes are more critical about their use, leading to high rates of wound dehiscence with subsequent local exposures and infections, and require a second surgery for its often removal [6, 9, 14].

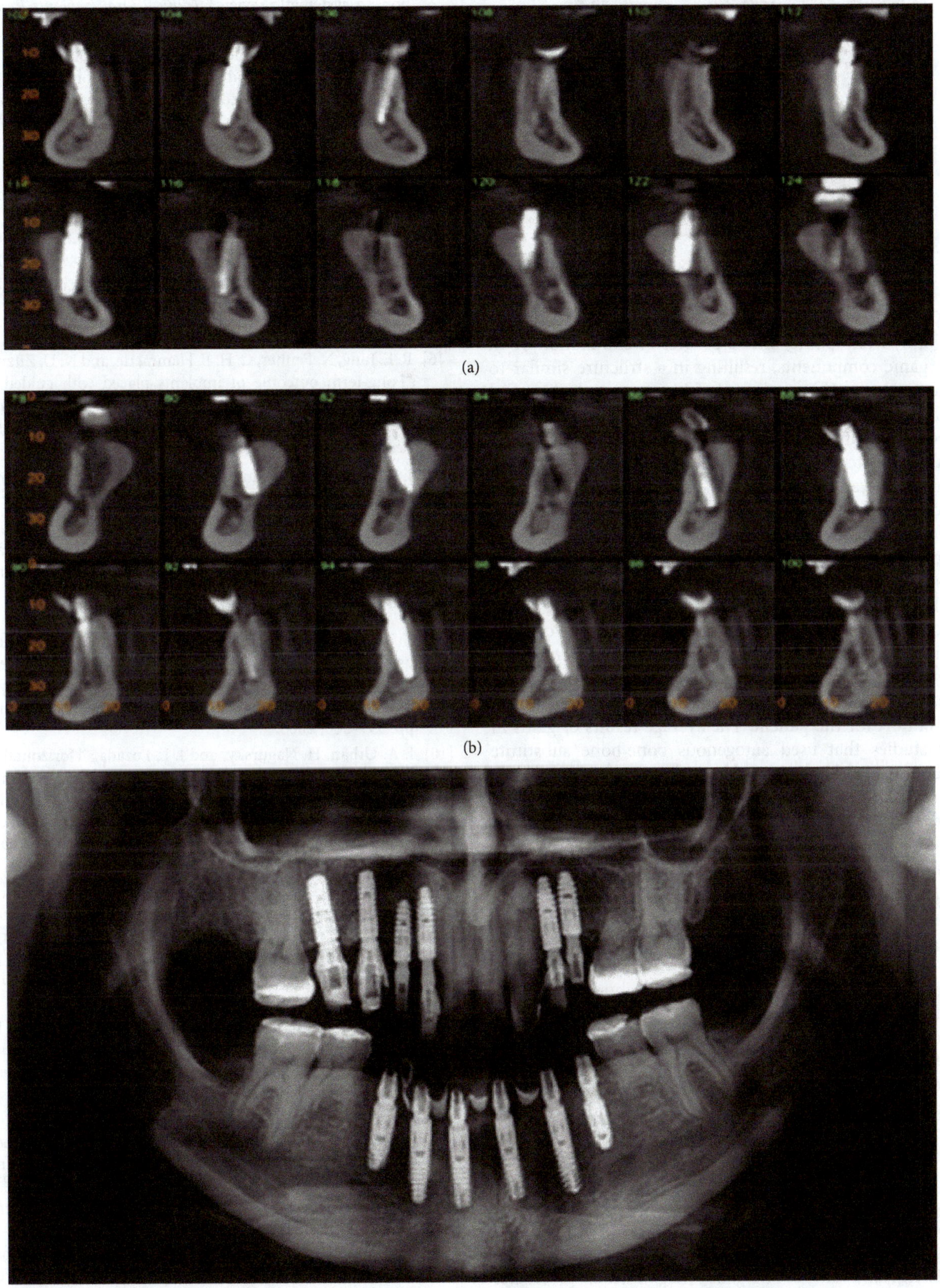

(a)

(b)

(c)

FIGURE 9: Four-year follow-up CT, showing the stability of the bone tissue around the implants (a, b). Panoramic radiograph of the 4-year follow-up (c).

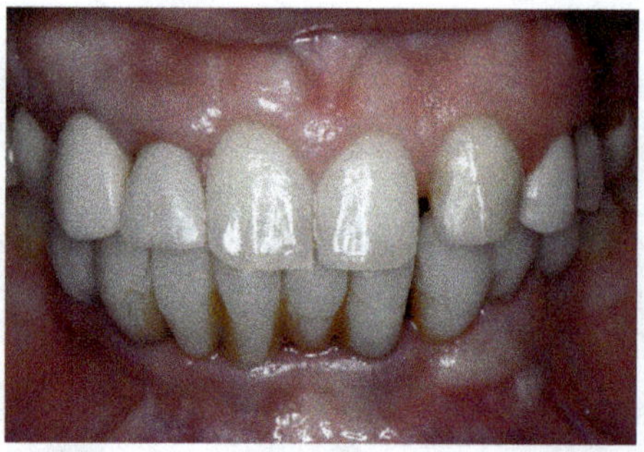

FIGURE 10: Buccal view of the four-year follow-up.

Xenogenous bovine bone substitutes are composed basically of hydroxyapatite, after a process of elimination of all the organic components, resulting in a structure similar to the human bone. Thus, at the end of this process, a biomaterial should be obtained where its particles may have interconnecting pores allowing thereby the penetration of new blood vessels and the osteoblast cellular migration into the graft [13].

In the literature, there are studies that used GBR protocols using collagen membranes and a mixture of autogenous bone/bone substitute [11]. The authors advocate the use of this mixture by the fact that autogenous bone particles add an osteogenic property to the graft.

However, one of the main advantages of the GBR approach using only bone substitutes is to avoid the complications of autogenous bone removal such as donor area morbidity, limited availability, and tooth sensitivity [1, 7, 9, 10]. Thus, the use of bone substitutes provides more satisfaction and comfort for the patient. The average results of gains in these studies that used autogenous bone/bone substitute mixture [10, 11] are comparable to this clinical case report. Other clinical studies [17, 18] showed similar results, as we found in this case report, with high rates of success on implant survival. Recent reviews also endorse the findings of this case report, with similar rates of horizontal bone augmentation [19–21].

4. Conclusion

Within the limitations of this report, the horizontal bone augmentation with the use of only a bovine bone substitute and a double layer collagen membrane seemed to be a feasible treatment option in the short term for promoting an increase in bone width of the alveolar ridge, allowing an appropriate size for predictable and successful placement of dental implants and a fixed oral implant-supported rehabilitation.

References

[1] B. Al-Nawas and E. Schiegnitz, "Augmentation procedures using bone substitute materials or autogenous bone – a systematic review and meta-analysis," *European Journal of Oral Implantology*, vol. 7, Supplement 2, pp. S219–S234, 2014.

[2] M. Chiapasco and M. Zaniboni, "Clinical outcomes of GBR procedures to correct peri-implant dehiscences and fenestrations: a systematic review," *Clinical Oral Implants Research*, vol. 20, Supplement 4, pp. 113–123, 2009.

[3] I. A. Urban, S. A. Jovanovic, and J. L. Lozada, "Vertical ridge augmentation using guided bone regeneration (GBR) in three clinical scenarios prior to implant placement: a retrospective study of 35 patients 12 to 72 months after loading," *The International Journal of Oral & Maxillofacial Implants*, vol. 24, no. 3, pp. 502–510, 2009.

[4] T. L. Aghaloo and P. K. Moy, "Which hard tissue augmentation techniques are the most successful in furnishing bony support for implant placement?," *The International Journal of Oral & Maxillofacial Implants*, vol. 22, pp. 49–70, 2007.

[5] M. Retzepi and N. Donos, "Guided bone regeneration: biological principle and therapeutic applications," *Clinical Oral Implants Research*, vol. 21, no. 6, pp. 567–576, 2010.

[6] R. E. Jung, N. Fenner, C. H. F. Hämmerle, and N. U. Zitzmann, "Long-term outcome of implants placed with guided bone regeneration (GBR) using resorbable and non-resorbable membranes after 12–14 years," *Clinical Oral Implants Research*, vol. 24, no. 10, pp. 1065–1073, 2013.

[7] J. H. Fu and H. L. Wang, "Horizontal bone augmentation: the decision tree," *The International Journal of Periodontics & Restorative Dentistry*, vol. 31, no. 4, pp. 429–436, 2011.

[8] M. O. Klein and B. Al-Nawas, "For which clinical indications in dental implantology is the use of bone substitute materials scientifically substantiated?," *European Journal of Oral Implantology*, vol. 4, pp. 11–29, 2011.

[9] T. von Arx and D. Buser, "Horizontal ridge augmentation using autogenous block grafts and the guided bone regeneration technique with collagen membranes: a clinical study with 42 patients," *Clinical Oral Implants Research*, vol. 17, no. 4, pp. 359–366, 2006.

[10] I. A. Urban, H. Nagursky, and J. L. Lozada, "Horizontal ridge augmentation with a resorbable membrane and particulated autogenous bone with or without anorganic bovine bone-derived mineral: a prospective case series in 22 patients," *The International Journal of Oral & Maxillofacial Implants*, vol. 26, no. 2, pp. 404–414, 2011.

[11] I. A. Urban, H. Nagursky, J. L. Lozada, and K. Nagy, "Horizontal ridge augmentation with a collagen membrane and a combination of particulated autogenous bone and anorganic bovine bone-derived mineral: a prospective case series in 25 patients," *The International Journal of Oral & Maxillofacial Implants*, vol. 33, no. 3, pp. 299–307, 2013.

[12] C. H. F. Hämmerle, R. E. Jung, D. Yaman, and N. P. Lang, "Ridge augmentation by applying bioresorbable membranes and deproteinized bovine bone mineral: a report of twelve consecutive cases," *Clinical Oral Implants Research*, vol. 19, no. 1, pp. 19–25, 2008.

[13] L. Ohayon, "Ridge enlargement using deproteinized bovine bone and a bioresorbable collagen membrane: a tomodensitometric, histologic, and histomorphometric analysis," *The International Journal of Periodontics & Restorative Dentistry*, vol. 31, no. 3, pp. 237–245, 2011.

[14] S. S. Jensen and H. Terheyden, "Bone augmentation procedures in localized defects in the alveolar ridge: clinical results with different bone grafts and bone-substitute materials," *The International Journal of Oral & Maxillofacial Implants*, vol. 24, pp. 218–236, 2009.

[15] A. Friedmann, K. Gissel, M. Soudan, B. M. Kleber, S. Pitaru, and T. Dietrich, "Randomized controlled trial on lateral aug-

mentation using two collagen membranes: morphometric results on mineralized tissue compound," *Journal of Clinical Periodontology*, vol. 38, no. 7, pp. 677–685, 2011.

[16] P. A. Fugazzotto, "GBR using bovine bone matrix and resorbable and nonresorbable membranes. Part 1: histologic results," *The International Journal of Periodontics & Restorative Dentistry*, vol. 23, no. 4, pp. 361–369, 2003.

[17] A. Patel, H. Greenwell, M. Hill, B. Shumway, and A. Radmall, "Ridge augmentation comparing an allograft plus autogenous bone chips to an osteoinductive demineralized bone Matrix," *Implant Dentistry*, vol. 28, no. 6, pp. 613–620, 2019.

[18] G. Mendoza-Azpur, A. de la Fuente, E. Chavez, E. Valdivia, and I. Khouly, "Horizontal ridge augmentation with guided bone regeneration using particulate xenogenic bone substitutes with or without autogenous block grafts: a randomized controlled trial," *Clinical Implant Dentistry and Related Research*, vol. 21, no. 4, pp. 521–530, 2019.

[19] M. Troeltzsch, M. Troeltzsch, P. Kauffmann et al., "Clinical efficacy of grafting materials in alveolar ridge augmentation: a systematic review," *Journal of Cranio-Maxillo-Facial Surgery*, vol. 44, no. 10, pp. 1618–1629, 2016.

[20] P. H. de Azambuja Carvalho, G. dos Santos Trento, L. B. Moura, G. Cunha, M. A. C. Gabrielli, and V. A. Pereira-Filho, "Horizontal ridge augmentation using xenogenous bone graft—systematic review," *Oral and Maxillofacial Surgery*, vol. 23, no. 3, pp. 271–279, 2019.

[21] L. Tolstunov, J. F. E. Hamrick, V. Broumand, D. Shilo, and A. Rachmiel, "Bone augmentation techniques for horizontal and vertical alveolar ridge deficiency in oral implantology," *Oral and Maxillofacial Surgery Clinics of North America*, vol. 31, no. 2, pp. 163–191, 2019.

15

Vertical Guided Bone Regeneration with Mineralized Cancellous Bone Allograft in a Severe Anterior Maxillary Defect: A Clinical Report with 14-Year Follow-Up

Gerardo La Monaca,[1] Nicola Pranno,[1] Giorgio Pompa,[1] Susanna Annibali,[1] Iole Vozza,[1] and Maria Paola Cristalli[2]

[1]*Department of Oral and Maxillo-Facial Sciences, Sapienza University of Rome, Rome, Italy*
[2]*Department of Biotechnologies and Medical Surgical Sciences, Sapienza University of Rome, Rome, Italy*

Correspondence should be addressed to Gerardo La Monaca; gerardo.lamonaca@uniroma1.it and Nicola Pranno; nicola.pranno@uniroma1.it

Academic Editor: Muawia A. Qudeimat

Purpose. To report the supracrestal bone regeneration of approximately 10 mm using solvent-dehydrated mineralized cancellous bone allograft and nonresorbable membrane in rehabilitation of unsuccessful implants in the anterior maxilla and stability of the regenerated bone at the 14th-year follow-up. *Case Presentation.* A 24-year-old female patient with a history of anterior dentoalveolar trauma resulting in the loss of upper left incisors and canine underwent rehabilitation several years ago with three implant-supported fixed prostheses. The prosthesis was both functionally and aesthetically inadequate, and the patient complained of gingival swelling, bleeding, and food impaction at the site of the implants. A staged approach for retreatment was planned, wherein the first surgical stage aimed at removing the existing implants and preparing the bone ridge and soft tissues for the augmentation procedure. The second stage was vertical ridge augmentation and simultaneous prosthetic-driven placement of two new implants at the sites of the left central incisor and canine. After nine months of uneventful healing, complete regeneration of the bony defect was achieved, and the new prosthetic rehabilitation satisfied both functional and aesthetic requirements. *Conclusion.* The therapeutic approach followed in the present case proved effective in achieving satisfactory functional and aesthetic results and in maintaining the stability of the regenerated bone at 14 years of follow-up.

1. Introduction

Clinical management of implant-supported restorations in the anterior maxillary region is complicated due to the requirement to achieve optimal aesthetic outcomes, such as suitable width and position of the keratinized soft tissue, convex buccal contour of the alveolar process, harmonious gingival margins around implants and adjacent teeth, and proper size and shape of the papillae [1, 2].

The aesthetics of the peri-implant soft tissues depends on not only the height and thickness of the underlying supporting bone and interproximal bone height of adjacent teeth but also the appropriate three-dimensional position and size of the implants [3–5].

Indeed, positioning the implant shoulder too far facially can result in a potential risk of soft tissue recession, while too far palatal placement can result in ridge-lap restorations [2, 3]. An implant positioned too close to the natural teeth causes resorption of the interproximal bone, affecting papillary support. Similarly, implants positioned too deep in the alveolar ridge can lead to increased bone loss, due to the microgap at the implant-abutment interface, which will require a long prosthetic crown, use of pink porcelain, or visible metal margins [2].

Furthermore, the extended edentulous gap and severe bone loss due to trauma present adjunctive problems, making it more questionable to achieve aesthetic results in the anterior maxillary region. In this situation, unsuccessful

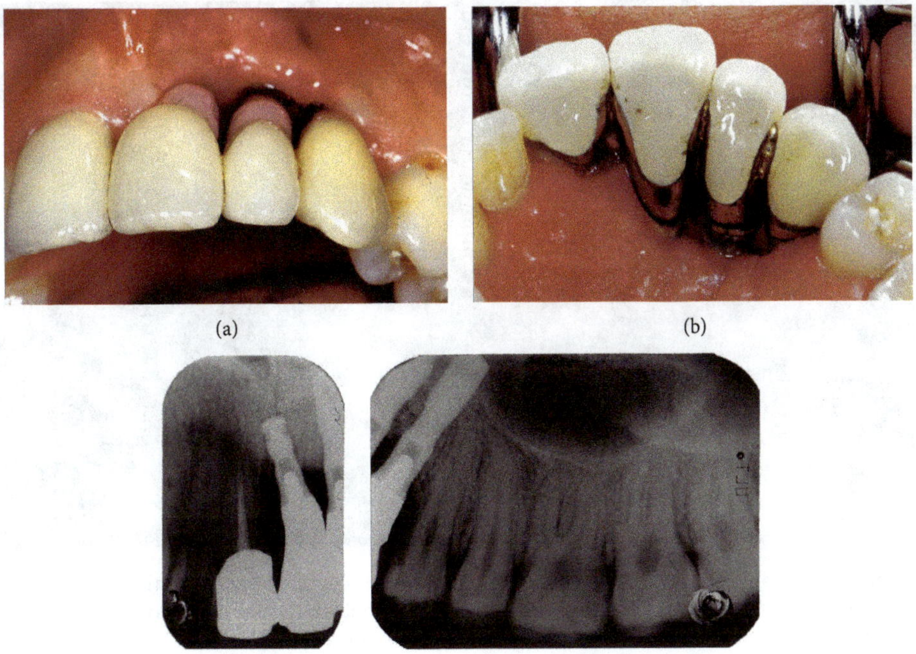

(a) (b)

(c) (d)

FIGURE 1: Preoperative clinical and radiographic views: (a) buccal aspect, (b) palatal aspect, (c) periapical radiograph of the right central incisor, (d) periapical radiograph of the left first premolar.

treatment outcomes can lead to clinical disasters, which require to be corrected with the removal of the implants and augmentation procedures to regenerate adequate volumes of bone in order to place new implants with a prosthetic-driven approach [2].

Among the different techniques proposed in the literature, vertical guided bone regeneration (v-GBR) has demonstrated predictable and effective outcomes of supracrestal bone regeneration in animal experiments and human clinical trials, allowing the correct positioning of implants [6–16].

The purpose of this case report is to report vertical bone regeneration of approximately 10 mm using solvent-dehydrated mineralized cancellous bone allograft and non-resorbable membrane in the rehabilitation of unsuccessful implants in the anterior maxilla and stability of the regenerated bone at 14 years of follow-up.

2. Clinical Report

A 24-year-old healthy female patient with a history of anterior dentoalveolar trauma resulting in loss of the upper left incisors and canine underwent rehabilitation several years ago with three implant-supported fixed prostheses. The prosthesis was both functionally and aesthetically inadequate, and the patient complained of gingival swelling, bleeding, and food impaction at the site of the implants (Figures 1(a) and 1(b)). Standard periapical dental radiographs taken to assess periodontal status of the right central incisor (Figure 1(c)) and left first premolar (Figure 1(d)) adjacent to the implants showed significant bone loss on the mesial aspect of the roots.

Computed tomography scans showed three-dimensional bone loss around implants, which were osseointegrated only in the apical portion. The remaining surfaces of the implants were covered by radiopaque biomaterial particles encapsulated in the soft tissue, and the implant in the region of the central incisor was inside the incisive canal (Figure 2).

Treatment planning involved removal of pre-existing prosthesis and implants, reconstruction of the bony ridge by a v-GBR procedure, and simultaneous insertion of two new implants with a prosthetic driven approach. As vertical ridge augmentation is affected by the interproximal height of the bone adjacent to the defect, the roots of the right central incisor and left first premolar were endodontically treated in order to be submerged under the membrane after decoronation, for utilizing the regenerative potential of their distal interproximal bone.

For all interventions, the patient received preoperative antibiotic and analgesic therapy with amoxicillin 875 mg +clavulanic acid 125 mg (Augmentin, GlaxoSmithKline S.P.A., Verona, Italy) and ibuprofen 600 mg (Brufen, Abbott, Rome, Italy) 1 hour prior to surgery and were repeated twice daily postoperatively.

Surgical procedures were performed after oral sedation with diazepam 0.25 mg/kg (Valium gtt 25 ml/5%, Roche S.P.A., Monza, Italy), administered 30 minutes preoperatively, under local anaesthesia with mepivacaine 2% with adrenalin 1 : 100,000 (Carbocaine, AstraZeneca, Italy).

The first surgical stage was aimed at removing the implants and preparing the bone ridge and soft tissues for augmentation procedure (Figures 3(a) and 3(b)). A full-thickness flap was raised, and the implants, grafting material (hydroxyapatite), and granulation tissue were removed. The

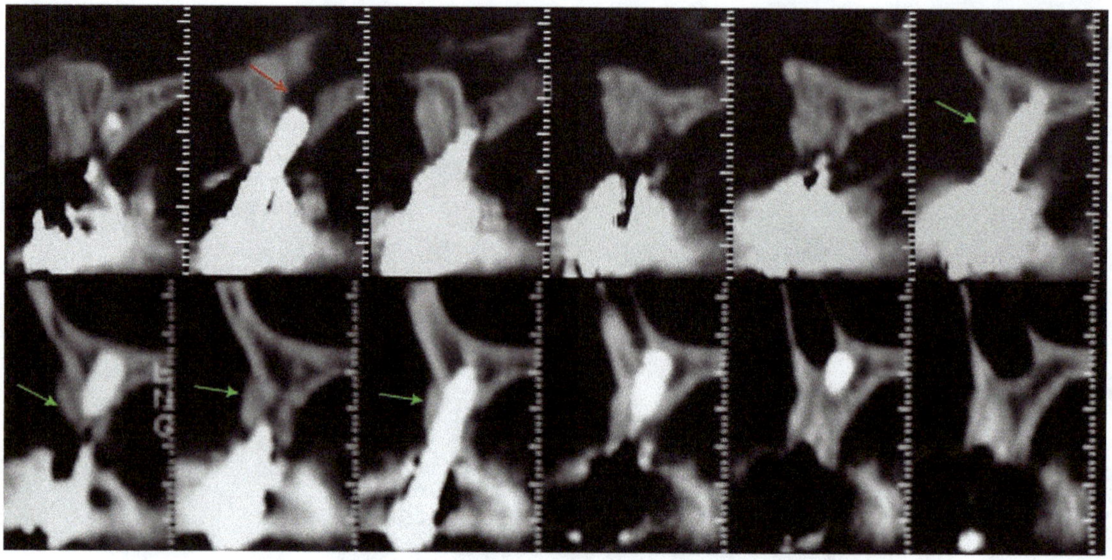

FIGURE 2: Computed tomography scans showed the implant in the region of the central incisor inside the incisive canal (red arrow) and the three-dimensional bone loss around the implants, which were osseointegrated only in the apical portion with the remaining surfaces being covered by radiopaque biomaterial particles encapsulated in the soft tissues (green arrows).

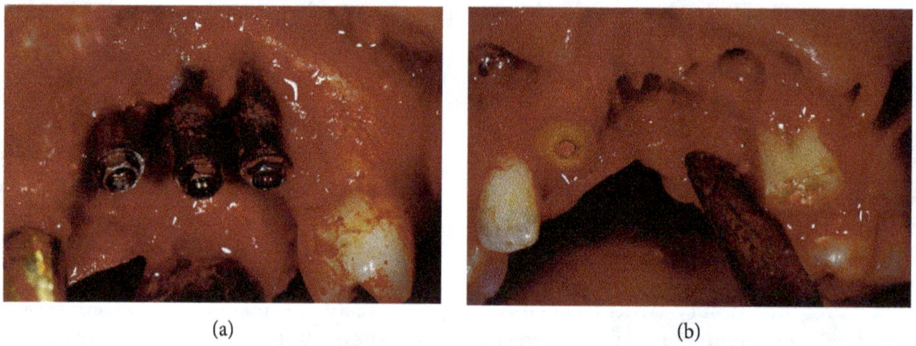

FIGURE 3: The first intervention: (a) clinical view of the implants and grafting material after flap elevation and (b) the bone ridge after removing implants and cutting the crowns of the adjacent teeth.

crowns of the adjacent teeth were cut, and the roots, after scaling and surface debridement, were submerged under the flap, which was coronally repositioned by means of periosteal releasing incisions. To support the aesthetic needs of the patient, a removable partial denture, with metal subframework and rests on posterior teeth, was provided to avoid transmucosal pressure on the surgical area.

After two months of uneventful healing (Figure 4(a)), wax-up of the prosthetic restoration was made on diagnostic/study mounted casts in order to identify the ideal three-dimensional position of the implants. A template was then fabricated to be used in the radiographic diagnosis of the selected implant sites and during surgery as a guide for correct insertion of the implants.

Postoperative computed tomography scans (Figure 4(b)) showed residual bone height of 5 mm and a three-dimensional bone defect of approximately 10 mm at the planned implant sites, corresponding to the radiopaque markers on the template. Spread of some hydroxyapatite granules into the soft tissues was also observed.

Based on clinical and radiographic information, the second intervention was planned for vertical ridge augmentation and simultaneous prosthetic driven placement of two implants at the sites of the left central incisor and canine.

A full-thickness trapezoidal flap (Figure 5(a)) with wide buccal base and palatal pedicle was performed in order to ensure good vascular supply to the grafted area and tension-free complete closure over the augmented ridge. The horizontal incision was performed within the mucosa of the buccal fold and was connected with two divergent vertical incisions, distal to the right canine and left second premolar. The incisions were extended intrasulcularly all around the teeth mesial to the defect. The flap was elevated with great caution to avoid perforations due to the presence of scar tissue from the previous surgery followed by the removal of fibrous tissue. The bony defect, as measured with two crossed-calibrated periodontal probes, extended 10 mm from its most apical portion to a line connecting the cementoenamel junction of the adjacent teeth (Figure 5(b)). Two implants (MKIV 4×15 mm, Branemark System®,

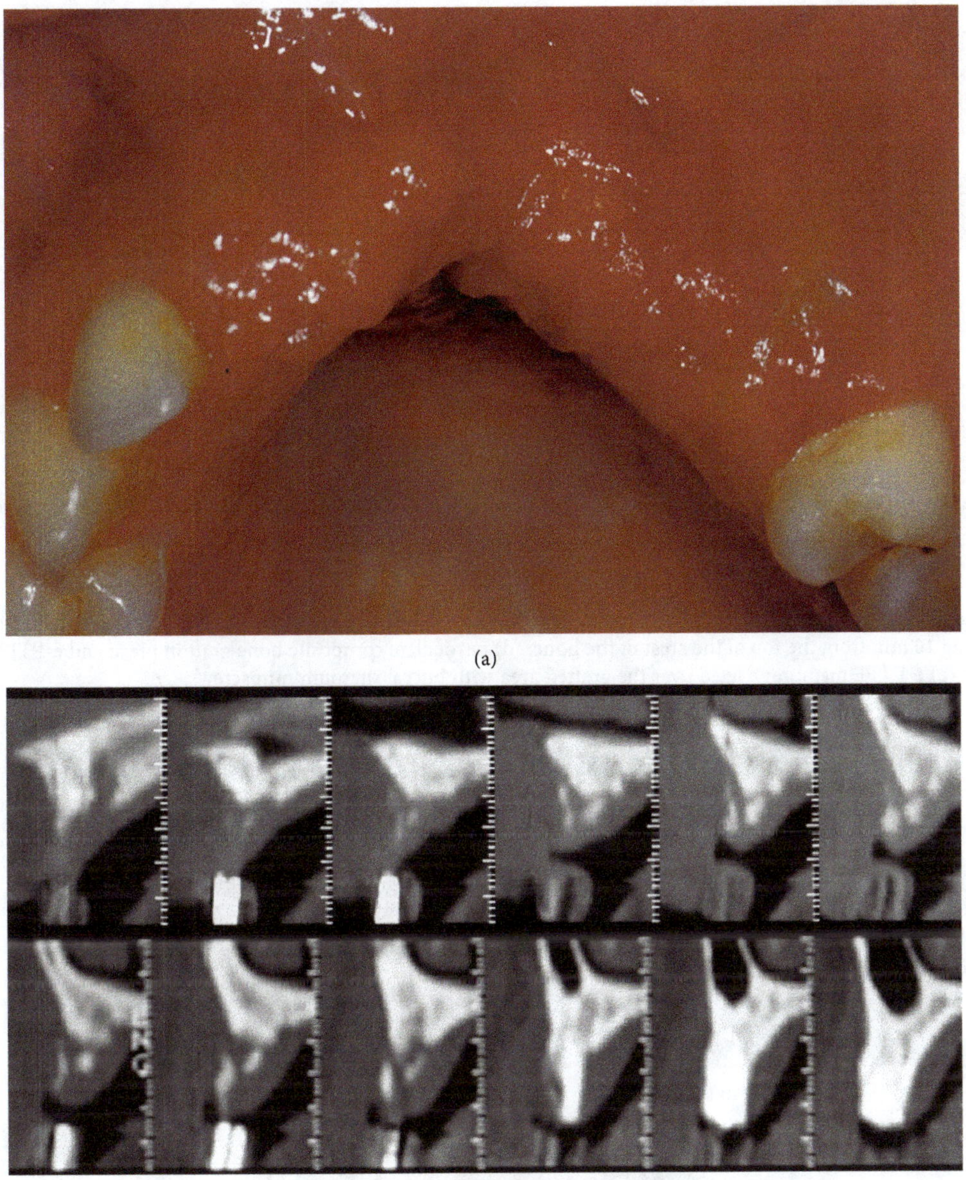

(a)

(b)

FIGURE 4: After two months of uneventful healing: (a) clinical view and (b) computed tomography scans showing the three-dimensional ridge defect and height of the available bone (5 mm) in the implant sites indicated by the template radiopaque markers.

Nobel Biocare), protruding for about 10 mm from the top of the bony crest, were placed in the three dimensionally corrected position using the radiographic/surgical template (Figure 5(c)). A nonresorbable titanium-reinforced e-PTFE membrane (W. L. Gore & Associates, Flagstaff, AZ, USA) was trimmed, adapted to the defect, and fixed on the palatal plate using two titanium miniscrews. Multiple perforations of the cortical bone were made with a small round bur in order to open the medullary spaces and increase bleeding. Following this, exposed implant threads were covered with autogenous bone chips that were harvested using a bone scraper (Safescraper; META, Reggio Emilia, Italy) from the mandibular ramus. The autograft was enhanced with a second layer of solvent-dehydrated mineralized cancellous bone allograft (Puros® allograft, Zimmer Dental) (Figure 5(d)). The membrane was stabilized over the augmented area with two additional buccal titanium self-tapping screws (Figure 5(e)). The flap was then coronally advanced by means of periosteal releasing incisions in the buccal fold and sutured with two lines of closure (GORE-TEX CV-5 Suture, W.L. Gore & Associates), to be removed on the fourteenth day. Horizontal mattress sutures were given on the horizontal incision facing at least 3 mm of the marginal connective tissue, in order to prevent exposure of the membrane. Interrupted sutures were given at a more coronal position on the horizontal and vertical incisions to seal the wound.

At the surgical re-entry after 9 months of uneventful healing (Figure 6(a)), the miniscrews and titanium-reinforced e-PTFE membrane were removed. Complete filling of the bony defect was observed with a hard regenerated

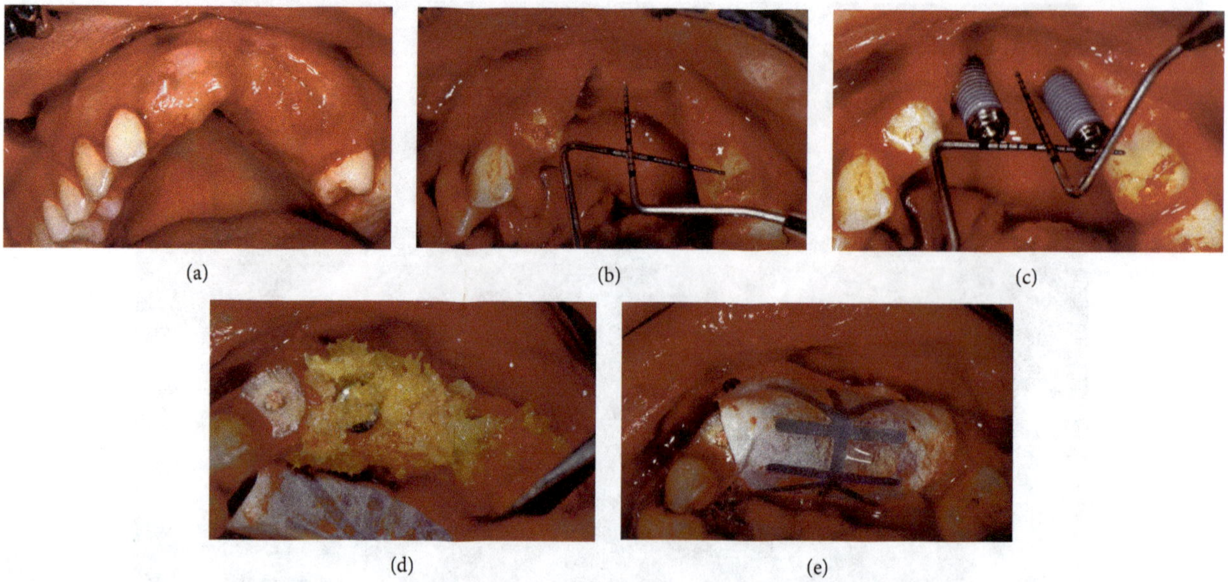

(a) (b) (c) (d) (e)

FIGURE 5: The second intervention: (a) the full-thickness trapezoidal flap, (b) buccal view of the vertical defect in the anterior maxilla, (c) the implants protruding 10 mm from the top of the crest of the bone; (d) particulate composite bone graft in place and e-PTFE membrane fixed on the palate, and (e) e-PTFE membrane fixed over the grafted area with buccal titanium miniscrews.

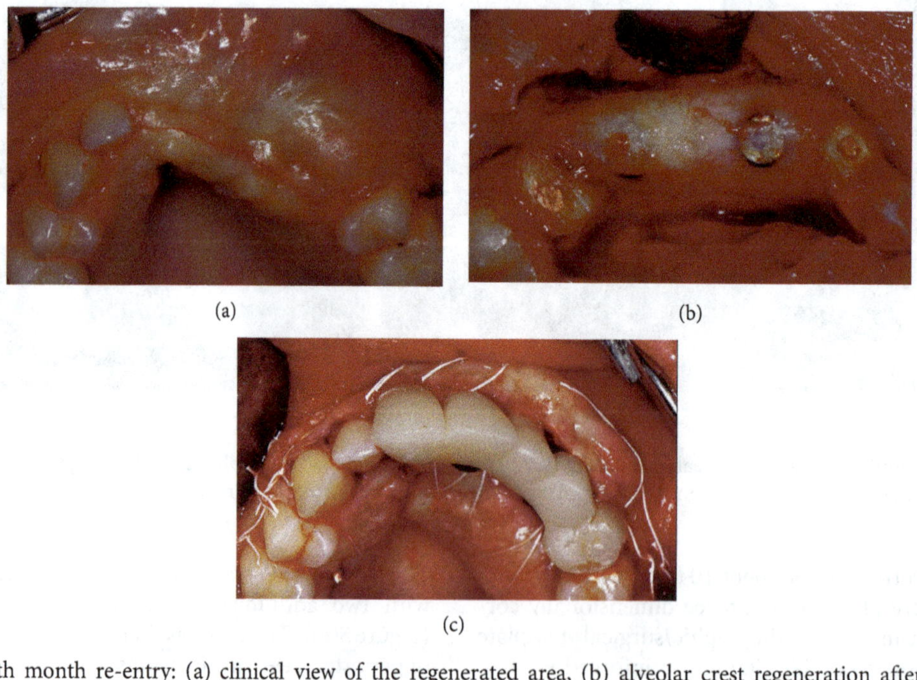

(a) (b) (c)

FIGURE 6: At the 9th month re-entry: (a) clinical view of the regenerated area, (b) alveolar crest regeneration after flap elevation and membrane removal, and (c) flap sutured after free connective tissue graft and first temporary bridges.

tissue clinically similar to bone, covered by a thin layer of firm connective tissue (Figure 6(b)). At the same time, healing abutments were connected to the implants, the right central incisor and left first premolar roots were prepared to receive gold-cast post and cores to support an interim bridge. The flap was apically repositioned to restore the vestibular depth lost during the second surgical stage, and a free connective tissue graft, harvested from the palatal mucosa, was performed to improve the aesthetics of the soft tissues (Figure 6(c)). After 2 weeks, the gold-cast post and cores were cemented inside the roots. A second temporary bridge with two single crowns supported by the teeth was fixed along with a three-unit bridge supported by two implants, to guide morphological maturation of the soft tissue and stamp the ovate pontic.

The definitive cemented prosthetic restoration in porcelain-fused-to-metal was fixed after 6 months with two single

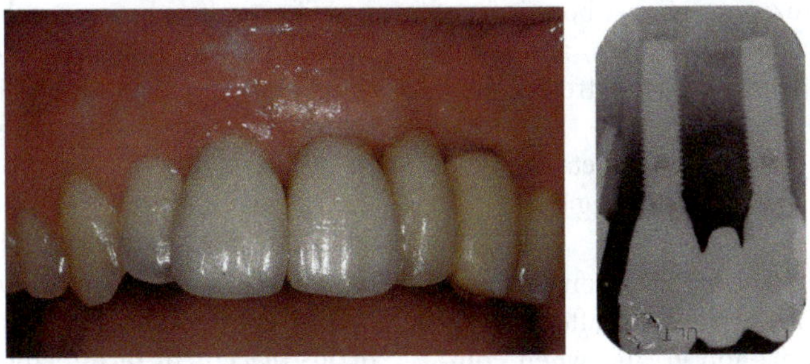

(a) (b)

FIGURE 7: Definitive cemented prosthetic restoration in porcelain-fused-to-metal: (a) clinical view and (b) periapical radiograph.

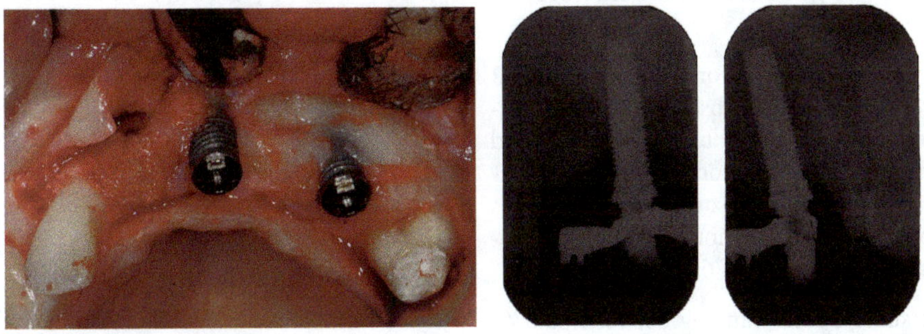

(a) (b) (c)

FIGURE 8: The regenerated bone after 14 years of loading, during surgery to treat the peri-implantitis lesions on the buccal surface of the implants and after extraction of the right central incisor: (a) clinical view, (b) periapical radiograph of mesial implant, and (c) periapical radiograph of distal implant.

crowns supported by the teeth and a three-unit implant-supported bridge (Figures 7(a) and 7(b)).

After 14 years of loading, the stability and quality of the regenerated bone was clinically and radiographically assessed during surgery to remove the right central incisor and treat peri-implantitis on the buccal surface of the implants (Figure 8).

3. Discussion

In the presented case, failure of the pre-existing implants in the anterior maxilla led to a complex clinical situation, which necessitated the removal of the implants. Additional bone and soft tissue augmentation procedures and new implant-prosthetic treatment were also indicated in order to achieve satisfactory aesthetics, function, and long-term stability of the reconstructed peri-implant tissues.

Keeping in mind the challenging site, the anterior maxillary aesthetic zone, anatomic and pathologic factors, such as the pre-existing unsuccessful implant rehabilitation and residual three-dimensional bone defect of approximately 10 mm, and surgical experience and skill of the surgeon, the decision-making process for the treatment planning was based on scientific evidence [2].

Among the different procedures proposed for vertical ridge augmentation (distraction osteogenesis, block graft, and guided bone regeneration), v-GBR with cancellous bone allograft and titanium-reinforced e-PTFE membrane was chosen for treatment in this clinical case [17, 18].

Clinical and histological data reported in the literature in the last decade appear to support the v-GBR procedure as an effective treatment to augment the lost bony structure and thus allow positioning of the implants [9–13].

In a review on augmentation procedures for rehabilitation of deficient edentulous ridges with oral implants, Chiapasco and coworkers reported bone gain of 2-7 mm following v-GBR. The study also reported an overall survival rate of 92% to 100% in implants placed in the augmented sites with nonresorbable barriers, while success rates ranged from 61.5% to 100% [9].

In another systematic review, Aghaloo and Moy reported more detailed documentation and long-term follow-up studies on GBR procedures than other alveolar ridge augmentation techniques. However, they reported that implant survival rates were not significantly different from those in nonaugmentated sites [10].

The results of the systematic review by Rocchietta and coworkers were consistent with those previously reported by Chiapasco and coworkers. The review reported vertical bone gain of 2-8 mm, implant survival rates of 92.1% to 100% over 1-7 years of follow-up, and success rates ranging from 61.5% to 97.5% [11].

In 2014, a systematic review by Milinkovic and Cordaro aimed at establishing the clinical indications for various bone augmentation procedures based on type and dimensions of the defect. The review reported an average linear bone gain of 3.04 mm, mean implant survival rate of 98.9%, and mean complication rate of 13.1% for vertical defects treated with simultaneous GBR [13].

In a more recent systematic review and meta-analysis, Urban and coworkers [12] reported the following data:

(i) The weighted mean clinical vertical bone gain of 4.18 mm after GBR was lower than that after distraction osteogenesis (8.4 mm) and greater when compared to bone blocks (3.46 mm). The main findings of the meta-analysis, based on the changes in baseline and final values, showed that in v-GBR technique, clinical bone gain was influenced by the type of particulate grafting material and nonresorbable membrane

(ii) The incidence of complications following GBR (12.1%) was lower than that observed after distraction osteogenesis and bone blocks (47.3% and 23.9%, respectively). Furthermore, in line with previous systematic reviews, resorbable membranes were more prone to complications than nonresorbable membranes (22.7% versus 6.9%)

(iii) The implant success rates ranging between 85.33% and 100% and the aggregated mean implant survival rate (98.95%, range: 90.5-100%) were comparable to previous studies that reported on implants placed in pristine sites

(iv) To obtain adequate vertical bone gain in large defects, e-PTFE membranes have proven effective in preventing migration of epithelial cells and fibroblasts, in maintaining space, and in stabilizing graft materials [19]

Although autogenous bone is considered the "gold standard," many bone substitutes have been used in augmentation procedures to decrease the extent of surgical invasion and postoperative discomfort. The efficacy of the bone allograft used in the present case in promoting bone formation has been reported in many studies and in different augmentation procedures [6, 7, 20–26]. Indeed, the processing of solvent-dehydrated mineralized cancellous bone, which preserves the natural collagen matrix, trabecular pattern, and porosity of human cancellous bone, would have better osteoconductive potential compared to freeze-dried bone allografts [19, 22]. Furthermore, the presence of calcium and phosphate would result in less reabsorption than demineralized bone allografts, thus maintaining the space for a longer period [23].

The rationale behind the combination of bone allograft and autologous bone chips was to associate the osteoconductive properties of mineralized cancellous allograft with osteogenic and osteoinductive properties of the autogenous bone. Bone allograft acts as a scaffold for space creation and maintenance and autologous bone initiates the regenerative process, releasing osteoblasts and growth factors [27]. Furthermore, the use of a bone scraper for harvesting bone chips minimizes donor site morbidity and shortens the collection time.

The two-stage approach, with removal of the existing prosthesis and implants prior to the augmentation procedure, was necessary to eradicate the infection and enhance the quality and quantity of soft tissues at the recipient site. In addition, tension-free complete soft tissue closure over the augmented area could be obtained, which is crucial for success of the procedure [28]. Furthermore, although studies have reported more bone gain with delayed implant placement after the GBR procedure, in the present case, simultaneous placement of implants insertion was chosen to avoid an additional surgical intervention.

Lastly, despite the increased risk of peri-implantitis in augmented sites compared with pristine sites, the peri-implantitis lesion in this case developed at the 14th year of follow-up [29]. This may be attributed to low compliance with the maintenance protocol and not to the augmentation technique or graft material used [28].

4. Conclusions

In the present case, the therapeutic approach to the severe anterior maxillary defect, based on v-GBR and mineralized cancellous bone allograft, resulted in satisfactory aesthetic and functional prosthetic rehabilitation. In addition, the clinical assessment at 14 years of follow-up showed the three-dimensional stability of the regenerated bone, despite the loss of the adjacent right central incisor and the onset of peri-implantitis.

The positive outcomes were closely related to the awareness of ridge anatomy, soft and hard tissue deficiencies, preoperative prosthetic planning, three-dimensional correct positioning of implants with a prosthetic driven approach, strict v-GBR surgical protocol, careful handling of soft tissues, and appropriate provisional and definitive prosthetic rehabilitation.

No ethical committee approval was sought to start this clinical report study since this was not required by national legislation or any ordinance of the local inspection authority.

References

[1] S. Annibali, I. Bignozzi, G. La Monaca, and M. P. Cristalli, "Usefulness of the aesthetic result as a success criterion for implant therapy: a review," *Clinical Implant Dentistry and Related Research*, vol. 14, no. 1, pp. 3–40, 2012.

[2] D. Buser, W. Martin, and U. C. Belser, "Optimizing esthetics for implant restorations in the anterior maxilla: anatomic and surgical considerations," *The International Journal of Oral & Maxillofacial Implants*, vol. 19, pp. 43–61, 2004.

[3] B. Leblebicioglu, S. Rawal, and A. Mariotti, "A review of the functional and esthetic requirements for dental implants," *The Journal of the American Dental Association*, vol. 138, no. 3, pp. 321–329, 2007.

[4] F. Higginbottom, U. Belser, J. D. Jones, and S. E. Keith, "Prosthetic management of implants in the esthetic zone," *The International Journal of Oral & Maxillofacial Implants*, vol. 19, pp. 62–72, 2004.

[5] S. Annibali, G. La Monaca, M. Tantardini, and M. P. Cristalli, "The role of the template in prosthetically guided implantology," *Journal of Prosthodontics*, vol. 18, no. 2, pp. 177–183, 2009.

[6] B. Le, M. D. Rohrer, and H. S. Prasad, "Screw "tent-pole" grafting technique for reconstruction of large vertical alveolar ridge defects using human mineralized allograft for implant site preparation," *Journal of Oral and Maxillofacial Surgery*, vol. 68, no. 2, pp. 428–435, 2010.

[7] M. Simion, S. A. Jovanovic, C. Tinti, and S. P. Benfenati, "Long-term evaluation of osseointegrated implants inserted at the time or after vertical ridge augmentation. A retrospective study on 123 implants with 1-5 year follow-up," *Clinical Oral Implants Research*, vol. 12, no. 1, pp. 35–45, 2001.

[8] C. H. F. Hammerle and R. E. Jung, "Bone augmentation by means of barrier membranes," *Periodontol 2000*, vol. 33, no. 1, pp. 36–53, 2003.

[9] M. Chiapasco, M. Zaniboni, and M. Boisco, "Augmentation procedures for the rehabilitation of deficient edentulous ridges with oral implants," *Clinical Oral Implants Research*, vol. 17, no. S2, pp. 136–159, 2006.

[10] T. L. Aghaloo and P. K. Moy, "Which hard tissue augmentation techniques are the most successful in furnishing bony support for implant placement?," *The International Journal of Oral & Maxillofacial Implants*, vol. 22, pp. 49–70, 2007.

[11] I. Rocchietta, F. Fontana, and M. Simion, "Clinical outcomes of vertical bone augmentation to enable dental implant placement: a systematic review," *Journal of Clinical Periodontology*, vol. 35, Supplement 8, pp. 203–215, 2008.

[12] I. A. Urban, E. Montero, A. Monje, and I. Sanz-Sánchez, "Effectiveness of vertical ridge augmentation interventions: a systematic review and meta-analysis," *Journal of Clinical Periodontology*, vol. 46, pp. 277–286, 2019.

[13] I. Milinkovic and L. Cordaro, "Are there specific indications for the different alveolar bone augmentation procedures for implant placement? A systematic review," *International Journal of Oral and Maxillofacial Surgery*, vol. 43, no. 5, pp. 606–625, 2014.

[14] M. Esposito, M. G. Grusovin, P. Felice, G. Karatzopoulos, H. V. Worthington, and P. Coulthard, "The efficacy of horizontal and vertical bone augmentation procedures for dental implants—a Cochrane systematic review," *European Journal of Oral Implantology*, vol. 2, no. 3, pp. 167–184, 2009.

[15] I. A. Urban, A. Monje, and H. L. Wang, "Vertical ridge augmentation and soft tissue reconstruction of the anterior atrophic maxillae: a case series," *The International Journal of Periodontics & Restorative Dentistry*, vol. 35, no. 5, pp. 613–623, 2015.

[16] S. Annibali, I. Bignozzi, G. Sammartino, G. La Monaca, and M. P. Cristalli, "Horizontal and vertical ridge augmentation in localized alveolar deficient sites: a retrospective case series," *Implant Dentistry*, vol. 21, no. 3, pp. 175–185, 2012.

[17] C. Tinti and S. Parma-Benfenati, "Vertical ridge augmentation: surgical protocol and retrospective evaluation of 48 consecutively inserted implants," *The International Journal of Periodontics & Restorative Dentistry*, vol. 18, no. 5, pp. 434–443, 1998.

[18] M. Simion, S. A. Jovanovic, P. Trisi, A. Scarano, and A. Piattelli, "Vertical ridge augmentation around dental implants using a membrane technique and autogenous bone or allografts in humans," *The International Journal of Periodontics & Restorative Dentistry*, vol. 18, no. 1, pp. 8–23, 1998.

[19] A. Khojasteh, S. Soheilifar, H. Mohajerani, and H. Nowzari, "The effectiveness of barrier membranes on bone regeneration in localized bony defects: a systematic review," *The International Journal of Oral & Maxillofacial Implants*, vol. 28, no. 4, pp. 1076–1089, 2013.

[20] H. L. Wang and Y. P. Tsao, "Histologic evaluation of socket augmentation with mineralized human allograft," *The International Journal of Periodontics & Restorative Dentistry*, vol. 28, no. 3, pp. 231–237, 2008.

[21] S. J. Froum, S. S. Wallace, N. Elian, S. C. Cho, and D. P. Tarnow, "Comparison of mineralized cancellous bone allograft (Puros) and anorganic bovine bone matrix (Bio-Oss) for sinus augmentation: histomorphometry at 26 to 32 weeks after grafting," *International Journal of Periodontics & Restorative Dentistry*, vol. 26, no. 6, pp. 543–551, 2006.

[22] E. S. Browning, B. L. Mealey, and J. T. Mellonig, "Evaluation of a mineralized cancellous bone allograft for the treatment of periodontal osseous defects: 6-month surgical reentry," *The International Journal of Periodontics & Restorative Dentistry*, vol. 29, no. 1, pp. 41–47, 2009.

[23] M. S. Block, I. Finger, and R. Lytle, "Human mineralized bone in extraction sites before implant placement: preliminary results," *The Journal of the American Dental Association*, vol. 133, no. 12, pp. 1631–1638, 2002.

[24] S. Annibali, G. Iezzi, G. L. Sfasciotti et al., "Histological and histomorphometric human results of HA-beta-TCP 30/70 compared to three different biomaterials in maxillary sinus augmentation at 6 months: a preliminary report," *BioMed Research International*, vol. 2015, Article ID 156850, 7 pages, 2015.

[25] S. Annibali, M. P. Cristalli, G. La Monaca et al., "Human maxillary sinuses augmented with mineralized, solvent-dehydrated bone allograft: a longitudinal case series," *Implant Dentistry*, vol. 20, no. 6, pp. 445–454, 2011.

[26] G. La Monaca, G. Iezzi, M. P. Cristalli, N. Pranno, G. L. Sfasciotti, and I. Vozza, "Comparative histological and histomorphometric results of six biomaterials used in two-stage maxillary sinus augmentation model after 6-month healing," *BioMed Research International*, vol. 2018, Article ID 9430989, 11 pages, 2018.

[27] S. S. Jensen, D. D. Bosshardt, R. Gruber, and D. Buser, "Long-term stability of contour augmentation in the esthetic zone: histologic and histomorphometric evaluation of 12 human biopsies 14 to 80 months after augmentation," *Journal of Periodontology*, vol. 85, no. 11, pp. 1549–1556, 2014.

[28] I. A. Urban, A. Monje, M. Nevins, M. L. Nevins, J. L. Lozada, and H. L. Wang, "Surgical management of significant maxillary anterior vertical ridge defects," *The International Journal of Periodontics & Restorative Dentistry*, vol. 36, no. 3, pp. 329–337, 2016.

[29] G. E. Salvi, A. Monje, and C. Tomasi, "Long-term biological complications of dental implants placed either in pristine or in augmented sites: a systematic review and meta-analysis," *Clinical Oral Implants Research*, vol. 29, no. S16, pp. 294–310, 2018.

16

Successful Management of Ludwig's Angina due to Dental Implant Displacement: A Rare Case Report

Lincoln Lara Cardoso,[1] Giovanni Gasperini ,[1] Leandro Carvalho Cardoso,[1] Guilherme Romano Scartezini,[1] Annika Ingrid Maria Soderberg Campos,[2] and Heloisa Fonseca Marão [2]

[1]*Department of Oral and Maxillofacial Surgery, Aparecida de Goiânia Hospital, Goiânia, Goiás, Brazil*
[2]*Department of Implantology, University of Santo Amaro, São Paulo, São Paulo, Brazil*

Correspondence should be addressed to Heloisa Fonseca Marão; heloisafonsecamarao@yahoo.com.br

Academic Editor: Daniel Torres-Lagares

Dental implant surgery is a common procedure in oral and maxillofacial surgery practices. Extensive training, skill, and experience allow this procedure to be performed with an atraumatic approach, but like any surgical technique, it is subject to accidents and complications. This is an unusual clinical case of an accidental displacement of an implant into the submandibular space that progressed to Ludwig's angina, and it has not yet been described in the literature. This case report describes a clinical case of dental implant displaced into the submandibular space after healing cap removal. After seven days, it progressed to Ludwig's angina. The removal was performed through extraoral access in the submandibular area by using hemostatic forceps and radioscopic technique. After implant removal, the clinical case showed a satisfactory repair emphasizing the importance of a meticulous clinical planning to achieve an appropriate treatment plan, which is essential for a favorable prognosis. Therefore, prevention and management of displaced objects requires proper planning and surgical technique.

1. Introduction

Implant-rehabilitation protocols are considered a treatment with good surgical and prosthetic predictability with high success rates [1]. Although dental implant surgery is a simple, predictable, and safe procedure, accidents and complications may occur [2]. The most frequent complications of titanium dental implant treatment are infection, implant rejection, and implant displacement. Displacement of implants into the maxillary sinus is a common complication encountered in oral and maxillofacial surgery, but the implant can also shift into the facial spaces, especially the infratemporal, buccal, sublingual, and submandibular fossae [3–5].

Ludwig's angina was originally described by the German army physician Wilhelm Frederick von Ludwig in 1836. This is a type of soft tissue infection (cellulitis) involving three compartments on the floor of the mouth [6]. The treatment of Ludwig's angina should consist of airway maintenance, adequate antibiotic therapy, and intraoral or extraoral surgical drainage when necessary [7]. Although displacement of objects may occur in the practice of almost all procedures performed in the oral and maxillofacial surgery, there is no report in the literature of dental implant displacement that had led to Ludwig's angina. Thus, the aim of this article is to present a rare case of Ludwig's angina due to displacement of dental implant into the submandibular space. Therefore, early treatment and correct management are recommended because this is a clinical diagnosis with unpredictable progression.

2. Case Report

A 47-year-old man underwent oral surgery in a private dental clinic for dental implant in the posterior region of the mandible. According to the surgeon's and patient's history, the implant (Titamax implants 3.75×11 mm, Neodent,

Curitiba, Paraná, Brazil) was placed at the region of the first lower right molar, but fenestration of the lingual cortical plate required simultaneous bone regeneration by using lyophilized bovine bone grafts (Genox Inorganic, Baumer, SP, Brazil) and collagen membrane (GenDerm, Baumer, SP, Brazil). The implant primary stability was checked with a torque wrench used at a force of 32 N·cm, and the healing cap was placed. There was no postoperative complication during the period of bone repair.

After 120 days, during the healing cap removal, the implant was accidentally displaced into the submandibular space. Although the lingual access was performed through intrasulcular flap in the same session, the implant was not localized. Therefore, the intraoral access was closed and the patient medicated with amoxicillin (500 mg, 08/08 h/07days), nimesulide (100 mg, 12/12 h/03days), and dipyrone sodium (500 mg, 06/06 h). The patient was instructed to undergo a computed tomography (CT) scan of the mandible for reassessment and removal of the implant.

Panoramic radiographic and CT scan examinations showed displacement of the dental implant into the submandibular space and fracture of the mandibular lingual cortical bone adjacent to the region of tooth #36 (Figures 1(a) and 1(b)). The patient was advised to return within 48 hours, but he did it only after seven days complaining of pain, swelling in the face, fever, and difficulty swallowing. After an initial evaluation, the patient was referred urgently to the Buccomaxillofacial Surgery Service of the Aparecida de Goiânia Hospital, Goiânia, Goiás, Brazil (Figures 2(a)–2(c)).

On physical examination, the patient presented consistent swelling in the submental region. In the submandibular and sublingual spaces, there was presence of painful symptomatology on local palpation bilaterally, trismus, mouth opening of approximately 20 mm, dysphonia, pain on cervical palpation, and intraoral purulent drainage, also affecting the floor of the mouth. In view of the clinical symptoms, laboratory tests and hospitalization were requested. Laboratory tests confirmed the infection, and Ludwig's angina was diagnosed.

After lingual flap retraction at the region of implant placement, detachment of the mucoperiosteum was performed for exploration of the area, but the dental implant was not found. Due to the failure of the intraoperative procedure, it was decided to use the surgical arch for radiographic shots in profile. At this time, it was verified that the implant had shifted to the submandibular space (Figure 3(a)). Following the treatment, extraoral access was performed in the submandibular area by using hemostatic forceps and radioscopic technique, thus allowing the dental implant to be clamped and removed (Figure 3(b)).

After removal, a Penrose drain was inserted into the bilateral submandibular region and the patient remained hospitalized for 72-hour follow-up, receiving ceftriaxone (1 g, 12/12 h), clindamycin (600 mg, 06/06 h), dexamethasone (5 mg, 12/12 h), tenoxicam (20 mg, 12/12 h), and sodium dipyrone (2 cc, 06/06 h). The Penrose drain was removed after 48 hours. The patient's postoperative recovery was uneventful, with regression of signs and symptoms, and he was discharged from the hospital with clindamycin (600 mg, 06/06 h for 7 days) prescription. After 7 days, the patient returned for reassessment. Clinical and radiographic examinations were performed, and the patient presented neither signs of infection nor limitation of mouth opening and pain complaints (Figure 4).

3. Discussion

Reports of accidental implant displacement often indicate that this is located in the upper craniofacial structures such as the maxillary sinus, the ethmoid sinus, or the orbital floor [8]. However, an implant displaced into the lower spaces with evolution for Ludwig's angina has not been reported in the literature.

Quality of bone tissue found in the posterior regions of the maxilla and mandible, anatomical variations, inadequate surgical technique, inexperienced surgeon, insufficient planning, bone resorption, improper occlusal forces, and bone deficiencies could all cause implant displacement complications [3, 9].

The submandibular fossa represents a high risk zone during placement of dental implants due to the possibility of fenestration or perforation of the lingual cortical plate. When the submandibular fossa is pronounced, the implants should be angled correctly for proper perforation [10, 11]. According to Kim et al. (2015), a dental implant can be dislodged between the alveolar bone and lingual flap when the mandibular lingual cortical bone is absent, resulting in the risk of it sinking into the lower soft tissue [12].

Thus, CT scan allows characterization of the submandibular fossa anatomy and provides important information to evaluate the posterior mandible region for implant placement [13]. Height and width of the bone, mandibular canal location, and anatomical characteristics of the submandibular fossa will define the implant length and diameter, as well as the preparation angle for implant [14]. In the present case report, the CT scan was not performed to plan the implant preparation, being only used after dental implant displacement into the submandibular space for location and surgical removal of it.

The infection evolution to Ludwig's angina is possibly related to factors such as lingual cortical plate fracture at the region of tooth #36, inadequate use of antibiotic therapy, no return within 48 hours, and patient's poor oral hygiene and insufficient rest.

Complications due to displacement of dental implants into the submandibular region can be avoided with a correct surgical planning through CT scan. Therefore, the placement of implants of inadequate length and diameter and in the wrong three-dimensional position should be avoided. In the present case report, we believe that the main cause for implant displacement was the surgeon's inexperience, resulting in a wrong surgical planning. The implant was placed very lingually (absence of CT), which caused fenestration and fracture of the lingual cortical plate. Consequently, there was no primary stability during the osseointegration period and the implant invaded the submandibular space when the healing cap procedure was performed.

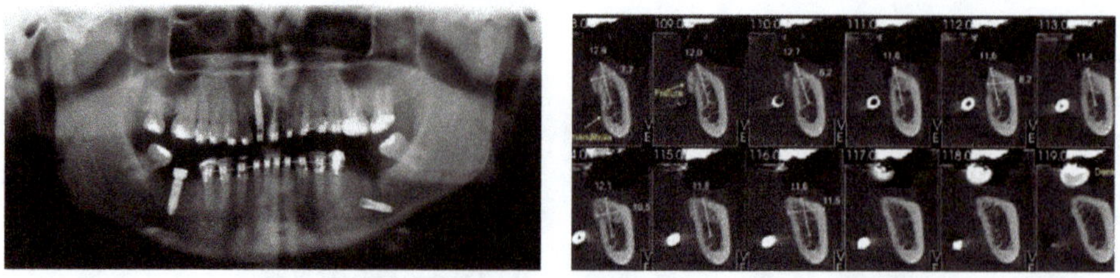

(a) (b)

Figure 1: (a) Panoramic radiographic image. (b) Cone beam computed tomographs in sagittal sections showing displacement of the dental implant and fracture of the mandibular lingual cortical bone adjacent to the region of tooth #36.

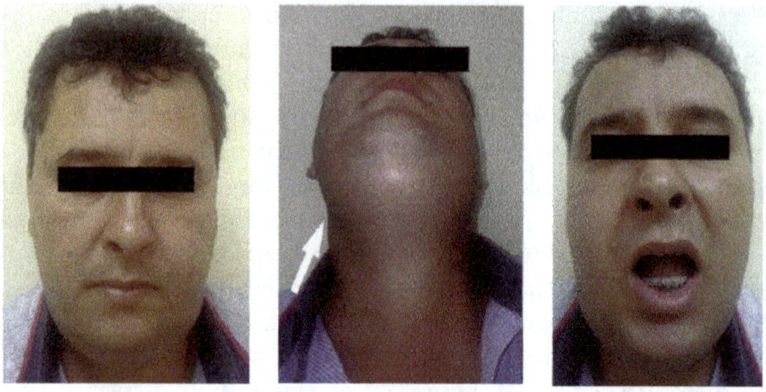

(a) (b) (c)

Figure 2: (a) Clinical aspect of the Ludwig's angina. (b) Arrow shows anterior neck edema. (c) Reduced mouth opening.

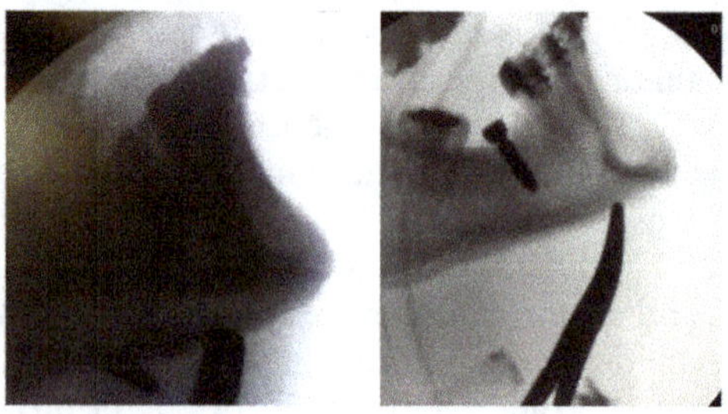

(a) (b)

Figure 3: (a) X-ray profile showing location of the dental implant in the submandibular region. (b) X-ray showing clamping and removal of the dental implant.

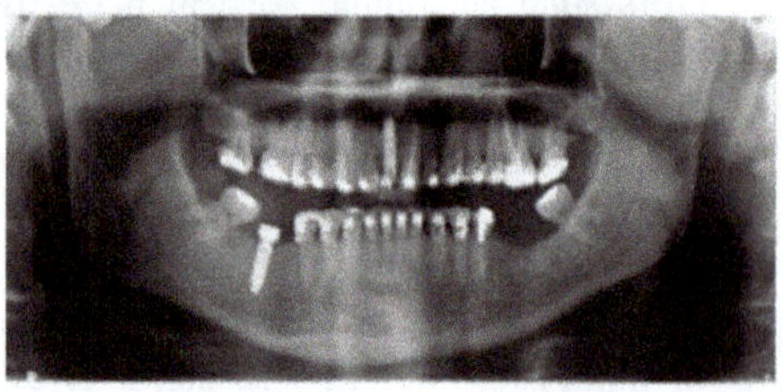

Figure 4: Postoperative panoramic radiograph without other complaints after 7 days.

4. Conclusion

In conclusion, the displacement of dental implants into the submandibular space evolving into Ludwig's angina is a rare complication in implant dentistry. Early intervention to maintain airways preserved, including drainage and removal of the dental implant, is mandatory in the treatment. In this case report, the radioscopic equipment has proved to be efficient for removal of the dental implant.

References

[1] L. Ardekian and T. B. Dodson, "Complications associated with the placement of dental implants," *Oral and Maxillofacial Surgery Clinics of North America*, vol. 15, no. 2, pp. 243–249, 2003.

[2] R. J. Silveira, R. R. Garcia, T. L. Botelho, A. Franco, and R. F. Silva, "Accidental displacement of third molar into the sublingual space: a case report," *Journal of Oral Maxillofacial Research*, vol. 5, no. 3, 2014.

[3] G. Alexander and H. Attia, "Oral maxillofacial surgery displacement complications," *Oral and Maxillofacial Surgery Clinics of North America*, vol. 23, no. 3, pp. 379–386, 2016.

[4] P. Cariati, J. Fernández-Solís, A. B. Marín-Fernández, A. Valencia-Laseca, and F. Monsalve-Iglesias, "Accidental displacement of a dental implant into the sublingual space: a case report," *Journal of Clinical and Experimental Dentistry*, vol. 8, no. 4, 2016.

[5] C. J. Goodacre, G. Bernal, K. Rungcharassaeng, and J. Y. K. Kan, "Clinical complications with implants and implant prostheses," *Journal of Prosthetic Dentistry*, vol. 90, no. 2, pp. 121–132, 2003.

[6] A. Shemesh, A. Yitzhak, J. Ben Itzhak, H. Azizi, and M. Solomonov, "Ludwig angina after first aid treatment: possible etiologies and prevention-case report," *Journal of Endodontics*, vol. 45, no. 1, pp. 79–82, 2019.

[7] S. S. S. Tavares, G. R. Tavares, M. O. A. Cavalcanti, P. F. S. Carreira, J. R. Cavalcanti, and M. A. F. de Paiva, "Ludwig's angina: literature review and a case report," *Revista de cirurgia traumatologia buco-maxilo-facial*, vol. 9, no. 3, pp. 9–14, 2009.

[8] S. Dundar, T. Karlidag, and E. Keles, "Endoscopic removal of a dental implant from maxillary sinus," *Journal of Craniofacial Surgery*, vol. 28, no. 4, pp. 1003-1004, 2017.

[9] M. Chiapasco, G. Felisati, A. Maccari, R. Borloni, F. Gatti, and F. Di Leo, "The management of complications following displacement of oral implants in the paranasal sinuses: a multicenter clinical report and proposed treatment protocols," *International Journal of Oral and Maxillofacial Surgery*, vol. 38, no. 12, pp. 1273–1278, 2009.

[10] C. Angelopoulos, S. L. Thomas, S. Hechler, N. Parissis, and M. Hlavacek, "Comparison between digital panoramic radiography and cone-beam computed tomography for the identification of the mandibular canal as part of presurgical dental implant assessment," *Journal of Oral and Maxillofacial Surgery*, vol. 66, no. 10, pp. 2130–2135, 2008.

[11] H. L. Chan, S. L. Brooks, J. H. Fu, C. Y. Yeh, I. Rudek, and H. L. Wang, "Cross-sectional analysis of the mandibular lingual concavity using cone beam computed tomography," *Clinical Oral Implants Research*, vol. 22, no. 2, pp. 201–206, 2011.

[12] B. H. Kim, B. C. Kim, and J. Lee, "Accidental displacement of a dental implant into the submandibular space during explantation," *British Journal of Oral and Maxillofacial Surgery*, vol. 54, no. 6, pp. 686–688, 2016.

[13] J. Herranz-Aparicio, J. Marques, N. Almendros-Marqués, and C. Gay-Escoda, "Retrospective study of the bone morphology in the posterior mandibular region. Evaluation of the prevalence and the degree of lingual concavity and their possible complications," *Medicina Oral Patolologia Oral y Cirurgía Bucal*, vol. 21, no. 6, pp. e731–e736, 2016.

[14] H. Watanabe, M. Mohammad Abdul, T. Kurabayashi, and H. Aoki, "Mandible size and morphology determined with CT on a premise of dental implant operation," *Surgical and Radiologic Anatomy*, vol. 32, no. 4, pp. 343–349, 2010.

17

Reverse Cast Metallic Core Based on the Original Prosthetic Crown

Eliana de Souza Bastos Mazuquelì Pereira,[1] **Fernando Accetturi**,[2] **Rachel Gomes Eleutério**,[1] **Daniela Vieira Buchaim**,[1,3] **Rogério Leone Buchaim**,[1,4] **and Juliana Trindade Clemente-Napimoga**[5]

[1]*School of Dentistry, University of Marília (UNIMAR), Marília 17525-902, Brazil*
[2]*Private Dental Clinic, Fernando Accetturi Implants and Aesthetic Dentistry, Marília 17525-170, Brazil*
[3]*Medical School, University Center of Adamantina (UniFAI), Adamantina 17800-000, Brazil*
[4]*Bauru School of Dentistry, University of São Paulo (FOB/USP), Bauru 17012-901, Brazil*
[5]*School of Dentistry, São Leopoldo Mandic (SLMANDIC), Campinas 13045-755, Brazil*

Correspondence should be addressed to Eliana de Souza Bastos Mazuqueli Pereira; elianabastosmsn@hotmail.com

Academic Editor: Daniel Torrés-Lagares

The dental crown can be restored using the root in clinical situations where the dental remnant allows adequate anchorage by the use of an intraradicular retainer. After endodontic treatment, reconstruction of the dental anatomy depends on correct planning and the type of restoration to be used. This requires reestablishment of form and function with creation of anchoring features, avoiding detachment and favoring the distribution of forces, thus preventing fracture of the remnant due to functional and parafunctional forces applied on the tooth. This paper reports the clinical case of a patient who sought dental care for a full metal-ceramic crown with a cast metallic core with reduced length that had been detached from tooth 24. After clinical and radiographic examination, root integrity was verified. The patient was offered reconstruction with a cast metallic core of satisfactory length, providing adequate retention and support, with reutilization of the original prosthetic crown, serving as a reverse template of the coronal portion of this new core, providing reduction in costs and operational time.

1. Introduction

Intraradicular posts and cores were originally designed to provide retention and mechanical resistance to the coronal restoration when the remaining dental structure is inadequate [1, 2]. The ability of the core to undergo stress, ease of placement and removal, compatibility with other restorative materials, and the health of supporting tissues are important factors that must be considered when their placement is required [3]. Endodontically treated teeth usually require core restorations for retention due to structural defects resulting from caries and extensive preparation for access, with significant decrease in their resistance due to the reduction of dentin moisture and compromise of strengthening structures such as marginal ridges, enamel bridge, and roof of the pulp chamber [4–6].

The dental restoration should be planned to protect the remaining structure from fractures and replace the lost dental structure and should ideally be done immediately after endodontic treatment [7–9]. The use of intraradicular retainers is indicated for esthetic and functional rehabilitation in endodontically treated teeth that have lost 50% or more of their coronal structure [10–12], requiring the use of prefabricated posts or cast metallic cores. The success of

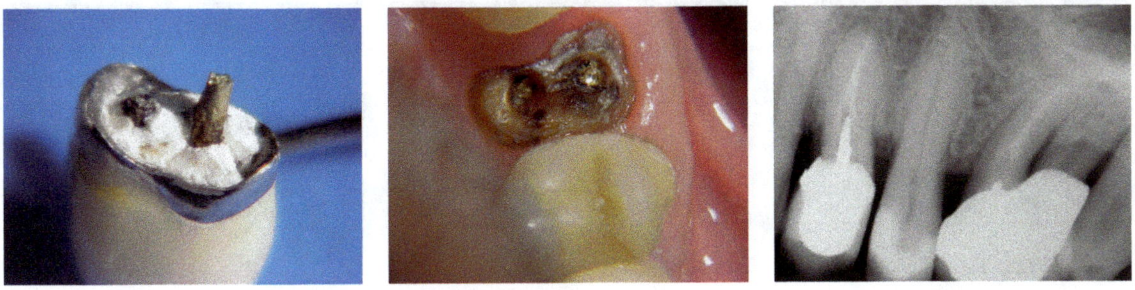

(a) (b) (c)

Figure 1: (a) Initial aspect of the metal-ceramic crown with a fractured cast core; (b) aspect of the fractured dental remnant of the cast core inside the root canal, which was later removed; (c) initial radiography.

reconstruction is more dependent on the remaining dental structure and its implantation than on the choice of the intraradicular retention system.

The clinical decision may be complicated due to factors that contribute to additional weakening of these teeth associated with the compromised root canal. Despite the constant criticism, cast metallic cores have been used for decades, since they are indicated for ordinary cases, where the extent of tooth structure loss is significant and maximum retention is required. They are also very versatile, allow better adaptation to the root canal despite differences in root configurations and angulations, and present satisfactory performance in many long-term clinical studies [13–15].

Ideally, the length of cast metallic cores should be two thirds of the total length of the dental remnant [16, 17], or when the tooth being restored presents bone loss, it must be equivalent to at least half of its bone support. In addition, a minimum amount of 4 mm of obturation material should be left in the apical root portion to ensure adequate sealing of this region [17]. However, this conventional restoration method has biological and mechanical disadvantages, such as excessive tooth structure reduction, retention loss, radical fractures, and high modulus of elasticity, which induce stress concentrations at the root apex [18–21]. Thus, this case report aims at presenting the clinical reuse of an original prosthetic crown serving as a reverse template of the coronal portion of a new cast metallic core.

2. Case Presentation

A 43-year-old male patient attended a dental clinic with the prosthetic crown of tooth 24 in hand, with the remaining fractured root core, part of which was inside the root canal (Figures 1(a) and 1(b)).

Clinical and radiographic examination revealed the absence of a root fracture, which might preclude maintenance of the tooth (Figure 1(c)). It was also observed that the root canal had not been submitted to removal of sealing material up to the adequate length of 2/3 of the dental remnant to the root apex [16, 17]; the cast metallic core was short, which impaired the intraradicular retention.

During clinical examination, it was observed that the dental remnant presented satisfactory conditions for a new rehabilitation with placement of an intraradicular core and a total prosthetic crown. It was proposed to remove the portion of the cast core that was inside the root canal for later accomplishment of a new intraradicular cast core, using the existing metal-ceramic crown as a reverse template for the coronal portion of this future core.

This alternative was possible because there was no need for additional preparation (wear) of the dental remnant at the cervical level, which would impair the adaptation and reuse of the original prosthetic crown. Initially, root canal preparation (buccal and palatal) was performed by instrumentation with Gates Glidden drills at the appropriate length (2/3 of the dental remnant in the largest (palatal root canal), 1/2 of the dental remnant in the other canal (buccal)) [16, 17].

Then, the prosthetic crown was internally ground with carbide drills to allow coronal adaptation of the new cast core. For that purpose, the prepared root canals were previously isolated with petroleum jelly and filled with fluid acrylic resin, supported by prefabricated resin rods (Pincanal®) in each canal. Polymerization of the acrylic resin was properly controlled to avoid adhesion of the resin pin inside the root canal (Figure 2(a)).

For preparation of the coronal portion of the core, the prosthetic crown was fitted on the coronal remnant and was internally isolated with petroleum jelly, filled with acrylic resin, and repositioned on the dental remnant with the core in place, thus serving as a reverse template for reconstruction of the coronal portion of this new core (Figures 2(b)–2(d)).

After completion of polymerization, the finished resin core was sent to the prosthesis laboratory for alloy casting (Figures 2(e) and 2(f)).

This new core was properly adjusted to the remaining root, and the adaptation of the metal-ceramic crown on it was also verified (Figures 3(a)–3(d)).

Finally, both pieces (core and crown) were cemented with definitive zinc phosphate cement (Figures 4(a) and 4(b)), and the occlusal contacts were adjusted (Figure 4(c)).

3. Discussion

In prosthesis and oral rehabilitation, correct reconstruction of the dental anatomy provides greater masticatory effectiveness, being a constant search of dental professionals [22]. Newman et al. stated that the need for placement of an intraradicular core is determined by two factors: the amount of remaining dentin to retain the core and the internal anatomy

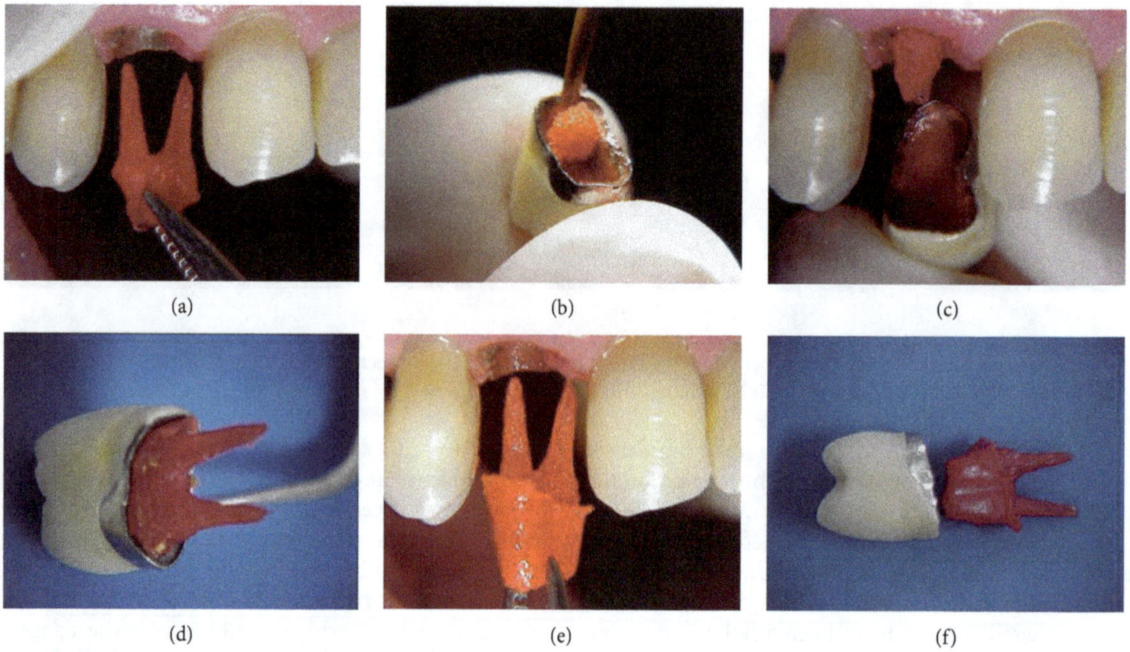

FIGURE 2: (a) Molding of the root canals with acrylic resin to make a new cast metallic core; (b) initiation of filling of the inner portion of the metal-ceramic crown with acrylic resin; (c) filling of the inner portion of the metal-ceramic crown with acrylic resin and placement on the coronal remnant of the core molded in resin; (d) fitting of the prosthetic crown on the dental remnant after placement of resin in the inner portion of the crown; (e, f) finished acrylic resin core.

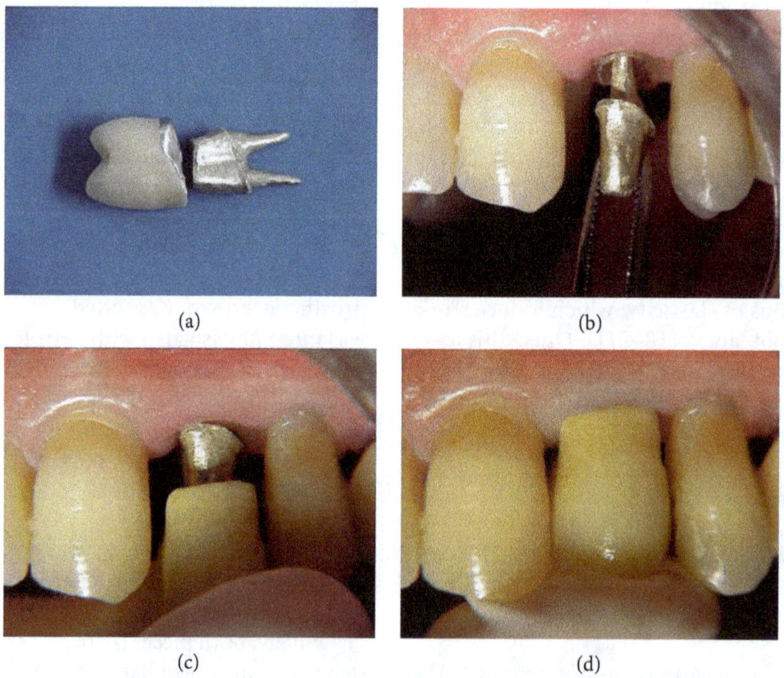

FIGURE 3: (a) Finished new cast metallic core; (b) fitting and adaptation of the cast metallic core on the dental remnant; (c) verification of adaptation of the original prosthetic crown on the new cast metallic core; (d) verification of adaptation of the original prosthetic crown on the new cast metallic core.

of the root; therefore, the professional should have the necessary knowledge to decide the best option to restore an endodontically treated tooth [23]. In this clinical case report, an alternative of reusing a metal-ceramic crown was demonstrated by performing an intraradicular reverse-cast core. This is clinically feasible when the dental remnant supports the masticatory forces applied on the tooth.

With the variety of options available to restore a tooth with great coronal destruction, it is increasingly necessary to know the main intraradicular retainer systems, so they

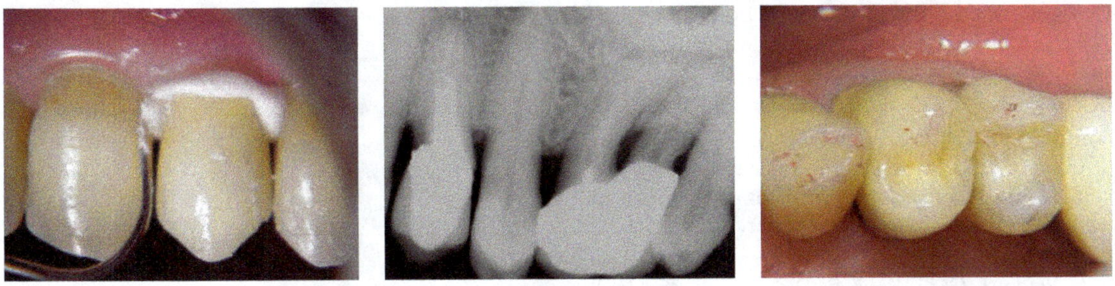

(a) (b) (c)

FIGURE 4: (a) Definitive cementation of prosthetic parts (core and crown); (b) final radiography; (c) verification and adjustments of occlusal contacts.

can be adequately indicated for each specific clinical situation. It is known that the cast metallic cores and titanium posts exhibit high modulus of elasticity and high flexural strength, which allow the core to withstand large amounts of stress before it flexes and transmits the load to the root of the restored tooth, providing great resistance to this core system [23]. The cast metallic cores, together with prefabricated metallic posts, represent a good prosthetic option when the teeth to be restored are weakened for any reason (wide root canals, lack of remnants); however, the protocol for fabrication and placement of these intraradicular cores must be respected to allow treatment predictability [24].

Removal of intraradicular cores is a safe procedure and should be indicated in most situations rather than endodontic surgery or dental extraction. When the need for removal and exchange of a cast intraradicular core is required, utilization of the prosthetic crown as a template for the resin coronal portion of the new core is a viable, less expensive, and more convenient option for dental reconstruction, taking advantage of the same definitive original crown for final restoration [25, 26].

As shown in this case report, the correct observation of criteria for its indication allows utilization of the prosthetic crown previously placed in the oral cavity. Reverse casting of the intraradicular metallic core leads to resolution in shorter clinical time with reduction in the number of sessions in which the patient should be treated, in addition to a lower operating cost.

Acknowledgments

The authors thank Gisele da Silva Dalben, expert in scientific English, for manuscript editing.

References

[1] B. Akkayan, "An in vitro study evaluating the effect of ferrule length on fracture resistance of endodontically treated teeth restored with fiber-reinforced and zirconia dowel systems," *The Journal of Prosthetic Dentistry*, vol. 92, no. 2, pp. 155–162, 2004.

[2] M. Schmitter, P. Rammelsberg, O. Gabbert, and B. Ohlmann, "Influence of clinical baseline findings on the survival of 2 post systems: a randomized clinical trial," *The International Journal of Prosthodontics*, vol. 20, no. 2, pp. 173–178, 2007.

[3] P. C. F. Santos-Filho, C. Veríssimo, L. H. A. Raposo, P. Y. Noritomi, MecEng, and L. R. Marcondes Martins, "Influence of ferrule, post system, and length on stress distribution of weakened root-filled teeth," *Journal of Endodontics*, vol. 40, no. 11, pp. 1874–1878, 2014.

[4] G. Heydecke and M. C. Peters, "The restoration of endodontically treated, single-rooted teeth with cast or direct posts and cores: a systematic review," *The Journal of Prosthetic Dentistry*, vol. 87, no. 4, pp. 380–386, 2002.

[5] R. Sarkis-Onofre, T. Pereira-Cenci, N. J. Opdam, and F. F. Demarco, "Preference for using posts to restore endodontically treated teeth: findings from a survey with dentists," *Brazilian Oral Research*, vol. 29, no. 1, pp. 1–6, 2015.

[6] A. C. L. Faria, R. C. S. Rodrigues, R. P. de Almeida Antunes, M. G. C. de Mattos, and R. F. Ribeiro, "Endodontically treated teeth: characteristics and considerations to restore them," *Journal of Prosthodontic Research*, vol. 55, no. 2, pp. 69–74, 2011.

[7] W. A. Fokkinga, C. M. Kreulen, E. M. Bronkhorst, and N. H. J. Creugers, "Up to 17-year controlled clinical study on post-and-cores and covering crowns," *Journal of Dentistry*, vol. 35, no. 10, pp. 778–786, 2007.

[8] G. E. Salvi, B. E. Siegrist Guldener, T. Amstad, A. Joss, and N. P. Lang, "Clinical evaluation of root filled teeth restored with or without post-and-core systems in a specialist practice setting," *International Endodontic Journal*, vol. 40, no. 3, pp. 209–215, 2007.

[9] R. D. Trushkowsky, "Esthetic and functional consideration in restoring endodontically treated teeth," *Dental Clinics of North America*, vol. 55, no. 2, pp. 403–410, 2011.

[10] C. Varlan, B. Dimitriu, V. Varlan, D. Bodnar, and I. Suciu, "Current opinions concerning the restoration of endodontically treated teeth: basic principles," *Journal of Medicine and Life*, vol. 2, no. 2, pp. 165–172, 2009.

[11] M. Zarow, W. Devoto, and M. Saracinelli, "Reconstruction of endodontically treated posterior teeth - with or without post? Guidelines for the dental practitioner," *The European Journal of Esthetic Dentistry*, vol. 4, no. 4, pp. 312–327, 2009.

[12] F. A. Guiotti, A. M. Guiotti, M. F. Andrade, and M. C. Kuga, "Contemporary vision of anatomic posts," *Archives of Health Investigation*, vol. 3, no. 2, pp. 64–73, 2014.

[13] A. Martinez-Gonzales, V. Amigo-Borras, A. Fons-Font, E. Selva-Otaolaurruchi, and C. Labaig-Rueda, "Response of

three types of cast posts and cores to static loading," *Quintessence International*, vol. 32, no. 7, pp. 552–560, 2001.

[14] D. A. Stewardson, "Non-metal post systems," *Dental Update*, vol. 28, no. 7, pp. 326–332, 334-336, 2001.

[15] L. B. Torcato, E. P. Pellizzer, M. R. Mendonça, M. B. Ferreira, A. P. Amoroso, and R. M. Flacon-Antenucci, "Inner root retention systems: theoretical considerations and biomechanical behavior," *Revista Odontológica de Araçatuba*, vol. 33, no. 1, pp. 9–17, 2012.

[16] M. A. A. Prado, J. C. M. Kohl, R. D. Nogueira, and V. R. Geraldo-Martins, "Retentores intraradiculares: Revisão da Literatura," *Unopar Científica Ciências Biológicas e da Saúde*, vol. 16, no. 1, pp. 51–55, 2014.

[17] M. E. Minguini, M. B. Mantovani, L. F. Lolli, C. O. Silva, P. Progiante, and F. C. Marson, "Estudo clínico de pinos intraradiculares diretos e indiretos na região anterior," *Revista Uningá Review*, vol. 20, no. 1, pp. 15–20, 2014.

[18] P. Bolhuis, A. De Gee, and A. Feilzer, "Influence of fatigue loading on four post-and-core systems in maxillary premolars," *Quintessence International*, vol. 35, no. 8, pp. 657–667, 2004.

[19] N. J. Scholz, M. D. Ribeiro, and J. Giacomini, "Núcleo de fragmento homogêneo em dente com estrutura radicular debilitada," *Jornal Brasileiro de Clinica Odontologica Integrada*, vol. 8, no. 44, pp. 96–100, 2004.

[20] C. M. E. Tait, D. N. J. Ricketts, and A. J. Higgins, "Weakened anterior roots - intraradicular rehabilitation," *British Dental Journal*, vol. 198, no. 10, pp. 609–617, 2005.

[21] P. C. Maccari, D. C. Cosme, H. M. Oshima, L. H. Burnett Jr., and R. S. Shinkai, "Fracture strength of endodontically treated teeth with flared root canals and restored with different post systems," *Journal of Esthetic and Restorative Dentistry*, vol. 19, no. 1, pp. 30–36, 2007.

[22] R. L. Buchaim, J. C. Andreo, A. C. Rodrigues et al., "Multidisciplinary approach in the teaching of dental sculpture and anatomy," *International Journal of Morphology*, vol. 32, no. 2, pp. 399–403, 2014.

[23] M. P. Newman, P. Yaman, J. Dennison, M. Rafter, and E. Billy, "Fracture resistance of endodontically treated teeth restored with composite posts," *The Journal of Prosthetic Dentistry*, vol. 89, no. 4, pp. 360–367, 2003.

[24] A. M. AL-Wahadni, S. Hamdan, M. Al-Omiri, M. M. Hammad, and M. M. Hatamleh, "Fracture resistance of teeth restored with different post systems: in vitro study," *Oral Surgery, Oral Medicine, Oral Pathology, Oral Radiology, and Endodontology*, vol. 106, no. 2, pp. e77–e83, 2008.

[25] G. R. Biacchi, B. Mello, and R. T. Basting, "The endocrown: an alternative approach for restoring extensively damaged molars," *Journal of Esthetic and Restorative Dentistry*, vol. 25, no. 6, pp. 383–390, 2013.

[26] C. Estrela, J. D. Pécora, C. R. A. Estrela et al., "Common operative procedural errors and clinical factors associated with root canal treatment," *Brazilian Dental Journal*, vol. 28, no. 2, pp. 179–190, 2017.

18

Customized Allogeneic Bone Augmentation Improves Esthetic Outcome in Anteromaxillary Dental Implantation

Manfred Nilius,[1,2] Minou Hélène Nilius,[1] Charlotte Mueller,[1] Bernhard Weiland,[2] Dominik Haim,[2] Anna Krahe,[1] and Guenter Lauer[2]

[1]*Niliusklinik, Londoner Bogen 6, D-44269 Dortmund, Germany*
[2]*Department of Oral and Maxillofacial Surgery, University Hospital "Carl Gustav Carus", Technische Universität Dresden, Fetscherstr 74, D-01307 Dresden, Germany*

Correspondence should be addressed to Manfred Nilius; manfrednilius@niliusklinik.de

Academic Editor: Alberto Delbem

Purpose. In cases of severe atrophic maxilla or maxillary involution, augmentation is necessary for implant-supported prosthetics. Using bone grafts is a standard procedure, and using customized allogeneic bone blocks may be a predictable alternative before dental implantation. *Clinical Findings.* This case study shows the digital workflow, including a preimplantological augmentation by a customized allogeneic block, followed by soft tissue optimization and template-based dental implantation, after six months of healing. It is part of a three-year follow-up study on the resorption rate of allogeneic bone blocks. *Outcomes.* Allogeneic bone augmentation is an alternative treatment option to autologous bone grafts. It allows predictable advanced backward planning (ABP) even in the maxillary esthetic zone. Diameter-reduced implants show long-term stability of a minimum of three years after loading and excellent results of prosthetic fixtures. *Conclusion.* Prefabricated customized allogeneic blocks for augmentation may increase the fitting accuracy of the graft, decrease morbidity, and reduce the operation time in esthetic maxillary rehabilitation.

1. Introduction

In the case of maxillary involution, augmentation is necessary for implant-supported prosthetics. Using bone grafts is a standard procedure, and using customized allogeneic bone blocks may be a predictable alternative before dental implantation.

An augmentative procedure for the hard or soft tissue is necessary and represents a critical success factor in implantology in around half of all implantological interventions. To decide which bone substitute material is the most suitable depends on the indication and the individual wishes of the patient and surgeon. Besides autologous bone, the focus is increasingly on allogeneic transplants, which have been used since 2007 [1].

Reduced morbidity and pain potential associated with the transplant removal are particular advantages of using an allogeneic transplant; thus, the process is more pleasant for the patient. Furthermore, we can avoid many complications such as wound healing disorders and uncontrolled resorption using an allogeneic transplant, and allogeneic materials, in contrast to autologous materials, are virtually unlimited [2]. They are similar to autologous bones in terms of requirements and functional profile, and the prerequisites for bone regeneration are met [3–6]. The overall rehabilitation in "backward planning" is based on the bony situation. Thus, the ideal positioning of the subsequent implants is known before augmentation.

2. Case Presentation

A 65-year-old female patient presented for an implantological consultation to replace the existing bridge and replace a missing lateral incisor (tooth 12), which had been in situ

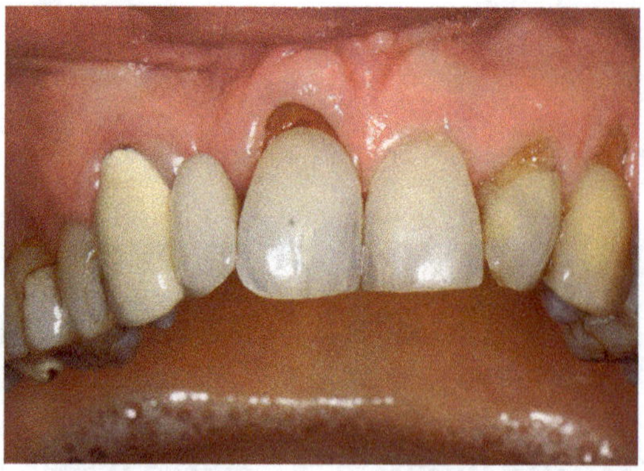

Figure 1: Initial situation with mesial trailer bridge on tooth 13 with missing tooth 12.

for 19 years, with a single-tooth restoration. Tooth 12 was lost due to cystectomy three decades earlier with subsequent bone regression.

3. Clinical Findings

Clinically, there was a mesial trailer bridge on tooth 13 with mesial support on tooth 11. A vestibular soft tissue recession and erosion at the enamel-cement junction were evident on this tooth. In region 12, a vertical and transverse bone deficit was already clinically evident, which was confirmed by the radiological diagnosis (Figures 1 and 2).

The orthopantomogram showed a bone defect in region 12 and moderate horizontal, molar bone loss without vertical fractures. Teeth 35 and 46 are missing, and teeth 34 and 47 had endodontic and prosthetic treatment. Cone-beam computed tomography (CB-CT) showed that the transverse width of the bone in region 12 was 4.5 mm.

4. Diagnostic Assessment

The patient wanted a single-tooth restoration. We recommended advanced backward planning (ABP), including preprosthetic bone and soft tissue augmentation. The alternatives would have been to renew with different material combinations, use removable dentures, or leave the extraction site without prosthetics ("courage to gap").

The concept of "ABP" means that one starts with the desired result and plans the work steps "backward" in a team with the dentist, implantologist, and dental laboratory. We decided for a treatment with a CAD/CAM manufactured allogenic bone block (maxgraft® bonebuilder, botiss biomaterials GmbH) and transferred CB-CT data to botiss biomaterials GmbH to virtually design the shape of a customized bone block to be able to maintain correct implant prosthetic planning, followed by ABP through digital wax-up of the future tooth crown 12. Next, we planned for Straumann implants (BLT Roxolid Ø 3.3 mm and length 12 mm; Narrow CrossFit platform). The ideal implant position and needed block volume was decided by determination of tooth axis and natural bone width for the upcoming implantation using 3D planning tools (Figures 3–8).

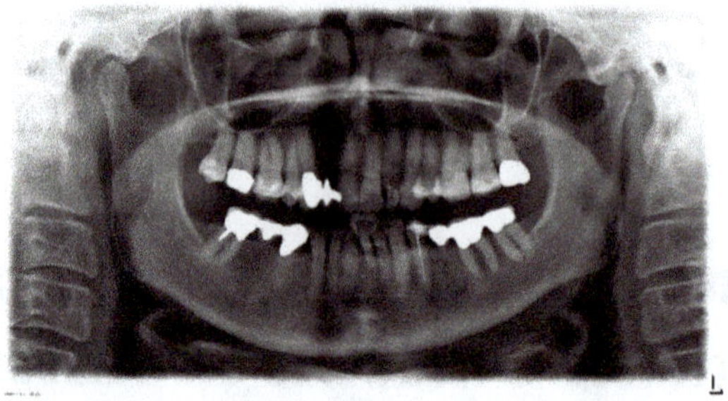

Figure 2: The orthopantomogram (OPT) shows a bone defect in the region of the right lateral incisor.

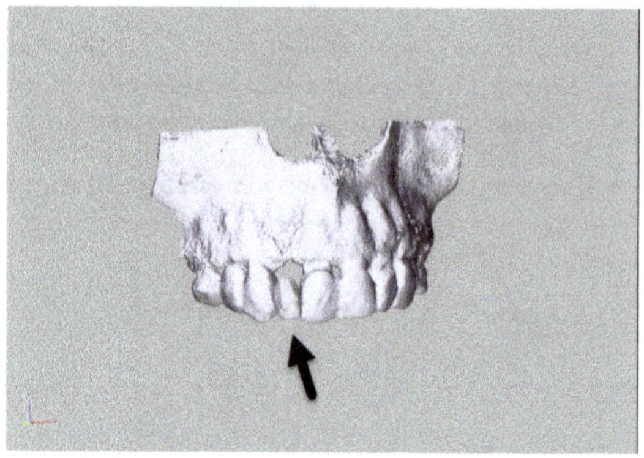

Figure 3: Rendered 3D planning model (STL file) showing a bony deficit in region 12.

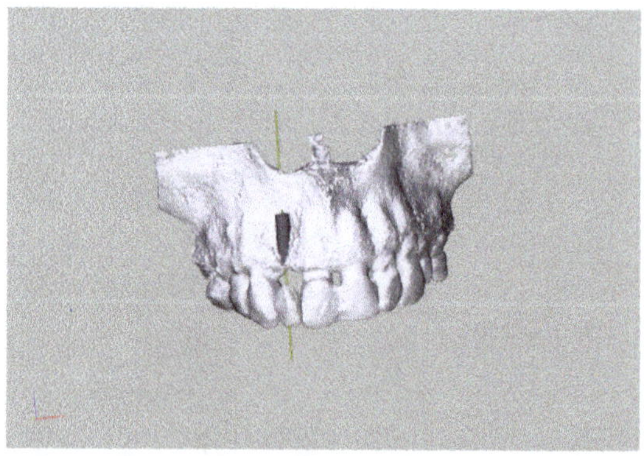

Figure 4: Rendered 3D planning model (STL file) showing a virtual implant in position 12.

Based on CB-CT, botiss used 3D planning software to construct a model of the jaw defect and created the 3D bone block (maxgraft bonebuilder®, botiss biomaterials GmbH). The virtually created bone graft has to be checked by the doctor before the milling process, using a 3D PDF document, and modified if necessary. Once released, the production of the customized block graft begins. Each customized block graft is milled out of a processed freeze-dried cancellous bone block, originating from femoral heads from living donors obtained during arthroplastic surgery (Allotec process, Cells + Tissuebank Austria, Krems an der Donau, Austria). The delivery time is about four weeks.

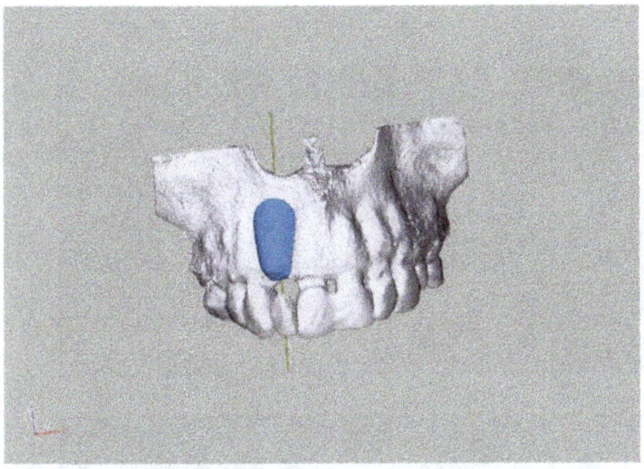

FIGURE 5: Rendered 3D planning model (STL file) with 3D bonebuilder block graft (3D BB) in position 12.

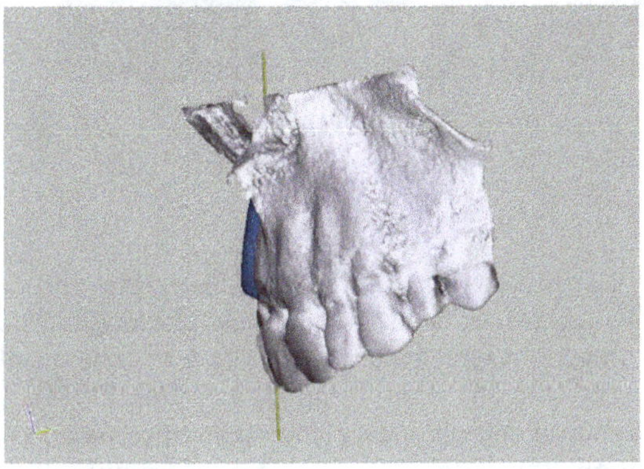

FIGURE 6: Rendered 3D planning model (STL file) with 3D BB in the transversal view.

5. Therapeutic Interventions/Timeline

5.1. Hard Tissue Augmentation (0–6 Months). After removing the bridge on tooth 13, we augmented the bone by approaching through the marginal incision with mesial relief to expose the bone defect. The customized block graft was previously soaked in metronidazole to ventilate. Punctiform drilling to provoke bleeding of the local cancellous bone is necessary after trying this on. We fixed the bone block using two osteosynthesis screws (1.5 × 10 mm). A resorbable porcine pericardium membrane (Jason® membrane, 15 × 20 mm) was used to protect the augmentation (Figure 8).

5.2. Soft Tissue Augmentation (4th Month). Soft tissue optimization is necessary after around four months from bony augmentation; thus, we recommended connective tissue transplantation due to the recession on tooth 11 and the deficit of the attached gingiva in region 12. Donor site incision was made palatally of teeth 23 to 26 (Figures 9 and 10).

We tunneled the recipient gingiva region 11 to 12 without a vertical incision. Next, to accommodate the soft tissue graft, we prepared a supraperiosteal pocket. We stabilized a connective tissue graft transmucosal through a suture (5/0 PTFE, nonabsorbable suture material made of polytetrafluoroethylene, Teflon). Finally, we covered the recession on tooth 11 by the graft and a coronal transposition flap using a double-crossed suture.

On the first day after the operation, the recessions were slightly excessively covered by the graft. However, the soft tissue conditions were stable at the checkup after one month so that stable transplant healing could be assumed.

5.3. Dental Implantation (9th Month). Six months after bone grafting and two months after soft tissue augmentation, dental implantation was performed. After opening the mucous membrane, we removed the osteosynthesis screws. The cancellous bleeding indicated that the bone had healed well.

As planned, we drilled a reduced-diameter bone level tapered implant (Straumann) made of Roxolid Ø 3.3 mm and length 12 mm, with a Narrow CrossFit platform with a maximum torque of 35 Ncm. Finally, we covered the implant region with particulate allogeneic bone substitute material (maxgraft® processed human allograft, botiss biomaterials GmbH) followed by saliva-tight wound closure. After intervention, we checked the dental implant's position using X-ray (Figures 11–13).

5.4. Implant Prosthetic Restoration (10th Month). We made a transgingival impression of the osseointegrated implant with an impression tray using the open impression technique three months after implantation. Then, to accommodate the future crown, we attached an individual abutment made of zirconium dioxide (Straumann CARES CAD/CAM) to the implant (Figures 14 and 15).

We checked the chewing function, phonetics, and aesthetic try-on with correcting the tooth shape, tooth color, and transparency. After completion, we incorporated the tooth crown using dual-curing cement (Figures 16–18) and made a final CB-CT (Figure 19.

6. Discussion

The efficacy of processed allografts is comparable to autogenic/autologous bone transplants [7, 8]. However, processed allografts belong to bone substitutes, so comparing other xenogeneic or synthetical origin substitutes is reasonable [9]. There are a few animal studies of allografts because human-processed bone substitutes in animals are classified as xenogeneic transplant (usually immunological reactions caused by remaining collagen) [10]. Schmitt et al. [11] compared different bone substitutes and reported that there is no significant difference in bone formation rates between allogeneic material (35.4 ± 2.8%) and autogenous bone (42.7% ± 2.1%) in the maxillary sinus lift.

Moreover, the advantage of mineralized allografts compared to the deproteinized xenogeneic bone matrix was reported by Froum et al. [12]. Both variants are superior to a bovine demineralized bone matrix (24.9 ± 5.67%). Furthermore, autogenous bone also showed higher bone formation rates compared with a biphasic synthetic bone substitute (30.3 ± 2.2%).

26–32 weeks after sinus floor elevation, there were apparent differences in bone formation rates between

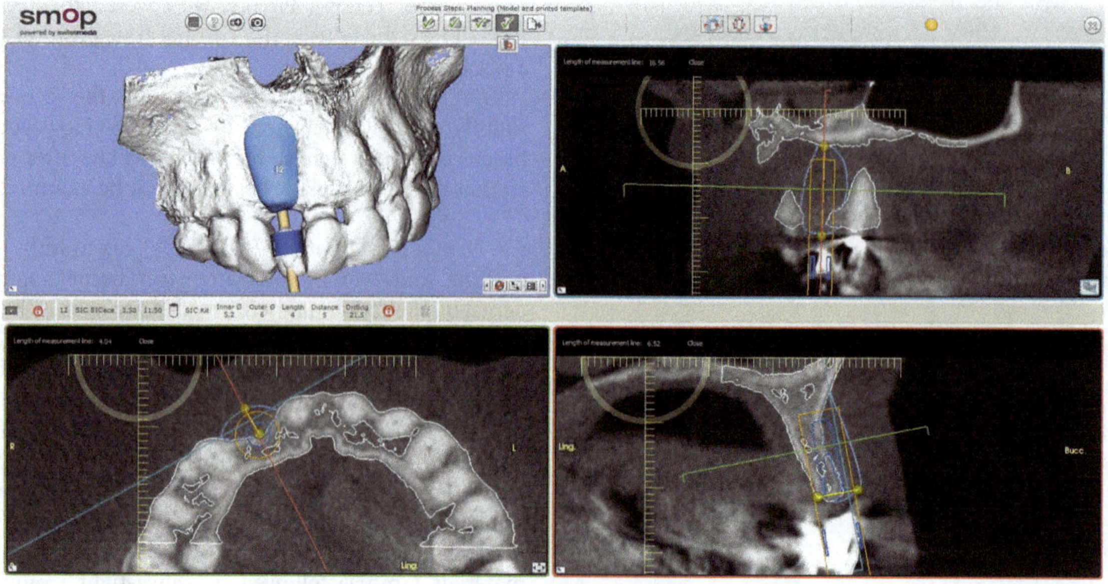

FIGURE 7: A planning tool for implant positioning and producing a SMOP template (Smop, Swissmeda, Baar, Switzerland) for navigated implant placement. Multiplanar view with 3D BB superimposed on the implant position.

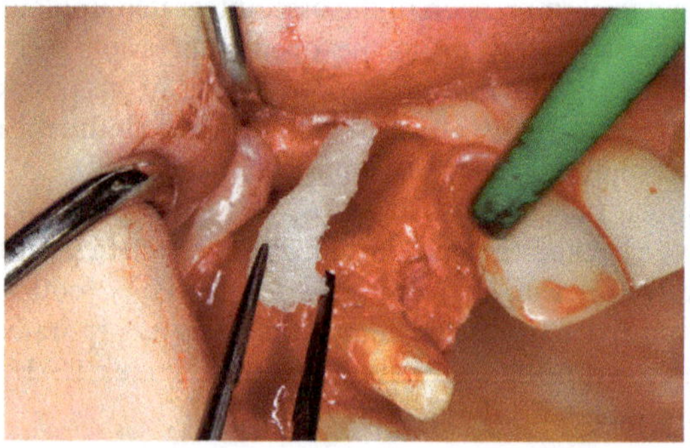

FIGURE 8: Intraoral view after opening the mucoperiosteal flap and inserting the individually CAD/CAM-milled block.

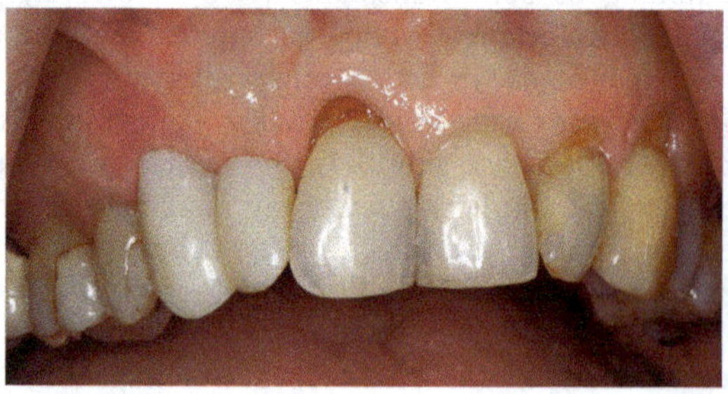

FIGURE 9: Intraoral view with long-term temporary prosthetics (PMMA) bridge 13-12 in situ.

allografts (28.3%) and xenografts (12.4%) [12]. Even the remaining nonvitalized bone substitute was better in allografts (33%) than that in xenografts (7.7%). Laino et al. [13] concluded that allogeneic blocks should be preferable because of the absence of extraction morbidity at the bone graft extraction site and less invasiveness. Their survey for sandwich osteotomy of the lateral lower jaw showed no notable differences between allogeneic blocks (30.6 ± 3.7%) and autogenous chin blocks (31.47 ± 2.2%). The results are consistent with the results from Laino et al. (2014). When comparing allogeneic sandwich osteotomies to onlay augmentation, the latter showed a higher complication rate due to increased soft tissue dehiscences.

When the healing period is uneventful and lasts longer (seven months), one can obtain a two-millimeter higher vertical augmentation using onlay plasty. Other authors confirmed these positive results [14–17].

Tallarico et al. [18] presented a fully digitized approach for the aesthetic zone using a customized 3D-printed titanium mesh. In analogy to 3D BB technology, they designed the scaffold according to the maxillary bone deficit by mirroring the contralateral and unaffected surface via marketed membrane by CB-CT. They used a 50 : 50 mixture of autogenous bone and bone substitute (Bio-Oss, Geistlich Biomaterials Italia, Thiene, Vicenza, Italy). An advantage of this method is simultaneous implant placement during augmentation. Additionally, a narrow-diameter implant helps avoid bone defects on the buccal side. After one year, the prosthetics became stable [18].

Nevertheless, removing the titanium mesh and the screws increases the surgical effort and makes the reapproach worse. A recently published case series with a 3-year follow-up period compared different methods of augmentation before dental implantation, including autologous bone graft (hip graft), 3D BB, and cortical plate [19]. They concluded that the use of allogeneic blocks for maxillary augmentation was comparable with autologous bone grafts. Bone height was stable for a minimum of three years after loading with resorption less than 10% in vertical, buccolingual, and mesiodistal directions. Short or narrow implants allow for the long-term stability of prosthetic fixtures.

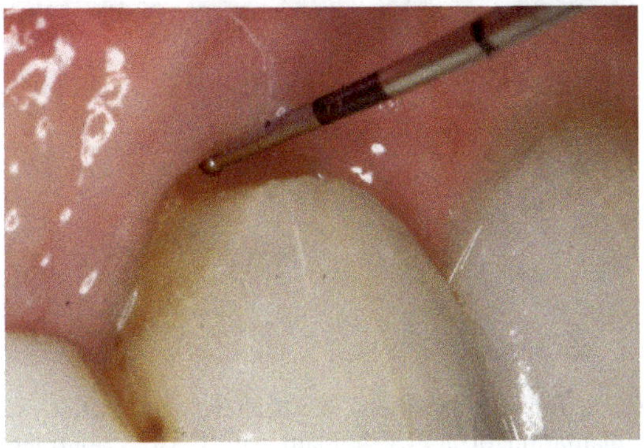

Figure 10: Intraoral view shows cervical recession of 2 mm on tooth 11.

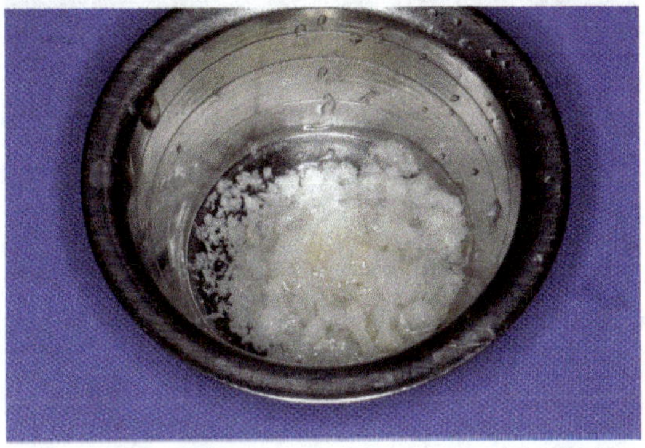

Figure 11: Processed human allograft (Maxgraft®; corticocancellous granules; Cells + Tissuebank Austria, Krems a. d. Donau, Austria).

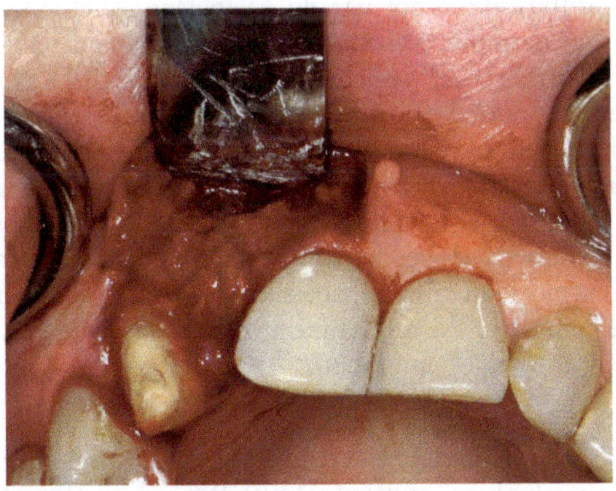

Figure 12: Superimposed processed human allograft covering the dental implant.

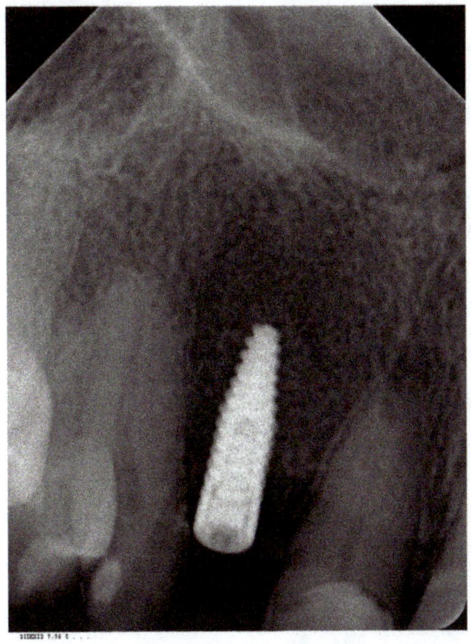

Figure 13: Dental X-ray after dental implantation.

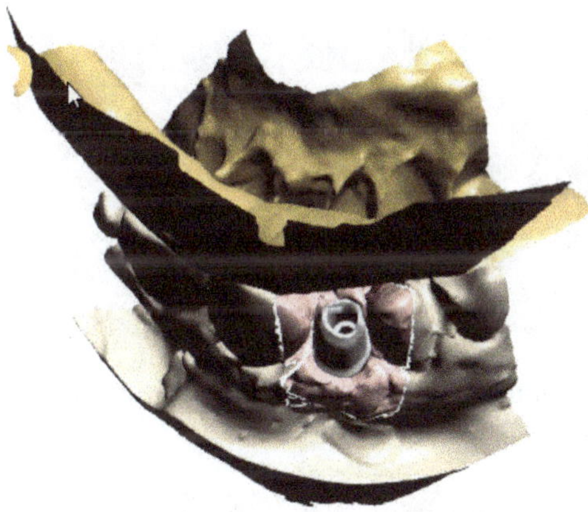

Figure 14: Design of the abutment/crown construction using 3Shape Dental Manager. Plaster model with the stationary scanner D2000 (3Shape, Trios). Antagonistic view.

Furthermore, filling up the scaffold maintenance of the mesh could also be a helpful method since there is no donor site comorbidity.

The risk assessment of mineralized processed allografts follows high standards. Producers must comply with providing security for the patient, including a protocol of the treatment process and the original harvested material. Industrial processing of the material is aimed at eliminating allergenic and infective parts. Different chemical techniques are used by tissue banks, such as peracetic acid-ethanol treatment, thermal disinfection (elimination of potentially contagious agents), lyophilization, osmotic treatment with saline solution, treatment with acetone, and oxygen (elimination of cellular components and fats), and gamma-sterilization to guarantee safe and sterile allografts. Risks (i.e., the transmission of infection and antigenicity) reduce significantly due to the processing and adverse reactions and events related to allografts are monitored worldwide [20, 21]. Fretwurst et al. reported in an in vitro study that there was no similar immunological reaction using allografts but they found isolated cell residues and DNA parts within the matrix structure of different mineralized, decellularized allografts in block shape [22]. However, it lacks the clinical implications of these findings. Apart from considering risks associated with the origin and processing of the tissue, one must also consider surgical as well as patient-related risks based on

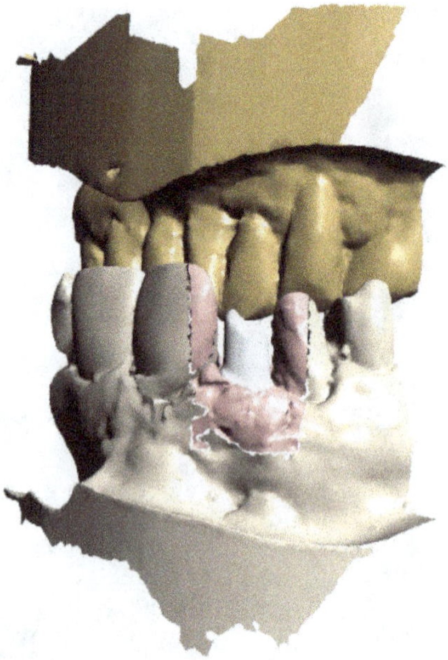

FIGURE 15: Design of the abutment/crown construction using 3Shape Dental Manager. Plaster model with the stationary scanner D2000 (3Shape, Trios). Lateral view.

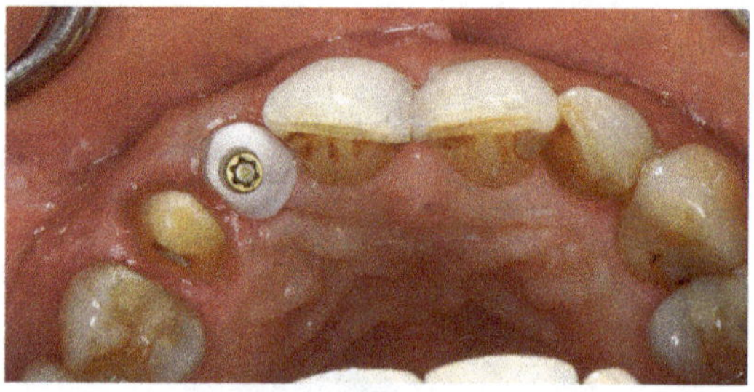

FIGURE 16: Custom-made implant abutment made of zirconium dioxide (Straumann CARES CAD/CAM).

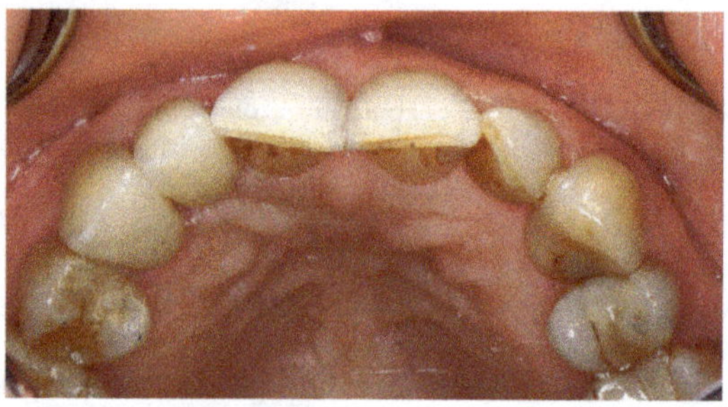

FIGURE 17: Implant prosthetic result after augmentation with 3D BB, implantation of a BLT implant with CARES abutment, and ceramic crown (top supervision).

the surgeons' experience or patients' compliance. Tension-free closure of the wound by "loop" or "pulley" vertical mattress suture is one of the criteria for the success of the treatment protocol and can lower the risk of complication because insufficient soft tissue can lead to opening of the incision line over the grafted bone [2]. We recommend ablating exposed allogenic areas spaciously.

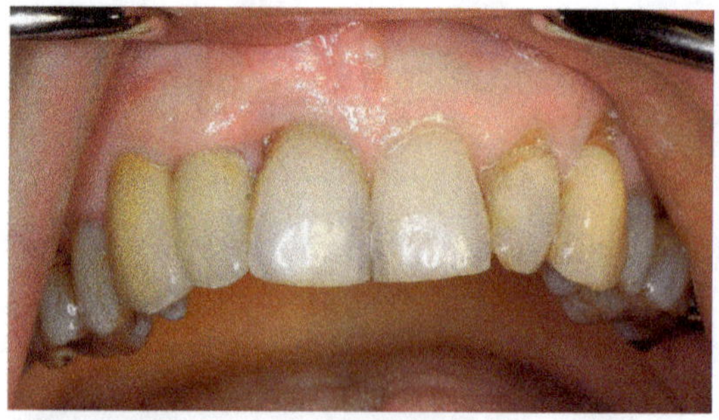

FIGURE 18: Implant prosthetic result after augmentation with 3D BB, implantation of a BLT implant with CARES abutment, and ceramic crown (anterior view).

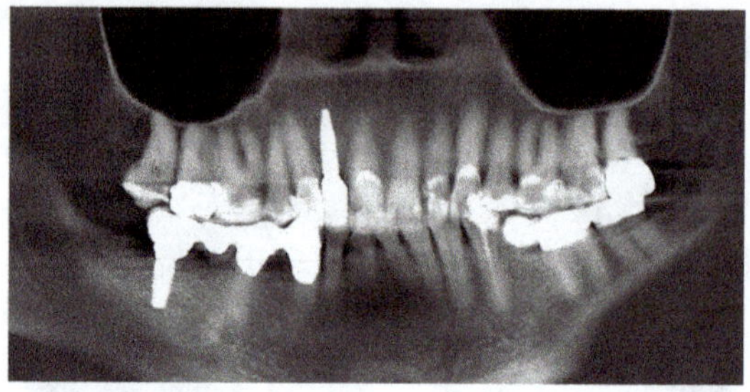

FIGURE 19: CB-CT after completion of the surgical and implant prosthetic rehabilitation.

The trabecular structure of the cancellous allogenic bone allows comparatively fast revascularization [23]. In this case here, reentry was performed after six months and the well-established bone was found, similar to other reports about allogenic bone blocks [6]. Today, nonabsorbable membranes made of 100% dense polytetrafluoroethylene (PTFE) are available. Furthermore, we recommend using titan-reinforced PTFE membranes, which have advantages for further implant-supported prosthetic planning. These membranes are an efficient barrier against cellular penetration and reduce wound dehiscence risk because of their small pore size. Long-time exposition of the membrane is possible. It is not comparable to fully developed keratinized soft tissue, but it protects the bone block. In this case, however, we opted for Jason membrane because at the same time a connective tissue graft was used for the neighboring tooth.

6.1. Dental Implantation. A drill template can be made based on the block planning data (3D BB). Bone resorption of allogenic bone blocks is reported to reach up to 5-10% after six months of healing; however, it can vary individually [24]. Six months after insertion, digital implant planning was done. The visualization of the bone was not ideal because of the incomplete vascularization. Allogeneic transplants' visibility is better after coverage by a radiopaque titan mesh membrane or a thin layer of radiopaque bone substitute in advance. Alternatively, by setting the Hounsfield units at the 200–400 HU range, differentiation of the reconstructed bone is relatively visible [19].

Usually, there is an attempt to insert the implants while using the local bone underneath the augmented area. Furthermore, there is a high risk of lifting the bone block during implant insertion because of the loose joint between the transplant and the local bone. Moreover, resorption, which is about 10 to 15%, is comparable with native bone grafts [1].

7. Conclusion

Allogeneic transplants are a suitable alternative to autologous bone. They enable a less invasive procedure compared to augmentations with the autologous bone, do not burden the patient with the removal of autologous bones, thereby reducing removal site morbidity and operating time, and are virtually unrestricted. In connection with the concept of backward planning, they enable aesthetically and functionally successful implant prosthetic results even in the aesthetically sensitive anterior region. Thus, the patient was very satisfied with the surgical procedure and the aesthetic result.

Consent

The patient gave written consent to participate in this study.

References

[1] M. Nilius, J. Kohlhase, J. Lorenzen, G. Lauer, and M. Schulz, "Multidisciplinary oral rehabilitation of an adolescent suffering from juvenile Gorlin-Goltz syndrome - a case report," *Head & Face Medicine*, vol. 15, no. 1, p. 5, 2019.

[2] G. Chaushu, O. Mardinger, M. Peleg, and O. Ghelfan, "Nissan J. Analysis of complications following augmentation with cancellous block allografts," *Journal of Periodontology*, vol. 81, no. 12, pp. 1759–1764, 2010.

[3] K. Al-Abedalla, J. Torres, and A. R. Cortes, "Bone augmented with allograft onlays for implant placement could be comparable with native bone," *Journal of Oral and Maxillofacial Surgery*, vol. 73, no. 11, pp. 2108–2122, 2015.

[4] M. Nevins, J. T. Mellonig, D. S. Clem, G. M. Reiser, and D. Buser, "Implants in regenerated bone: long-term survival," *The International Journal of Periodontics & Restorative Dentistry*, vol. 18, no. 1, pp. 34–45, 1998.

[5] J. Nissan, M. Vered, O. Gross, O. Mardinger, and G. Chaushu, "Histomorphometric analysis following augmentation of the posterior mandible using cancellous bone-block allograft," *Journal of Biomedical Materials Research. Part A*, vol. 97, no. 4, pp. 509–513, 2011.

[6] M. Schlee, J. F. Dehner, K. Baukloh, A. Happe, O. Seitz, and R. Sader, "Esthetic outcome of implant-based reconstructions in augmented bone: comparison of autologous and allogeneic bone block grafting with the pink esthetic score (PES)," *Head & Face Medicine*, vol. 10, no. 1, pp. 1–10, 2014.

[7] M. Nevins and J. T. Mellonig, "The advantages of localized ridge augmentation prior to implant placement: a staged event," *International Journal of Periodontics & Restorative Dentistry*, vol. 14, no. 2, pp. 96–111, 1994.

[8] J. Nissan, V. Marilena, O. Gross, O. Mardinger, and G. Chaushu, "Histomorphometric analysis following augmentation of the posterior mandible using cancellous bone-block allograft," *Journal of Biomedical Materials Research Part A*, vol. 97A, no. 4, pp. 509–513, 2011.

[9] K. Krasny, K. Krasny, A. Kaminski, and P. Fiedor, "Global maxillary ridge augmentation with frozen radiation-sterilised bone blocks followed by implant placement: a case report," *Cell and Tissue Ban*, vol. 16, no. 1, pp. 35–41, 2015.

[10] D. Rothamel, F. Schwarz, M. Herten et al., "Vertical augmentation of the mandible using cortico-spongious xenoblocks. A histomorphometrical study in dogs," *Schweizer Monatsschrift für Zahnmedizin*, vol. 118, no. 12, pp. 1162–1169, 2008.

[11] C. M. Schmitt, H. Doering, T. Schmidt, R. Lutz, F. W. Neukam, and K. A. Schlegel, "Histological results after maxillary sinus augmentation with Straumann® BoneCeramic, Bio-Oss®, Puros®, and autologous bone. A randomized controlled clinical trial," *Clinical Oral Implants Research*, vol. 24, no. 5, pp. 576–585, 2013.

[12] S. J. Froum, S. S. Wallace, N. Elian, S. C. Cho, and D. P. Tarnow, "Comparison of mineralized cancellous bone allograft (Puros) and anorganic bovine bone matrix (Bio-Oss) for sinus augmentation: histomorphometry at 26 to 32 weeks after grafting," *The International Journal of Periodontics & Restorative Dentistry*, vol. 26, no. 6, pp. 543–551, 2006.

[13] L. Laino, G. Lezzi, A. Piattelli, L. Lo Muzio, and M. Cicciu, "Vertical Ridge augmentation of the atrophic posterior mandible with sandwich technique: bone block from the chin area versus corticocancellous bone block allograft—clinical and histological prospective randomized controlled study," *BioMed Research International*, vol. 2014, Article ID 982104, 7 pages, 2014.

[14] S. Vastardis and R. A. Yukna, "Evaluation of allogeneic bone graft substitute for treatment of periodontal osseous defects: 6-month clinical results," *The Compendium of Continuing Education in Dentistry*, vol. 27, pp. 38–44, 2006.

[15] C. Tudor, S. Srour, M. Thorwarth et al., "Bone regeneration in osseous defects-application of particulated human and bovine materials," *Oral Surgery, Oral Medicine, Oral Pathology, Oral Radiology, and Endodontics*, vol. 105, no. 4, pp. 430–436, 2008.

[16] M. Yacker, J. Ricci, I. C. Matei, B. Hu, and S. Mamidwar, "Treatment of a mandibular cyst before implant placement: case report," *The New York State Dental Journal*, vol. 80, no. 4, pp. 41–44, 2014.

[17] L. Tolstunov and J. Chi, "Alveolar ridge augmentation: comparison of two socket graft materials in implant cases," *The Compendium of Continuing Education in Dentistry*, vol. 32, pp. e16–e24, 2011.

[18] M. Tallarico, C.-J. Park, A. I. Lumbau et al., "Customized 3D-printed titanium mesh developed to regenerate a complex bone defect in the aesthetic zone: a case report approached with a fully digital workflow," *Materials*, vol. 13, no. 17, p. 3874, 2020.

[19] M. Nilius, C. Mueller, M. H. Nilius, D. Haim, B. Weiland, and G. Lauer, "Advanced backward planning with custom-milled individual allogeneic block augmentation for maxillary full-arch osteoplasty and dental implantation: a 3-year-follow-up," *Cell and Tissue Banking*, vol. 23, no. 3, 2021.

[20] A. Pruss, C. Perka, P. Degenhardt et al., "Clinical efficacy and compatibility of allogeneic avital tissue transplants sterilized with a peracetic acid/ethanol mixture," *Cell and Tissue Banking*, vol. 3, no. 4, pp. 235 243, 2002, PMID: 15256872.

[21] M. Hinsenkamp, L. Muylle, T. Eastlund, D. Fehily, L. Noël, and D. M. Strong, "Adverse reactions and events related to muscu-

loskeletal allografts: reviewed by the World Health Organisation Project NOTIFY," *International Orthopaedics*, vol. 36, no. 3, pp. 633–641, 2012.

[22] T. Fretwurst, A. Spanou, K. Nelson, M. Wein, T. Steinberg, and A. Stricker, "Comparison of four different allogeneic bone grafts for alveolar ridge reconstruction: a preliminary histologic and biochemical analysis," *Oral Surgery, Oral Medicine, Oral Pathology, Oral Radiology*, vol. 118, no. 4, pp. 424–431, 2014.

[23] S. C. Wen, S. Barootchi, W. X. Huang, and H. L. Wang, "Time analysis of alveolar ridge preservation using a combination of mineralized bone-plug and dense-polytetrafluoroethylene membrane: a histomorphometric study," *Journal of Periodontology*, vol. 91, no. 2, pp. 215–222, 2019.

[24] J. Nissan, O. Ghelfan, O. Mardinger, S. Calderon, and G. Chaushu, "Efficacy of cancellous block allograft augmentation prior to implant placement in the posterior atrophic mandible," *Clinical Implant Dentistry and Related Research*, vol. 13, no. 4, pp. 279–285, 2011.

19

Bone Remineralization around Dental Implants following Conservative Treatment after Peri-Implantitis

Algirdas Puisys ,[1,2] Viktorija Auzbikaviciute ,[1,2] Renata Simkunaite-Rizgeliene,[3] Dainius Razukevicius,[4] Rokas Linkevicius,[2,4] and Tomas Linkevicius[2,3]

[1]*Vilnius Implantology Center, Vilnius, Lithuania*
[2]*Vilnius Research Group, Vilnius, Lithuania*
[3]*Vilnius University, Vilnius, Lithuania*
[4]*Lithuanian University of Health Science, Kaunas, Lithuania*

Correspondence should be addressed to Algirdas Puisys; algirdas@vicklinika.lt

Academic Editor: Miguel Peñarrocha

The aim of this case report is to show that bone remineralization around dental implants with a history of peri-implantitis is possible after irritant factors are removed and only conservative treatment is performed. Patient came to the clinic after three years of dental implant placement complaining about swelling, sensitivity and gingiva color changes at the posterior part of the maxilla. During radiographic and intraoral examinations peri-implantitis of the #24 implant site was diagnosed. The surgical treatment method was rejected and performed conservative treatment instead. The outcome is promising; periapical radiographs three months later showed bone remineralization as well as stable bone after 10 years. *A key clinical message*: Bone remineralization around dental implants with a history of peri-implantitis is possible after irritant factors are removed and conservative treatment performed.

1. Introduction

Biological complications predisposed by undetected cement remnants are receiving much attention recently. It was shown that excess cement might be responsible not only for quick peri-implantitis development but also for delayed or chronic manifestation of the disease many years after cementation [1, 2]. In vitro and clinical studies show that it is very difficult or in some cases even impossible to completely clean up cement excess from subgingival margins—the most popular position of a cementation line—when cement-retained restorations are fabricated [3–5]. The outcome of biological complications due to cement excess may vary from temporary inflammation of soft peri-implant tissues without serious esthetic and functional consequences to implant loss. There is a variety of scientific evidence that described treatment modalities to prevent or suppress the disease. However, there is still the lack of information about nonsurgical treatment and bone remineralization around implants.

This case report describes peri-implantitis caused by residual cement and the solution of the complications and provides a nonsurgical approach of the treatment.

2. Case History

A patient presented in 2009 with the main complaint of a fistula and tenderness on chewing and touching of the tissues above the implant restoration (Figure 1). Anamnesis revealed that this case was restored approximately 3 years before.

The patient's history chart showed that a regular connection two-piece implant (BioHorizons Internal, Birmingham, AL, USA) was placed and achieved successful integration. A standard abutment was used to support metal ceramic restoration, which was cemented with glass-ionomer modified

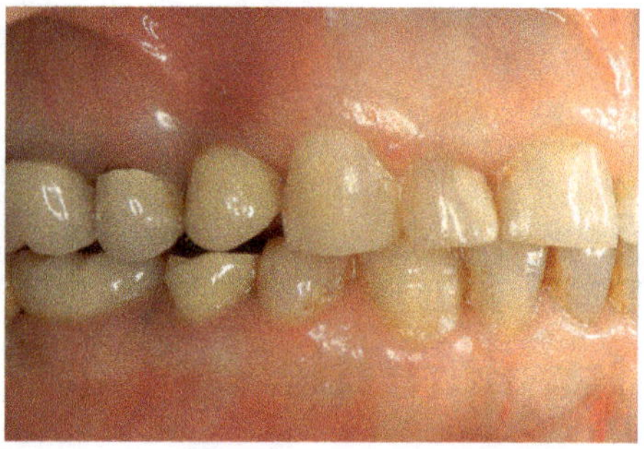

FIGURE 1: Draining sinus tract over implant-supported restoration.

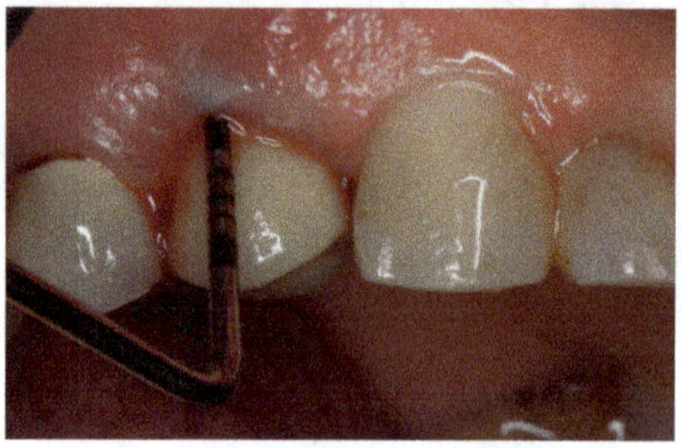

FIGURE 2: Bleeding on probing.

with a resin luting agent (Fuji Plus, GC, Tokyo, Japan). It was recorded in that cement remnants were cleaned, and radiographic examination did not show any residue. The treatment was considered being finished; the patient was satisfied and did not seek any consultation or intervention after the treatment.

Intraoral observation revealed deep pockets up to 8 mm; also, profuse bleeding on probing was recorded (Figure 2). However, general periodontal condition around other teeth was good; BOP and PI around other teeth were ≤15%.

Radiographic examination showed severe crestal bone loss till the third thread of the implant. The bone loss pattern was characteristic to peri-implantitis. No cement remnants could be noticed; also, the bone level of adjacent teeth indicated that the patient is not periodontally involved (Figures 3(a) and 3(b)). Clinical and radiological evaluation helped to determine the diagnosis of chronic peri-implantitis.

Initial treatment plan included removal of the restoration and evaluation of the peri-implant tissues. The restoration occlusal surface was swirled through to get the access to the abutment screw. The screw was loosened, and restoration was removed. Surprisingly, a big piece of cement rest was located in the buccal site of the implant, thus invisible to radiographic examination (Figures 4(a) and 4(b)).

An extensive undercut between the cementation line on the standard abutment (lower arrow) and emergence profile of the restoration in the buccal side (upper arrow) was present (Figure 4(b)). Exactly on this side cement remnant was located in peri-implant mucosa. Thus, undercut can be described as the distance between the cementation (cement extrusion) line and the emergence profile of the restoration. It was shown that a bigger undercut results in worse cement remnant removal (Vindasiute et al. 2013).

The cement rest was removed, and peri-implant tissues were abundantly rinsed with chlorhexidine-digluconate 0.12% solution (PerioAid, Dentaid, Barcelona, Spain). There was a bedsore in peri-implant tissues, where cement remnants were resting (Figure 5(a)). Then, chlorhexidine gel (PerioAid Gel, Dentaid, Barcelona, Spain) was applied on the healing abutment, and it was tightened to the implant (Figures 5(b) and 5(c)). The excess of the gel was washed away. The patient was instructed to rinse the infected site with the same chlorhexidine-digluconate solution twice a day for 1 week.

The patient presented at 1 week after removal of the cement excess. The fistula was not present; the patient did not report any tenderness of the site. Clinically, soft tissues appeared healthy; there was restricted blushing of the gingiva in the place of previous fistula. The removed restoration was screwed back to the implant, and occlusal entrance was isolated with polytetrafluorethylene tape and adhesively covered with composite (Figure 6). The decision was made not to proceed with any kind of antibacterial, surgical, or regenerative treatment of peri-implantitis, and the patient was scheduled for observation visits every 6 months.

3. Follow-Up

The patient presented after 1 year post removal of the cement excess without any complains. Radiological examination showed bone remineralization of the previously infected implant (Figure 7(b)). After 2 years, a full regrowth of the crestal bone around the implant was observed (Figure 7(c)). During this time, the patient had an adjacent tooth replaced with an implant. In 2019, 10 years after, a new periapical X-ray reveals stable bone around implant #24 (Figure 7(d)).

Clinically soft tissues were healthy; the bone contour was improved, compared to the previous situation, and only a minor change in soft tissue color remained (Figure 8).

4. Discussion

There was a visible crestal bone resorption due to cement remnants in this clinical case. It was shown that an individual abutment does not guarantee total cement excess cleaning at the subgingival margin [6, 7].

However, after the elimination of the residue, not only the soft tissue inflammation resolved but also bone remineralization occurred. This might be compared to remineralization of the alveolar bone around the tooth, which also can be expected. It was shown that bone regeneration occurs in infrabony pockets in patients maintained on an optimal standard of oral hygiene [8]. When infection and irritants are removed, remineralization of the bone organic matrix occurs. It can be speculated that a similar situation occurred in this implant case. Cement excess was acting like "artificial calculus," which predisposed peri-implant disease. This case report could suggest that surgical intervention is not always

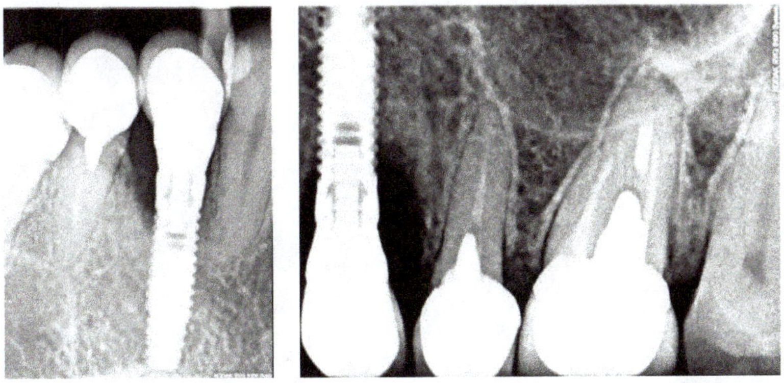

(a) (b)

FIGURE 3: (a, b) Radiographic examination with different positions of the holder.

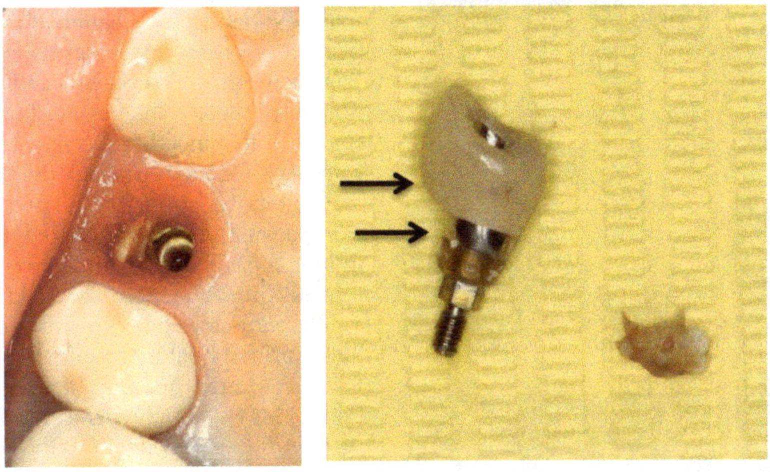

(a) (b)

FIGURE 4: (a) Undetected cement remnants in peri-implant sulcus; (b) removed cement excess and size of undercut of the restoration.

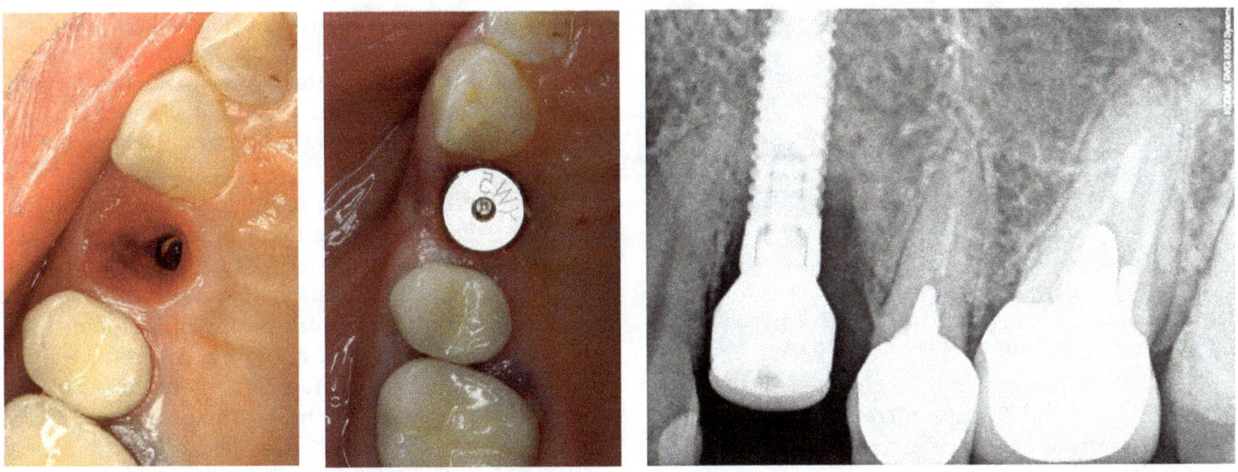

(a) (b) (c)

FIGURE 5: (a) Peri-implant sulcus after removal of cement excess, (b) healing abutment connection, and (c) radiographic verification.

necessary as a part of cement-related peri-implantitis treatment. When cement rest is removed and the patient is not periodontally compromised, remineralization of the crestal bone can occur.

The bone loss around a dental implant due to cement remnants is not direct bone loss but rather demineralization. The question arises: how long should it take to destroy all organic matrix and when to predict bone remineralization

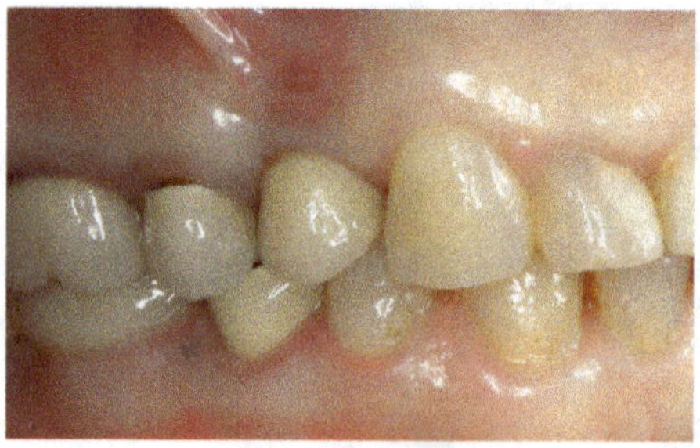

FIGURE 6: Sinus tract has healed.

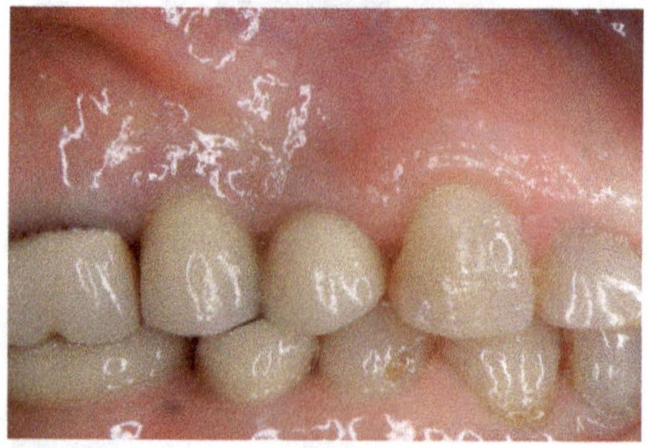

FIGURE 8: Clinical appearance of implant-supported restoration 10 years after treatment.

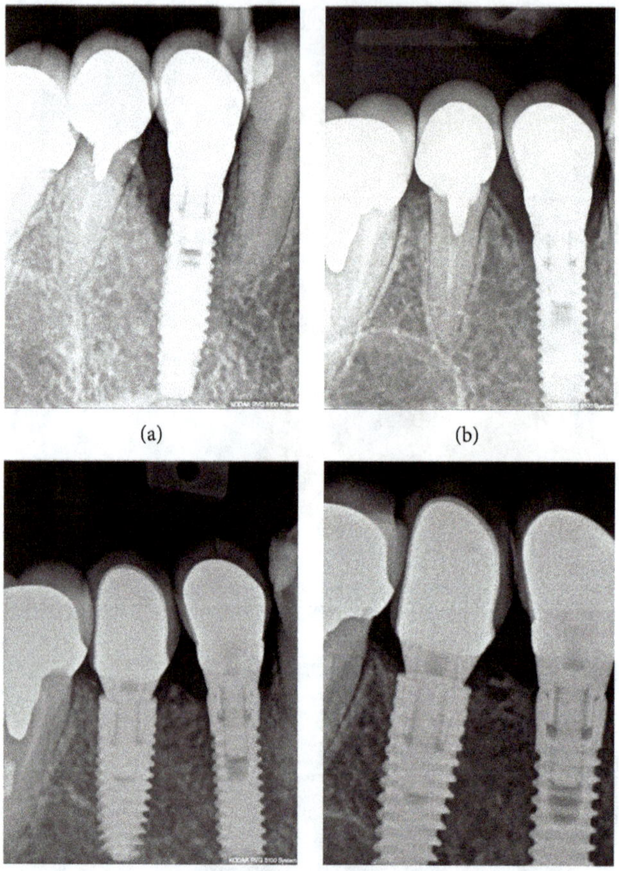

(a) (b) (c) (d)

FIGURE 7: (a) Reference radiograph in 2009; (b) partial remineralization of the bone defect in 2010; (c) full reestablishment of the bone level in 2012; (d) stable bone after 10 years.

around dental implant? Perhaps, there is strong probability for a direct correlation between host response and microbiota of peri-implant sulcus.

The lack of information about bone demineralization and remineralization kinetics is also observed. It can only be speculated as a process similar to periodontal tissue changes.

Demineralization is the process caused by inflammation when mineral ions of hydroxyapatite (HA) are removed from the hard tissues, particularly in the bone [9]. Even though HA is one of the most stable calcium phosphate salts [10], the inflammation process might lead to the bone matrix changes following bone loss. Inflammation is related to the overproduction of various cytokines and bone cells [11]. It initiates hyperactivation of osteoclasts and leads to the bone degradation; also, some cytokines negatively affect osteoblast function [12]. Remineralization might be achieved by increasing osteoblast function; particularly, these cells promote crystal formation of hydroxyapatite, propagate growth in the interior part of membrane-limited matrix vesicles [13], and induce crystals in the collagenous extracellular matrix thus mineralizing bone matrix overall [14].

Recent publications regarding peri-implantitis treatment have various treatment methods in order to obtain bone remineralization, but most of them contain surgical interventions [15–19]. A study performed by Froum et al. proposed a regenerative approach for peri-implantitis treatment [16] with a consecutive series of 170 implants in 100 patients up to a 10-year follow-up. The treatment consisted of flap elevation, surface decontamination, use of enamel matrix derivative (EMD) or platelet-derived growth factor (PDGF), and guided bone regeneration with mineralized freeze-dried bone and/or organic bovine bone (with PDGF or EMD) and covered with an absorbable membrane or subepithelial connective tissue graft. In the results, it was stated that probing depth reduction averaged 5,1 mm and bone level gain averaged 1,77 mm.

While taking a look in scientific articles reporting nonsurgical treatment for peri-implantitis, the mean differences were evaluated between either presence or absence of bleeding and changes in probing depth. From the existing literature on nonsurgical therapy of peri-implantitis, it seems that limited clinical improvements have been found following mechanical therapy with ultrasonic devices or carbon-fiber curettes. In the controlled study by Karring et al. [20], peri-implantitis treatment was performed with either carbon-fiber tip with aerosol spray with hydroxylapatite or carbon-fiber curette. None of these methods in the randomized split-mouth study resulted in healing of the peri-implantitis lesions. In a randomized controlled trial comparing the use of either titanium curettes or ultrasonic device for implants, a significant reduction in bleeding and plaque scores was noted after six months, but probing depths were not improved [21]. In the clinical study performed by Sahm et al., it was noted that air-abrasive treatment resulted in significantly higher bleeding on probing reduction compared with mechanical debridement with carbon-fiber curette [22]. In the Büchter and coworker study, it is already stated that local antimicrobial treatment gives positive results in reduction of pocket probing depth of about 1,15 mm [23]. A number of case series and clinical trials have reported similar results in terms of enhancing effectiveness of peri-implantitis treatment supplemented with local antimicrobials [24–27]. The question arises: does conservative treatment of peri-implantitis lead not only to absence of inflammation and reduction of probing depth but also to remineralization around the implant site?.

The main limitation to any human clinical study is the lack of histology needed to determine the newly formed bone of the remineralization process. There is still considerable uncertainty with regard to effectiveness of the proposed treatment; in fact, further experimental investigations are needed to estimate the accurate results.

Additional Points

A Key Clinical Message. Bone remineralization around dental implants with a history of peri-implantitis is possible after irritant factors are removed and conservative treatment is performed.

References

[1] T. G. Wilson Jr., "The positive relationship between excess cement and peri implant disease: a prospective clinical endoscopic study," *Journal of Periodontology*, vol. 80, no. 9, pp. 1388–1392, 2009.

[2] T. Linkevicius, A. Puisys, E. Vindasiute, L. Linkeviciene, and P. Apse, "Does residual cement around implant-supported restorations cause peri-implant disease? A retrospective case analysis," *Clinical Oral Implants Research*, vol. 24, no. 11, pp. 1179–1184, 2013.

[3] J. R. Agar, S. M. Cameron, J. C. Hughbanks, and M. H. Parker, "Cement removal from restorations luted to titanium abutments with simulated subgingival margins," *The Journal of Prosthetic Dentistry*, vol. 78, no. 1, pp. 43–47, 1997.

[4] T. Linkevicius, E. Vindasiute, A. Puisys, and V. Peciuliene, "The influence of margin location on the amount of undetected cement excess after delivery of cement-retained implant restorations," *Clinical Oral Implants Research*, vol. 22, no. 12, pp. 1379–1384, 2011.

[5] T. Linkevicius, E. Vindasiute, A. Puisys, L. Linkeviciene, N. Maslova, and A. Puriene, "The influence of the cementation margin position on the amount of undetected cement. A prospective clinical study," *Clinical Oral Implants Research* vol. 24, no. 1, pp. 71–76, 2013.

[6] G. Wasiluk, E. Chomik, P. Gehrke, M. Pietruska, A. Skurska, and J. Pietruski, "Incidence of undetected cement on CAD/-CAM monolithic zirconia crowns and customized CAD/CAM implant abutments. A prospective case series," *Clinical Oral Implants Research*, vol. 28, no. 7, pp. 774–778, 2017.

[7] S. Kappel, C. Eiffler, J. Lorenzo-Bermejo, T. Stober, and P. Rammelsberg, "Undetected residual cement on standard or individualized all-ceramic abutments with cemented zirconia single crowns - a prospective randomized pilot trial," *Clinical Oral Implants Research*, vol. 27, no. 9, pp. 1065–1071, 2016.

[8] B. Rosling, S. Nyman, and J. Lindhe, "The effect of systematic plaque control on bone regeneration in infrabony pockets," *Journal of Clinical Periodontology*, vol. 3, no. 1, pp. 38–53, 1976.

[9] E. A. Neel, A. Aljabo, A. Strange et al., "Demineralization–remineralization dynamics in teeth and bone," *International Journal of Nanomedicine*, vol. Volume 11, pp. 4743–4763, 2016.

[10] E. E. Machtei, Y. Mayer, J. Horwitz, and H. Zigdon-Giladi, "Prospective randomized controlled clinical trial to compare hard tissue changes following socket preservation using alloplasts, xenografts vs no grafting: clinical and histological findings," *Clinical Implant Dentistry and Related Research*, vol. 21, no. 1, pp. 14–20, 2019.

[11] A. Kantarci, L. Will, and S. Yen, Eds., *Tooth Movement. Frontiers of Oral Biology, Vol 18*, Karger, Basel, 2016.

[12] A. Insua, A. Monje, H.-L. Wang, and R. J. Miron, "Basis of bone metabolism around dental implants during osseointegration and peri-implant bone loss," *Journal of Biomedical Materials Research Part A*, vol. 105, no. 7, pp. 2075–2089, 2017.

[13] T. Hasegawa, "Ultrastructure and biological function of matrix vesicles in bone mineralization," *Histochemistry and Cell Biology*, vol. 149, no. 4, pp. 289–304, 2018.

[14] L. Hessle, K. A. Johnson, H. C. Anderson et al., "Tissue-non-specific alkaline phosphatase and plasma cell membrane glycoprotein-1 are central antagonistic regulators of bone mineralization," *Proceedings of the National Academy of Sciences*, vol. 99, no. 14, pp. 9445–9449, 2002.

[15] A. C. Wetzel, J. Vlassis, R. G. Caffesse, C. H. F. Hammerle, and N. P. Lang, "Attempts to obtain re-osseointegration following experimental peri-implantitis in dogs," *Clinical Oral Implants Research*, vol. 10, no. 2, pp. 111–119, 1999.

[16] S. Froum, S. Froum, and P. Rosen, "A regenerative approach to the successful treatment of peri-implantitis: a consecutive series of 170 implants in 100 patients with 2- to 10-year follow-up," *The International Journal of Periodontics & Restorative Dentistry*, vol. 35, no. 6, pp. 857–863, 2015.

[17] S. Froum and P. Rosen, "Reentry evaluation following treatment of peri-implantitis with a regenerative approach," *The International Journal of Periodontics & Restorative Dentistry*, vol. 34, no. 1, pp. 47–59, 2014.

[18] S. Renvert and I. N. Polyzois, "Clinical approaches to treat peri-implant mucositis and peri-implantitis," *Periodontology 2000*, vol. 68, no. 1, pp. 369–404, 2015.

[19] S.-Y. Park, K.-H. Kim, S.-H. Rhee et al., "An immediate peri-implantitis induction model to study regenerative peri-implantitis treatments," *Clinical Oral Implants Research*, vol. 28, no. 1, pp. 36–42, 2017.

[20] E. S. Karring, A. Stavropoulos, B. Ellegaard, and T. Karring, "Treatment of peri-implantitis by the VectorR system. A pilot study," *Clinical Oral Implants Research*, vol. 16, no. 3, pp. 288–293, 2005.

[21] S. Renvert, E. Samuelsson, C. Lindahl, and G. R. Persson, "Mechanical non-surgical treatment of peri-implantitis: a double-blind randomized longitudinal clinical study. I: clinical results," *Journal of Clinical Periodontology*, vol. 36, no. 7, pp. 604–609, 2009.

[22] N. Sahm, J. Becker, T. Santel, and F. Schwarz, "Non-surgical treatment of peri-implantitis using an air-abrasive device or mechanical debridement and local application of chlorhexidine: a prospective, randomized, controlled clinical study," *Journal of Clinical Periodontology*, vol. 38, no. 9, pp. 872–878, 2011.

[23] A. Büchter, U. Meyer, B. Kruse-Lösler, U. Joos, and J. Kleinheinz, "Sustained release of doxycycline for the treatment of peri-implantitis: randomised controlled trial," *British Journal of Oral and Maxillofacial Surgery*, vol. 42, no. 5, pp. 439–444, 2004.

[24] M. de Araujo Nobre, C. Capelas, A. Alves et al., "Non-surgical treatment of peri-implant pathology," *International Journal of Dental Hygiene*, vol. 4, no. 2, pp. 84–90, 2006.

[25] E. E. Machtei, S. Frankenthal, G. Levi et al., "Treatment of peri-implantitis using multiple applications of chlorhexidine chips: a double-blind, randomized multi-centre clinical trial," *Journal of Clinical Periodontology*, vol. 39, no. 12, pp. 1198–1205, 2012.

[26] G. R. Persson, G. E. Salvi, L. J. A. Heitz-Mayfield, and N. P. Lang, "Antimicrobial therapy using a local drug delivery system (ArestinR) in the treatment of peri-implantitis. I: microbiological outcomes," *Clinical Oral Implants Research*, vol. 17, no. 4, pp. 386–393, 2006.

[27] G. E. Salvi, G. R. Persson, L. J. A. Heitz-Mayfield, M. Frei, and N. P. Lang, "Adjunctive local antibiotic therapy in the treatment of peri-implantitis II: clinical and radiographic outcomes," *Clinical Oral Implants Research*, vol. 18, no. 3, pp. 281–285, 2007.

20

Root Membrane Replantation as an Alternative Technique for the Socket Preservation

Francesco Campione,[1] **Ludovica Campione**,[1] **Mario Francesco Campione**,[1] **Michele Melillo**,[2] **Claudia Arena**,[2] **Francesc Abella**,[3] **and Luca Boschini**[4]

[1]*Dottor Francesco Campione Clinic, via de Caro 104 Catania, Italy*
[2]*Department of Experimental and Clinical Medicine–University of Foggia, Italy*
[3]*Department of Endodontics, Universitat Internacional de Catalunya, Sant Cugat del Vallès, Barcelona, Spain*
[4]*Ambulatorio Polispecialistico Dottor Boschini Srl, Rimini, Italy*

Correspondence should be addressed to Luca Boschini; luca.boschini76@gmail.com

Academic Editor: Darko Macan

Background and Overview. Socket shield is a technique that allows the maintenance of tissue volumes. In the reported clinical case, the replantation of the buccal root fragment mistakenly extracted during a socket shield surgery is performed. We present a follow-up to 5 years with an unexpected healing.*Case Description.* An 88-year-old patient underwent an immediate loading implant placement associated with the replantation of the mistakenly extracted root fragment. The shaping of the fragment was performed extraorally, and the replantation was done so that the fragment protruded above the crest margin.*Conclusions and Practical Implications.* The 5-year follow-up shows an uneventful healing of the implant. At 48 months, postoperative CBCT exam reports images compatible with the regeneration of the bone over the portion of root that protruded over the margin. The outcome suggests clinical implications, as the opportunity to easily shape the fragment extraorally and replant sound portion of the root (not necessary the buccal) in buccal socket with bone defect.

1. Introduction

Maintenance or reconstruction of peri-implant soft tissues is still one of the main challenges for implant therapy in esthetic areas [1, 2]. Despite a high survival rate, the esthetic outcome is often compromised, especially by alveolar bone remodeling [3]. The resorption of the alveolar ridge after tooth extraction is more pronounced on the buccal than on the lingual side of the extraction socket, causing a soft tissue deficiency that can interfere with the esthetic outcome of implant supported prosthesis [4]. Several treatment approaches have been proposed in literature to maintain the tissues volume after tooth extraction [5], which is essential to preserve an esthetically pleasant soft tissue contour; among them, there are socket preservation, socket shield, gingival grafts, guided bone regeneration with membrane, and/or grafting materials [6–11]. Numerous studies show that socket preservation is a viable technique to maintain alveolar ridge volume and height. Hurzeler et al. first described the socket shield technique in 2010 [12] and the literature about this technique was reviewed by Gharpure and Bhatavadekar in 2017 [13] and by Ogawa et al. in 2021 [14]. This technique is based on the preservation of the vestibular fragment of the extracted tooth to prevent the alveolar bone resorption of the buccal side [12].

On the other hand, tooth autotransplantation is a treatment option in which a tooth is surgically moved from one site to another [15, 16]. If performed in accordance to biological principles, it ensures maintenance and regeneration of alveolar bone through physiological stimulation of periodontal ligament formation [17].

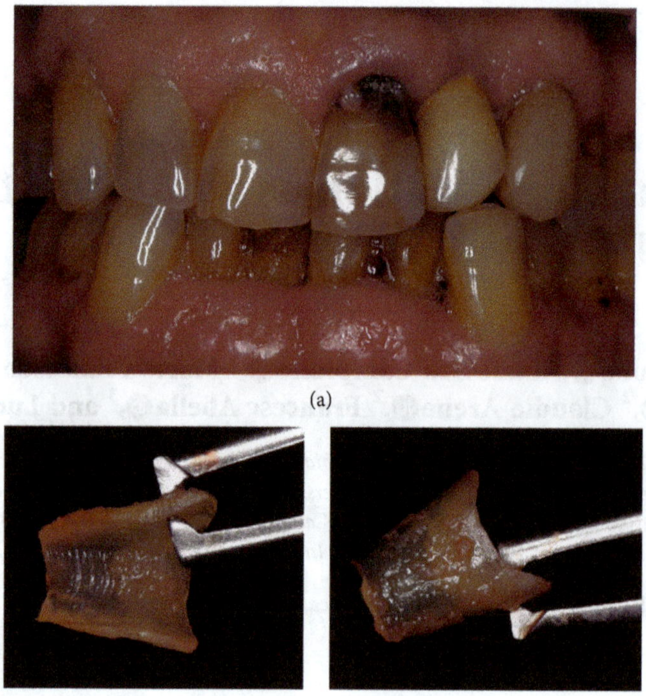

(a)

(b) (c)

Figure 1: (a) Clinical aspect of the central left incisor with a great decay on the cementoenamel junction. (b and c) Portion of the root after being shaped extraorally. The periodontal ligament fibers on the root remain untouched and visible on the buccal side.

This case report shows a clinical case of a socket shield technique performed in combination with principles of teeth autotransplantation.

2. Case Description

An 88-year-old man with a noncontributory medical history presented at private dental clinic in Catania, Italy, with a large cervical carious lesion on an endodontically treated upper left central incisor (Figure 1(a)). Patient requested a prompt rehabilitation of his anterior area, and therefore, extraction with placement of an immediate loaded implant was proposed. Periodontal clinical parameters recording showed no bleeding on probing. Pocket probing depth (PPD) was measured at six points for each tooth. The left central incisor showed 4 mm PPD in all the buccal points and 2 mm PPD in all the palatal points. The gum was firm and dimpled in texture; the gingival margin showed a recession of 2,5 mm due to the carious lesion affecting the cementum-enamel junction.

Cone beam computed tomography analysis was executed before surgery for the case study, to rule out the presence of periapical lesions and to evaluate the bundle bone plate volume. According to the tomography, the buccal bone was very thin, and a recession of 4 mm from the cementum-enamel junction was measured; no periradicular lesion was found.

After approval to perform immediate implant placement, the patient also gave his consent to perform the socket shield technique and signed informed consent. One hour before surgery, the patient received antibiotic prophylaxis with 2 g amoxicillin (Zimox; Pfizer). Surgery was performed under local anesthesia. The extraction was performed flapless. After crown removal with a coarse-grained diamond bur, the pulp chamber and the root canal were used as a guide to section the root in two parts following a mesiodistal direction. Then, during the luxation of the palatal fragment, the buccal portion of root was accidentally extracted. After careful examination of the avulsed fragment, the surgeons decided to replant it in the original site. Since the fragment was now extracted, the final shaping was performed extraorally. After the shaping, the root fragment measurement performed with an Iwanson caliper registered a 1 mm thickness, 4,5 mm height, and 3,5 mm width (Figures 1(b) and 1(c)). The root fragment was placed in saline solution in a sterile container.

The implant site was prepared with standard drills following the palatal bony wall as a guide. The fixture was placed 3 mm beneath the palatal level of the bone crest. A morse-taper implant ($3,8 \times 10$ mm, 3P Implafavourite, Torino, IT) was used. Primary implant stability assessment with resonance frequency analysis revealed an ISQ value of 70 and a Torque insertion value of 60 N/cm^2.

After implant placement, the root membrane was repositioned about 3 mm apical to the gingival margin leaning against the buccal wall of the site and 2,5 mm above the bone crest as revealed by the postoperative computed tomography. No filling material was used to fill the void between the fragment and the implant. The stabilization of the fragment was obtained with the positioning of the provisional restoration.

The provisional restoration was obtained by rebasing the natural sectioned crown on a Ti-base abutment using a hybrid composite (Optifil – IDS Spa).

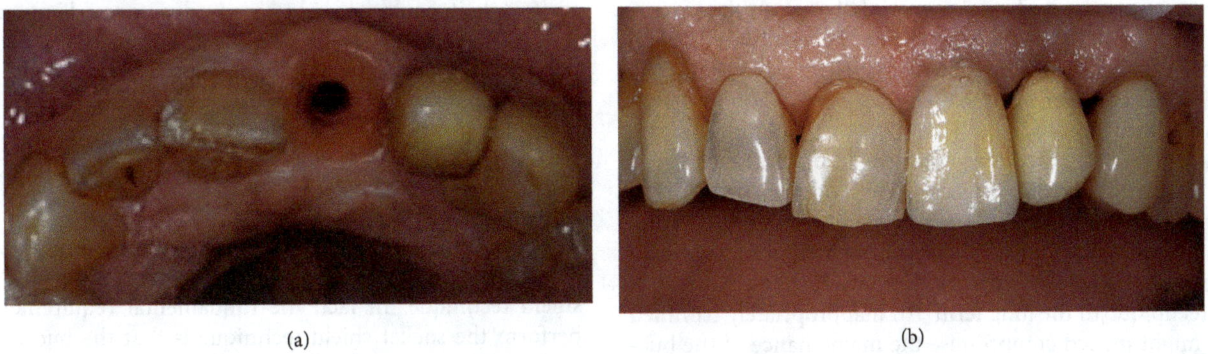

FIGURE 2: (a) Final tissue healing after 6-month follow-up. No signs of inflammation or rejection of the fragment were observed. (b) The final definitive restoration 5-year follow-up; the gingival tissues are healed and preserved.

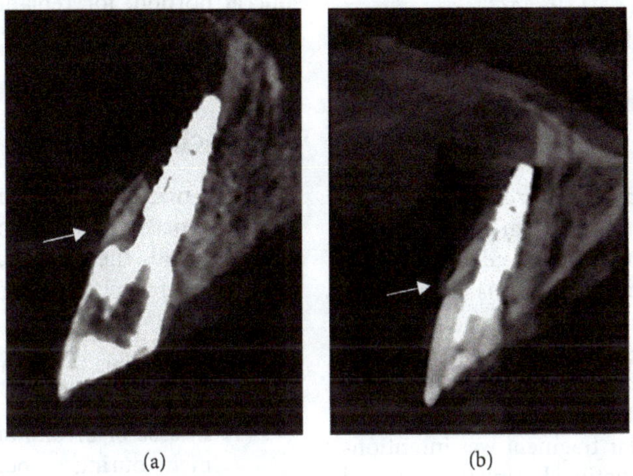

FIGURE 3: (a) At 6-month follow-up, CBCT images show the replanted root membrane in strict contact with the implant abutment and the bundle bone. The arrow indicates the portion of root not covered by bone. (b) At 48 months, CBCT images are compatible with the complete covering of the root membrane (see the arrow), as if there had been migration of the bone over all the root membrane surface.

Care was taken to remove all centric and eccentric functional contacts.

The patient was recommended to follow a soft diet and instructed in proper oral hygiene. Postoperative evaluation was performed after 2 weeks and showed uneventful healing. Six months after implant placement, provisional restoration was removed showing the complete healing of the implant site. At this time a final optical impression was taken with CEREC CAD-CAM technology (Dentsply-Sirona), and a definitive lithium disilicate screw retained crown (IPS e.max - Ivoclar Vivadent) was realized (Figure 2(b)).

Follow-up visits were scheduled at 6 and 12 months; all the following follow-up visits were annual (the last follow-up is at 5 years without complication). At every follow-up, clinical parameters were recorded showing an uneventful healing; no clinical signs of inflammation or plaque accumulation were recorded. Intraoral pictures were taken at every follow-up examination (Figure 2(a)).

A CBCT exam was performed at 6- and 48-month follow-up to evaluate healing or any tissue alteration (Figure 3). The root-membrane appeared well integrated in the context. Moreover, the CBCT images are suggestive of the buccal bone growth over the portion of root membrane which initially protruded beyond the margin of the bone crest (Figure 3(b)).

3. Discussion

Delayed implant placement has a high survival and success rate in both posterior and anterior areas [18, 19]. This kind of treatment is often more time demanding and requests multiple surgical sessions [20]. On the other hand, the resorption of the buccal bundle bone after tooth extraction and immediate implant placement can have a negative esthetic impact [21].

A buccal bone of at least 2 mm thickness seems to be required to perform a successful restoration [22].

Socket shield technique is an effective technique to prevent alveolar-ridge alterations that occur after tooth extraction reducing the possibility of a buccal bone resorption and improving the aesthetic outcome of the final restoration. This technique is also called partial extraction therapy [23] or root membrane technique [24]. It is particularly suitable for teeth in anterior areas, mainly in the maxilla, but it is achievable only in selected cases [23].

Success of this technique is mainly based on the preservation of the periodontal ligament on the vestibular portion of the root. Moreover, it is a minimally invasive procedure that reduces time of treatment and the need of soft and hard tissue grafting procedures. However, this technique is still highly operator experience sensitive [23]. Studies showed that accessing the apical aspect of the root during sectioning might be difficult, due to the poor visibility of the apical fragment, thus increasing the risk of leaving behind fragments of the root apex [25]. This might compromise the efficacy of this technique in the long term. An inappropriately trimmed root might indeed compromise the maintenance of the buccal alveolar bone volume [24]. The conventional socket shield technique can be applied only if the remaining parts of the root are periodontally healthy and if the socket is well conserved in particular on the buccal site [26].

The periodontal ligament is the success key of other well documented surgical therapies: tooth autotransplantation and replantation. Tooth autotransplantation consists in the movement of an extracted tooth from a donor site to another defined receiving socket [27–30].

This technique provides the maintenance and the regeneration of the alveolar bone volume through stimulation of viable cells of periodontal ligament preserved on the root surface [31, 32]. The same healing mechanisms were implemented in intentional replantation in which the donor and the receiving socket are the same; in fact, this technique consists in the repositioning of an extracted tooth in its socket after the extraoral management of endodontic problems [33, 34]. In this case, the vestibular fragment was intentionally replanted according to intentional replantation and transplantation protocol [33]. The rationale behind the choice of surgeons, experts in dental transplantations, is that if it is possible to extract and reposition a periodontally healthy tooth, then it will be possible to do the same with a portion of it. When the buccal root fragment dislocated and was extracted, the operators made the decision to replant the fragment rather than resorting to other surgical techniques, such as socket preservation, which would have required longer time. Having the root membrane in hand, the surgeons had the opportunity to shape the fragment more easily, taking care not to leave the apex or portion of endodontics spaces. In addition, the surgeons had the possibility to replant the fragment more coronally than the crest margin, leaving only the apical half of the fragment in contact with the wall socket; the other half of the root membrane protrude beyond the bone margin. After 48 months, CBCT images suggest a complete healing of the buccal bone; indeed, the images are compatible with the complete covering of the root membrane, as if there had been migration of the bone over all the root membrane surface. This healing is documented in tooth autotransplantation where it is possible to observe the bone regeneration of bone defect by the sound periodontal ligament present on the roots of the donor tooth [34]. The outcome was better than the surgeons would have expected, suggesting some clinical implication. The root membrane replantation technique requires some insights to be scientifically validated, unlike the socket shield technique for which the literature is abundant, but if approved, it could provide some advantages. First of all, the shaping of the root membrane can be carried out extraorally, avoiding the cited complications due to a lack of visibility during the intra oral modelling [23, 25].

In addition, the surgeon can decide to replant the root membrane in a more convenient position compared to the original.

Therefore, the root membrane replantation might allow to overcome several limitations of the conventional socket shield technique. In fact, the fundamental requirement to perform the socket shield technique is that the buccal wall of the socket is conserved. Considering the outcome of this case report, we can hypothesize the effectiveness of using a portion of periodontally healthy root, not necessarily the buccal portion, for replantation in the buccal wall of the socket even if it has a bone defect.

4. Conclusions

The replantation of a root membrane accidentally extracted during a socket shield technique surgery gave an unexpected outcome with the regeneration of bone over a portion of root fragment not submerged under the bone margin.

Although it is necessary to scientifically validate this technique, it is possible to hypothesize some clinical implications:

(1) In case of involuntary extraction of the buccal fragment during a socket shield surgery, it is possible to replant the fragment without diverting to other surgical techniques

(2) The possibility of extraoral shaping making the procedure easier than performing it intraorally

(3) The possibility of replantation of root fragment other than the buccal even in the case of a buccal bone defect of the socket, favoring its regeneration

References

[1] M. G. Araujo, F. Sukekava, J. L. Wennstrom, and J. Lindhe, "Ridge alterations following implant placement in fresh extraction sockets: an experimental study in the dog," *Journal of Clinical Periodontology*, vol. 32, no. 6, pp. 645–652, 2005.

[2] M. H. Amler, P. L. Johnson, and I. Salman, "Histological and histochemical investigation of human alveolar socket healing in undisturbed extraction wounds," *Journal of the American Dental Association (1939)*, vol. 61, no. 1, pp. 32–44, 1960.

[3] R. Fürhauser, D. Florescu, T. Benesch, R. Haas, G. Mailath, and G. Watzek, "Evaluation of soft tissue around single-tooth implant crowns: the pink esthetic score," *Clinical Oral Implants Research*, vol. 16, no. 6, pp. 639–644, 2005.

[4] J. Pietrokovski and M. Massler, "Alveolar ridge resorption following tooth extraction," *The Journal of Prosthetic Dentistry*, vol. 17, no. 1, pp. 21–27, 1967.

[5] G. H. Lin, H. L. Chan, and H. L. Wang, "Effects of currently available surgical and restorative interventions on reducing

midfacial mucosal recession of immediately placed single-tooth implants: a systematic review," *Journal of Periodontology*, vol. 85, no. 1, pp. 92–102, 2014.

[6] D. Botticelli, T. Berglundh, and J. Lindhe, "Hard-tissue alterations following immediate implant placement in extraction sites," *Journal of Clinical Periodontology*, vol. 31, no. 10, pp. 820–828, 2004.

[7] D. Carmagnola, P. Adriaens, and T. Berglundh, "Healing of human extraction sockets filled with bio-Oss," *Clinical Oral Implants Research*, vol. 14, no. 2, pp. 137–143, 2003.

[8] V. Lekovic, P. M. Camargo, P. R. Klokkevold et al., "Preservation of alveolar bone in extraction sockets using bioabsorbable membranes," *Journal of Periodontology*, vol. 69, no. 9, pp. 1044-9, 1998.

[9] M. Araujo, E. Linder, and J. Lindhe, "Effect of a xenograft on early bone formation in extraction sockets: an experimental study in dog," *Clinical Oral Implants Research*, vol. 20, no. 1, pp. 1–6, 2009.

[10] M. Araujo, E. Linder, J. Wennstrom, and J. Lindhe, "The influence of bio-Oss collagen on healing of an extraction socket: an experimental study in the dog," *The International Journal of Periodontics & Restorative Dentistry*, vol. 28, no. 2, pp. 123–135, 2008.

[11] S. Matic and N. Krakar, ""Socket shield" technique (partial tooth extraction) - case report. Abstracts of 7th International Congress of the Croatian Society of Dental Implantology, 12 - 14 October 2017, Osijek, Croatia," *Acta Stomatologica Croatica*, vol. 51, no. 4, pp. 362-363, 2017.

[12] M. B. Hürzeler, O. Zuhr, P. Schupbach, S. F. Rebele, N. Emmanouilidis, and S. Fickl, "The socket-shield technique: a proof-of-principle report," *Journal of Clinical Periodontology*, vol. 37, no. 9, pp. 855–862, 2010.

[13] A. S. Gharpure and N. B. Bhatavadekar, "Current evidence on the socket-shield technique: a systematic review," *The Journal of Oral Implantology*, vol. 43, no. 5, pp. 395–403, 2017.

[14] T. Ogawa, R. M. Sitalaksmi, M. Miyashita et al., "Effectiveness of the socket shield technique in dental implant: A systematic review," *Journal of Prosthodontic Research*, vol. 66, no. 1, pp. 12–18, 2022.

[15] W. C. Chung, Y. K. Tu, Y. H. Lin, and H. K. Lu, "Outcomes of autotransplanted teeth with complete root formation: a systematic review and meta-analysis," *Journal of Clinical Periodontology*, vol. 41, no. 4, pp. 412–423, 2014.

[16] L. Boschini, M. Melillo, and F. Mastrangelo, "Dental autotransplantation for the replacement of lost teeth," *Journal of Osseointegration*, vol. 11, no. 1, pp. 64-65, 2019.

[17] L. A. Machado, R. R. do Nascimento, D. M. T. P. Ferreira, C. T. Mattos, and O. V. Vilella, "Long-term prognosis of tooth autotransplantation: a systematic review and meta-analysis," *International Journal of Oral and Maxillofacial Surgery*, vol. 45, no. 5, pp. 610–617, 2016.

[18] T. Lindh, J. Gunne, A. Tillberg, and M. Molin, "A meta-analysis of implants in partial edentulism," *Clinical Oral Implants Research*, vol. 9, no. 2, pp. 80–90, 1998.

[19] D. Buser, R. Mericske-stern, J. P. Pierre Bernard et al., "Long-term evaluation of non-submerged ITI implants. Part 1: 8-year life table analysis of a prospective multi-center study with 2359 implants," *Clinical Oral Implants Research*, vol. 8, no. 3, pp. 161–172, 1997.

[20] N. P. Lang, L. Pun, K. Y. Lau, K. Y. Li, and M. C. Wong, "A systematic review on survival and success rates of implants placed immediately into fresh extraction sockets after at least 1 year," *Clinical Oral Implants Research*, vol. 23, Suppl 5, pp. 39–66, 2012.

[21] H. Gluckman, J. Du Toit, and M. Salama, "The pontic-shield: partial extraction therapy for ridge preservation and pontic site development," *The International Journal of Periodontics & Restorative Dentistry*, vol. 36, no. 3, pp. 417–423, 2016.

[22] D. Buser, V. Chappuis, U. C. Belser, and S. Chen, "Implant placement post extraction in esthetic single tooth sites: when immediate, when early, when late?," *Periodontology 2000*, vol. 73, no. 1, pp. 84–102, 2017.

[23] A. Mourya, S. K. Mishra, R. Gaddale, and R. Chowdhary, "Socket-shield technique for implant placement to stabilize the facial gingival and osseous architecture: a systematic review," *Journal of Investigative and Clinical Dentistry*, vol. 10, no. 4, article e12449, 2019.

[24] K. D. Siormpas, M. E. Mitsias, E. Kontsiotou-Siormpa, D. Garber, and G. A. Kotsakis, "Immediate implant placement in the esthetic zone utilizing the "root-membrane" technique: clinical results up to 5 years postloading," *The International Journal of Oral & Maxillofacial Implants*, vol. 29, no. 6, pp. 1397–1405, 2014.

[25] Y. Gandhi and N. Bhatavadekar, "Inappropriate socket shield protocol as a probable cause of peri-implant bone resorption: a case report," *Journal of Maxillofacial and Oral Surgery*, vol. 19, no. 3, pp. 359–363, 2020.

[26] O. Zuhr, S. Rebele, D. Schneider, P. Schupbach, and M. Hürzeler, "The socket-shield technique: first histological, clinical, and volumetrical observations after separation of the buccal tooth segment - a pilot study," *Clinical Implant Dentistry and Related Research*, vol. 17, no. 1, pp. 71–82, 2015.

[27] J. O. Andreasen, H. U. Paulsen, Z. Yu, R. Ahlquist, T. Bayer, and O. Schwartz, "A long-term study of 370 autotransplanted premolars. Part I. Surgical procedures and standardized techniques for monitoring healing," *European Journal of Orthodontics*, vol. 12, no. 1, pp. 3–13, 1990.

[28] J. O. Andreasen, H. U. Paulsen, Z. Yu, and T. Bayer, "A long-term study of 370 autotransplanted premolars. Part IV. Root development subsequent to transplantation," *European Journal of Orthodontics*, vol. 12, no. 1, pp. 38–50, 1990.

[29] J. O. Andreasen, H. U. Paulsen, Z. Yu, T. Bayer, and O. Schwartz, "A long-term study of 370 autotransplanted premolars. Part II. Tooth survival and pulp healing subsequent to transplantation," *European Journal of Orthodontics*, vol. 12, no. 1, pp. 14–24, 1990.

[30] J. O. Andreasen, H. U. Paulsen, Z. Yu, and O. Schwartz, "A long-term study of 370 autotransplanted premolars. Part III. Periodontal healing subsequent to transplantation," *European Journal of Orthodontics*, vol. 12, no. 1, pp. 25–37, 1990.

[31] J. H. Park, K. Tai, and D. Hayashi, "Tooth autotransplantation as a treatment option: a review," *The Journal of Clinical Pediatric Dentistry*, vol. 35, no. 2, pp. 129–135, 2010.

[32] L. Boschini, M. Melillo, and F. Berton, "Long term survival of mature autotransplanted teeth: a retrospective single center analysis," *Journal of Dentistry*, vol. 98, article 103371, 2020.

[33] M. Tsukiboshi, "Autotransplantation of teeth: requirements for predictable success," *Dental Traumatology*, vol. 18, no. 4, pp. 157–180, 2002.

[34] P. C. Gault and R. Warocquier-Clerout, "Tooth autotransplantation with double periodontal ligament stimulation to replace periodontally compromised teeth," *Journal of Periodontology*, vol. 73, no. 5, pp. 575–583, 2002.

21

Using the Digital Flow to Increase Efficiency in Complex Partial Rehabilitation with Dental Implants

Andrew Sotirios Melenikiotis,[1] **Camila Pereira Vianna**,[2] **Waleska Caldas**,[3] **Larissa Carvalho Trojan**,[4] **and Rubens Moreno de Freitas**[5]

[1]*Implantology at Ilapeo College, Curitiba, Brazil*
[2]*Pathology, Curitiba, Brazil*
[3]*Orthodontics, Curitiba, Brazil*
[4]*Biomechanics, Curitiba, Brazil*
[5]*Ilapeo College, Curitiba, Brazil*

Correspondence should be addressed to Waleska Caldas; waleska.caldas@alumni.usp.br

Academic Editor: Giuseppe Colella

Background. This report presents a clinical case in which the CAD-CAM technology was applied to optimize a complex partial rehabilitation with implant-supported prostheses of a patient with several functional and aesthetic issues. *Case presentation.* A 40-year-old patient with several complaints due to the absence of multiple teeth and great dissatisfaction regarding his oral health was referred to a Dental College (Curitiba, Brazil). Guided surgery of 11 implants was planned. Digital flow and immediate loading protocol were applied. The patient was followed up for 2 years presenting good clinical and radiographic outcomes. *Conclusions.* The digital flow brought agility and precision to implant placement, immediate provisionalization added to satisfaction in the provisional phase, and CAD/CAM technology provided predictability and comfort to deliver the definite restorations.

1. Introduction

Computer-aided design and manufacturing (CAD-CAM) was developed in the 1960s and first applied in automotive industries. Later, it started to be used in dentistry, increasing digital flow popularity in dental offices every year, contributing to the preliminary stages of dental implant treatment such as diagnosis and planning, and the actual surgical and prosthetics procedures [1]. Among the advantages of its use are reduced time and production costs, high-quality restorations due to consistent precision, and reproducible results [2].

The integration of this technology with rapid prototyping methods made surgical guide fabrication possible, and its use for dental implant placement is referred to as guided implant surgery [3]. Guided surgeries allow predictability in the relationship between planned restorations and the underlying bony anatomy, providing the placement of multiple dental implants, according to surrounding anatomy and principles of ideal implant positioning and spacing. Thereby, this technology is especially beneficial in situations of multiple units or full arch immediate rehabilitation, with or without extractions [4].

The aim of this report is to present a clinical case in which the CAD-CAM technology was applied to optimize a complex partial rehabilitation with implant-supported prostheses of a patient with the absence of multiple teeth and several functional and aesthetic issues.

2. Case Presentation

A 40-year-old patient in good general health was referred to a Dental College (Curitiba, Brazil) with chief complaints of difficulty in eating/chewing due to the absence of multiple teeth, altered speech due to use of a removable provisional partial prosthesis with palatal extension, and low self-

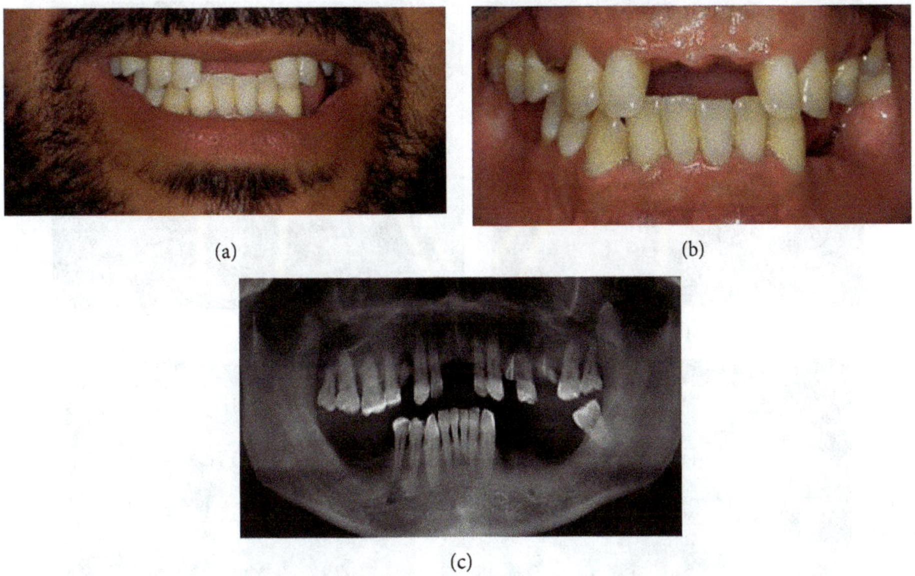

FIGURE 1: Patient's initial photos (a, b) and panoramic radiography (c) showing the absence of several elements in both arches.

esteem due to dissatisfaction with smile's aesthetics and bad breath. After careful anamnesis and clinical and radiographic evaluation, it was also possible to diagnose the loss of teeth 11 due to caries and failed endodontic and restorative treatments (Figure 1). Verbal explanations of treatment options like a removable partial denture, conventional nonguided implant surgery, and rehabilitation with dental implants using the guided surgery technique were given, and the latter was the patient's choice due to enhanced comfort and reduced surgery time and morbidity. The patient gave written consent, and ethics approval was not necessary for this study.

2.1. Case Planning. Superior and inferior impressions were taken and later digitized with a lab TRIOS scanner and the STL files, together with the DICOM files of a full mouth CBCT, and were uploaded to Neodent website for guided surgery planning. These were processed in Dental Wings program of coDiagnostix software (Chemnitz, Germany) by a third party, who virtually planned the case according to instructions given by the oral surgeon (Figure 2). Once this plan was reviewed and approved by the oral surgeon, the surgical guide was fabricated with a 3D printer (Rapid Shape GmbH, Heimsheim, Germany).

2.2. Surgical and Prosthetic Procedures. The patient was medicated and prepared for surgery, and after local anesthesia, the residual roots of teeth 14, 24, and 26 were carefully extracted with minimally invasive techniques, after which the tooth-supported surgical guide was installed (Figure 3 (a)), verifying a perfect fitting through the inspection windows. To increase the stability of the guide, stabilizing pins were screwed through the sleeves into the implant connection with the specific Guided Surgery Surgical kit for Helix GMimplants (Neodent, Curitiba, Brazil), and each bed was prepared following the sequence recommended by the manufacturer for bone type III, with the compensated drills through the corresponding drill guide and sleeve, whereas the drills have laser markings, the depth is controlled visually, and the implant drivers are fabricated with stoppers (Figure 3(b)). Once those touch the sleeve, they indicate that the implant has reached its planned position, which for this case was 2 mm subcrestal for all implants. Hydrophilic Morse cone tapered with 3.75 mm of diameter implants (Helix GMAcquaimplants, Neodent) and lengths between 8 and 13 mm were inserted in the sequence #14, 24,11,12,and 26. Once concluded, the stabilizing pins were removed as was the surgical guide, showing very little bleeding. The torque was measured with the torque wrench, and since all presented torques above 32 N/cm, indicating ideal primary stability for immediate loading, definitive screw-retained abutments were selected for each position, by means of measuring the transgingival height, with the aid of the GM height measurer and the abutment selection kit, and installed according to the specifications and torques recommended by the manufacturer (Neodent, Curitiba, Brazil). After this, and as previously planned, a technique for connective tissue graft in # 14 and xenograft fill was performed. Following the same steps as with the upper arch, implants in positions #35, 36, 37, 46, and 47 were placed using the surgical guide.

In order to follow the one abutment-one time philosophy [5] and since a compatible digital impression coping (scan body) was not available at the time, the abutment impression copings were inserted for a conventional impression of both arches with addition silicone material (Kulzer, Hanau, Germany). Then, with the bite registration, it was sent to the lab for fabrication of the temporary crowns and bridges. The patient returned the following day to install the temporary acrylic restorations. The maxillary prostheses were single crowns, either screw-retained or with the click abutment for temps, and the mandibular ones were screw-retained multiunit acrylic prostheses (Figures 4 and 5).

Three months thereafter, clinical and radiographic evaluation of the implants, abutments, and temporary prosthesis

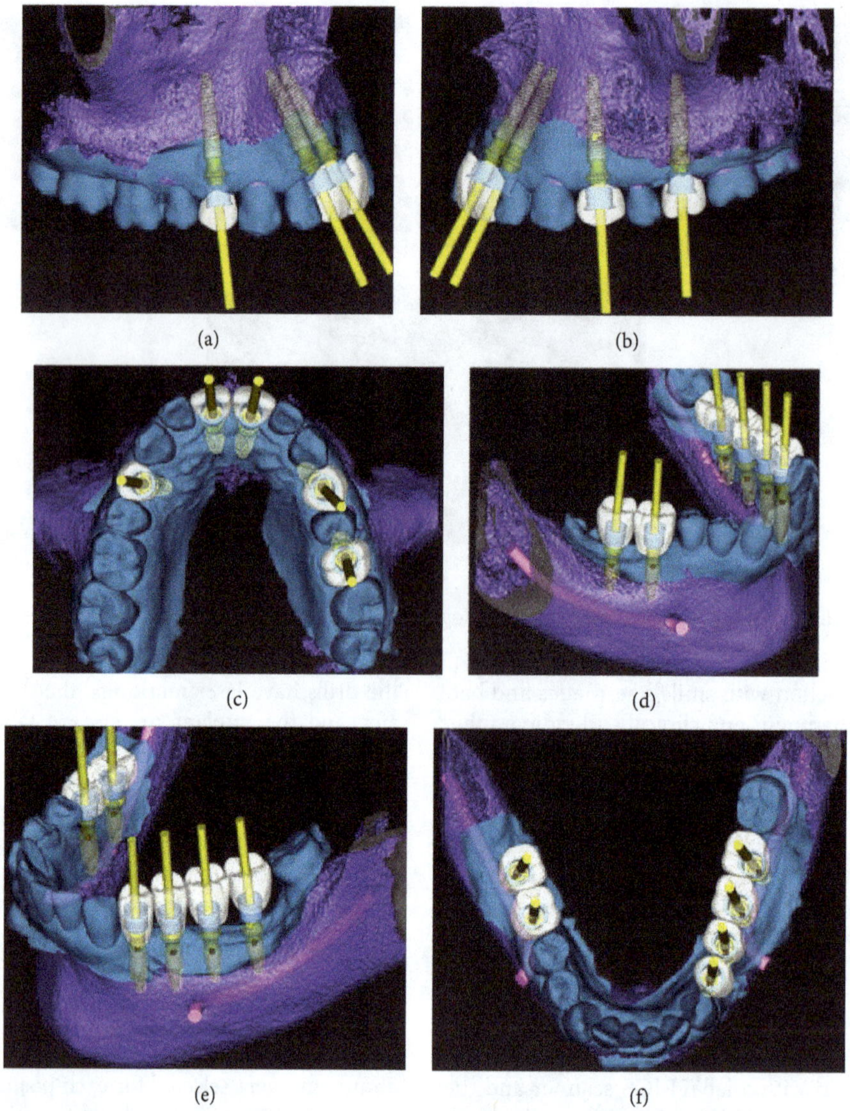

FIGURE 2: Virtual planning of maxillary (a)–(c) and mandibular (d)–(f) implants position considering the planned prosthesis rehabilitation.

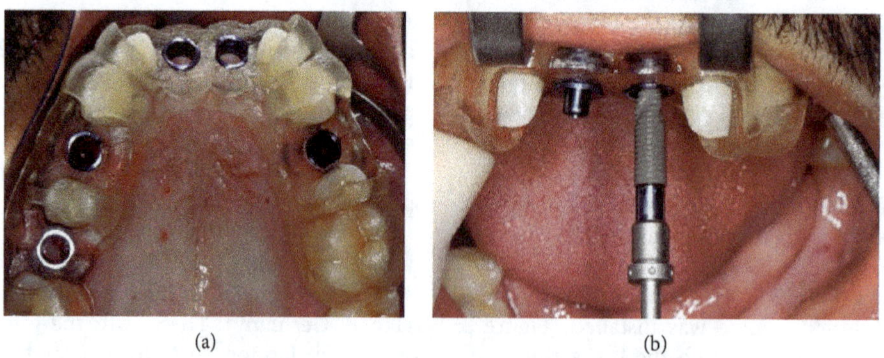

FIGURE 3: Tooth-supported surgery guide positioned in maxilla (a). Implant driver with stopper that indicates when the implant reaches the planned position (b).

revealed adequate regeneration of peri-implant bone and soft tissues and, thus, the procedures for the confection of the final metal-ceramic restorations were followed through. Since the scan body for the GM conical abutment was not yet available, the GM conical abutments were replaced for GM Titanium Bases in positions # 14 and 26, to allow obtaining digital impressions. The scan bodies were inserted, and an intraoral scan was performed. Next, the metal coping

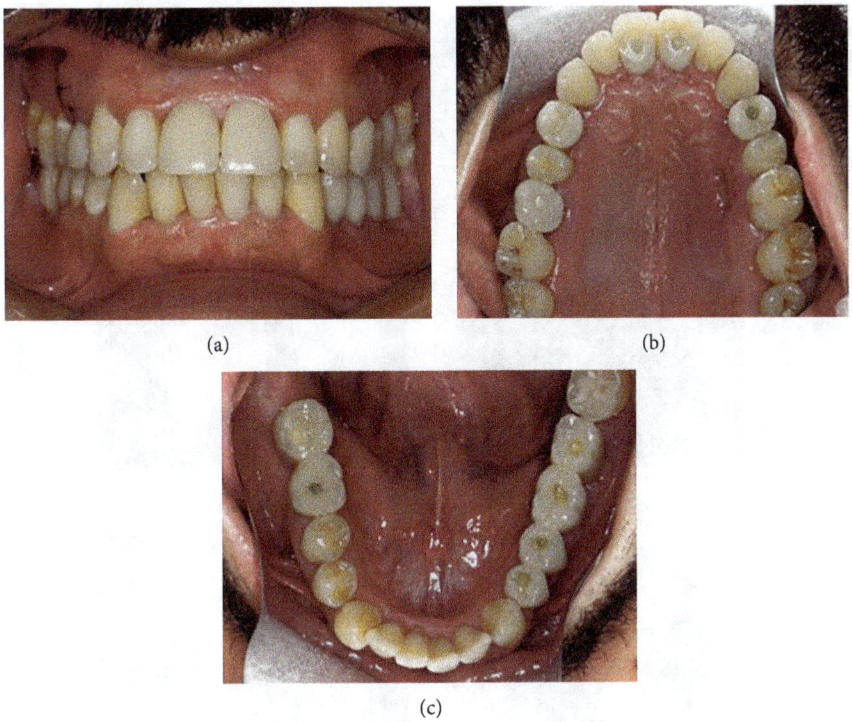

FIGURE 4: Clinical aspects at the time of immediate loading. Frontal view in occlusion (a), maxillary (b), and mandibular (c) occlusal view of acrylic resin temporary crowns.

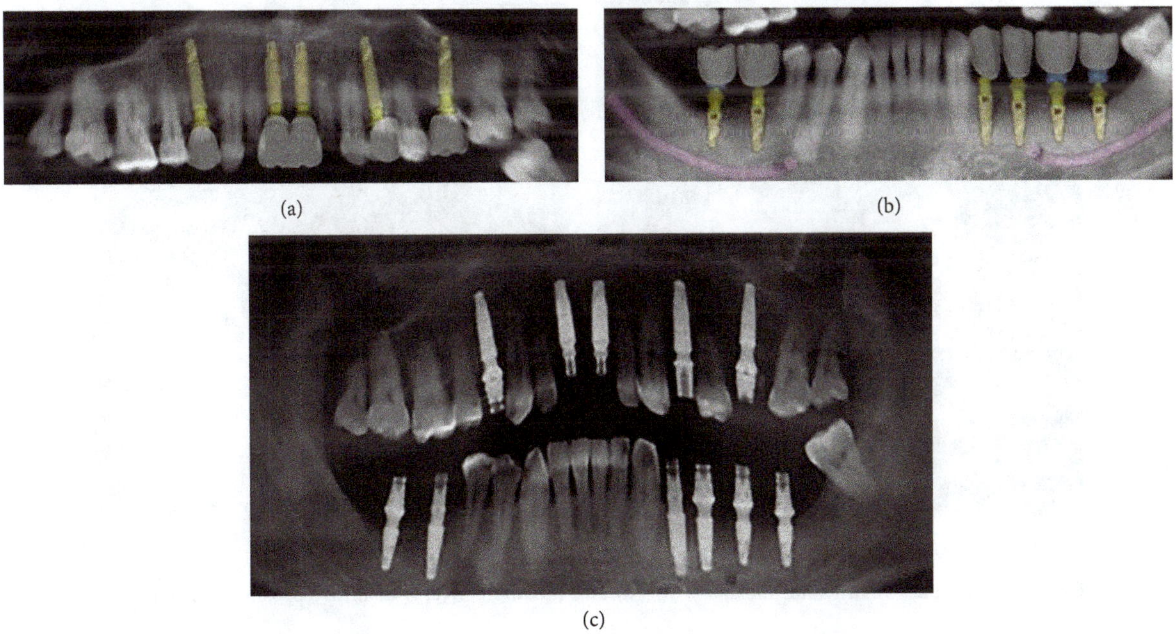

FIGURE 5: Virtual planning of implants and abutments (a, b) and immediate loading panoramic radiography (c).

try-in was conducted with radiographic verification, registration with red pattern resin (GC America, Alsip, USA), and repositioning of the temporaries. The metal copings were correctly positioned on the hybrid analogs in the printed models, with the resin registration and sent to the lab for porcelain build-up. After crownstry-in to adjust contact points and occlusal contacts, they were cemented onto the Tibases and then were installed (Figure 6).

The Portuguese translation of OHIP–14 (Oral Health Impact Profile) questionnaire [6, 7] was used to evaluate the quality of life related to oral health, as a measure of patient satisfaction during the treatment. The patient was

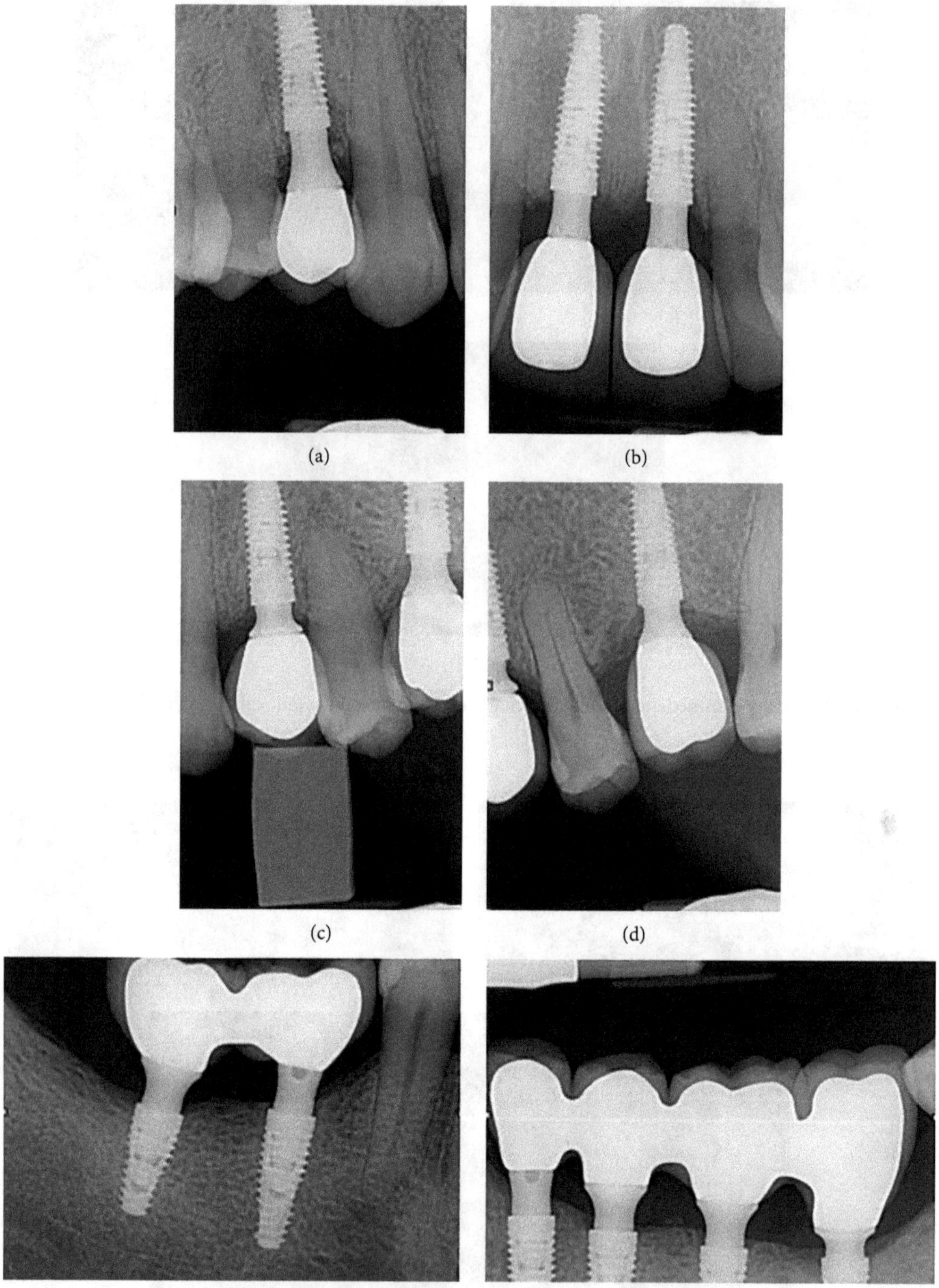

(a) (b) (c) (d) (e) (f)

Figure 6: Periapical X-rays after maxillary (a)–(d) and mandibular (e, f) definitive prosthesis installation.

asked before treatment, and after 6, 12, and 24 months postsurgery, how often, in the prior 6 months, he presented the problems evaluated by the questionnaire.

2.3. Clinical Follow-Up and Outcomes. The advantage of conducting the presented treatment using the guided surgery technique was mainly the ideal positioning of the implants, according to what was virtually planned, through evaluation of the virtual wax-up and available bone volume. Second, the ease and speed for site preparation and insertion of multiple implants, which, in conventional open-flap surgery, would have probably taken up to 4 sessions. Also, by having the virtual planning on the computer, communication with the patient by means of understanding the treatment plan was optimized, and the fascination factor by an innovative technology was decisive for this patient. During the surgery, the flapless technique resulted in little bleeding, the patient reported no postsurgical pain, and no edema was evidenced the days after, as well as other adverse events.

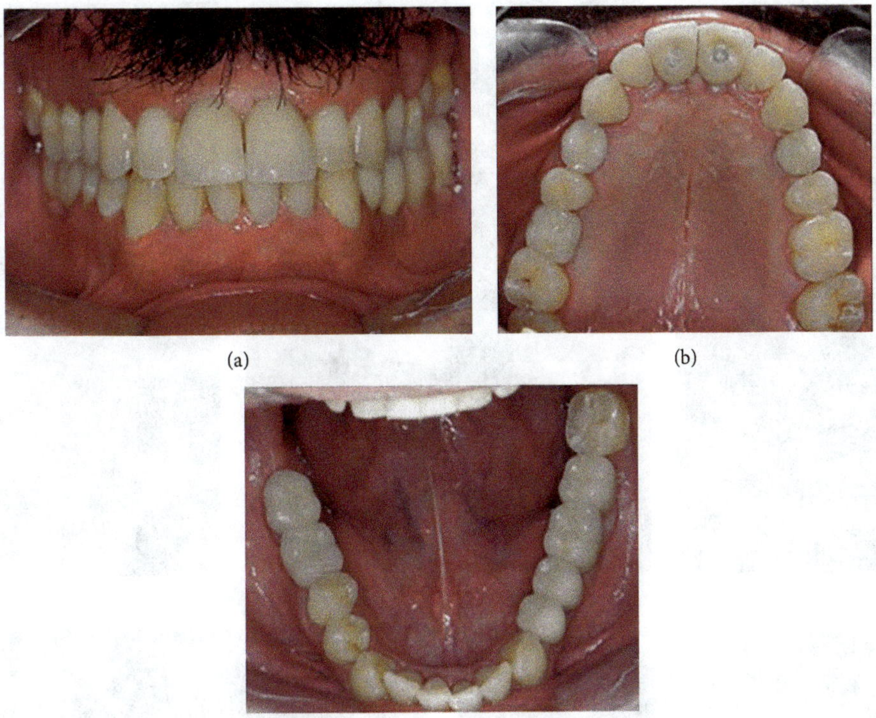

(a) (b) (c)

FIGURE 7: Clinical aspects at 2 years follow-up visit. Frontal view in occlusion (a), maxillary (b), and mandibular (c) occlusal photos.

Regarding patient's satisfaction, at the screening visit, the subject reported to have had fairly often trouble pronouncing words and discomfort to eat. Besides that, life was considered less satisfied by him. Self-consciousness, tenseness, unsatisfactory diet, and embarrassment were reported by him to happen very often due to his teeth problems. Occasionally, the patient has had painful aching in his mouth, according to the questionnaire. Therefore, OHIP-14 score was 14.9, showing how unsatisfied the patient was with his oral health. However, after 6 months of treatment start, OHIP-14 decreased to 0, revealing great satisfaction, which remained at the 2 years follow-up visit.

Also, good aesthetic outcomes remained 24 months after surgery, and soft tissue was clinically healthy (Figure 7). Moreover, no significant bone loss was observed at periapical X-rays, and thereby, all implants were considered as successful (Figure 8).

3. Discussion

The use of virtual planning and digital workflow has shown to improve preoperative planning and patients' comprehension of the proposed procedures, in addition to increased predictability and reduced surgical morbidity [3]. Moreover, the CAD/CAM technology makes a possible complex rehabilitation, like the one presented, to be completed with fewer appointments by anticipating surgical challenges and providing high quality restorations with consistent precision [1]. Also, regarding digital flow time-efficiency, it has been demonstrated that the entire clinical and laboratory process for single-unit crown production can take 16% less time than conventional prosthetic flow [8] Fewer clinical adjustments in digitally produced crowns have also been reported [2] and since these usually demand some time, digital flow can be very helpful, especially in complex cases with several prostheses to be installed.

Even though the present case was a guided surgery, surgeon's experience with conventional open flap free-hand surgeries, as well as passing through a good learning curve in the guided technique, was fundamental for the adequate management of the treatment. The understanding of the various steps and that errors in each step can accumulate and lead to the lack of precision of the final implant positioning, compared to the virtual planning, needs to be considered. First, careful image acquisition and reconstruction of CBCT and scanning, as well as segmentation and superpositioning of these images in the planning software, are performed. Then, adequate virtual wax-up, positioning of implants in relation to the wax-up, and choosing sleeves, followed by the design of the surgical guide, were also performed. After that, the virtual planning should be meticulously reviewed by the surgeon for approval. It is also important to assure careful maintenance of the 3D printer and correct printing and insertion of sleeves in the surgical guide, especially for these not to get loosen during the surgical procedure. Finally, previous disinfection/sterilization of the surgical guide without causing deformation should be made ,and the perfect fit of the tooth supported surgical guide should be verified through the inspection windows.

In comparison to conventional open-flap free-hand surgery, other advantages include during surgery, less bleeding, greater precision, and absence of suture; in the

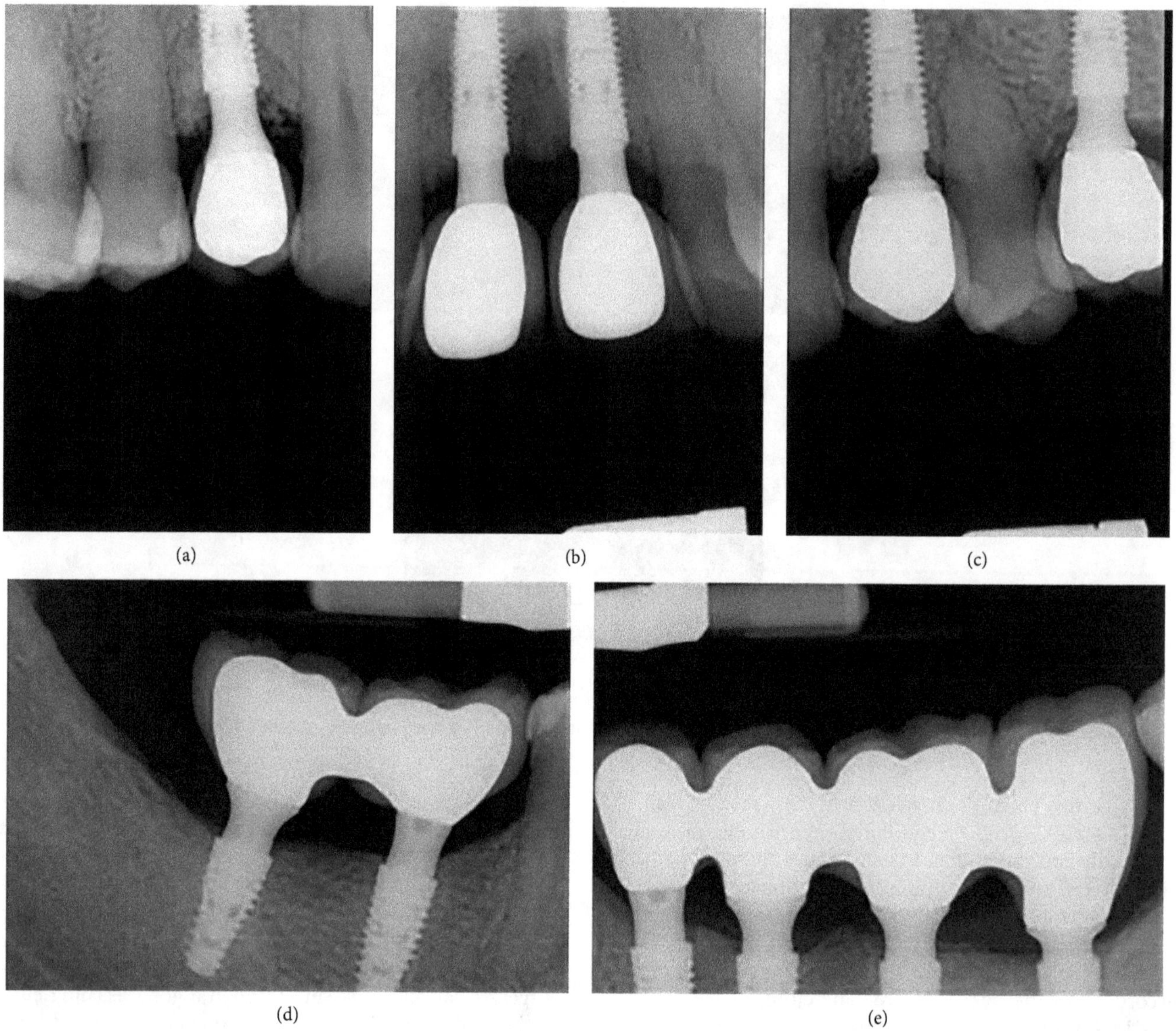

FIGURE 8: Periapical X-rays of maxillary (a)–(c) and mandibular (e, e) implants at the 24 months follow-up visit.

postoperative, less edema and pain, and consequently fewer medications leading to greater patient comfort and satisfaction; and in the healing process, since the periosteum is displaced, maintaining the blood supply, there is less bone and soft tissue, leading to an excellent prognosis and predictability [9], whereas some authors have shown that flapless surgery resulted in less crestal bone loss than when flaps are elevated [10]; other studies have reported that there was no statistically difference in bone loss between different techniques [11].

Flapless surgery has some drawbacks reported in the literature as the real condition of the underlying bone cannot be observed due to gingival tissue not being raised, which could lead to unwanted perforations and fenestration [12]. Another disadvantage that has been discussed is the potential for thermal damage due to reduced access for external irrigation [10]. However, even in the absence of flap, limited vision, and access to the bone bed, none of the aforementioned events occurred in the present case.

Finally, at the screening visit, the patient's OHIP-14 score was very high, revealing that his oral problems had a significant impact on function and social well-being, as reported in the literature [13]. However, after surgery, and being maintained for the 2 years of follow-up, the patient's great satisfaction showed how the implant-supported rehabilitation improved his quality of life.

4. Conclusion

With the use of technology and the digital flow, the prosthetically driven virtual planning for the correct 3D positioning of the implants provided the surgeon with a clear understanding of the outcome of this complex case with multiple implants in both arches, whereas the images generated an efficient communication with the patient. The guided surgery technique for implant placement, combined with the immediate loading concept with immediate provisionalization, brought agility and great comfort to both the patient and the professional. The intra-oral scanning for digital impression and CAD/CAM technology for design and fabrication of the definite restorations contributed to greater efficiency in re-establishing function and aesthetics to this oral rehabilitation case. A learning curve is necessary to understand all the steps involved in the digital flow.

Acknowledgments

The implants and abutments used in this case were provided by Neodent.

References

[1] G. Davidowitz and P. G. Kotick, "The use of CAD/CAM in dentistry," *Dental Clinics of North America*, vol. 55, no. 3, pp. 559–570, 2011.

[2] T. Joda, F. Zarone, and M. Ferrari, "The complete digital workflow in fixed prosthodontics : a systematic review," *BMC Oral Health*, vol. 17, no. 1, pp. 1–9, 2017.

[3] V. N. Viegas, C. Gustavo, S. Lacroix, R. M. Pagnoncelli, and M. G. De Oliveira, *Virtual planning for dental implant placement using guided surgery*, Implant Dentistry: The Most Promising Discipline of Dentistry, London, United Kingdom: IntechOpen, 2011, https://www.intechopen.com/chapters/21560.

[4] G. Orentlicher and M. Abboud, "Guided surgery for implant therapy," *Oral and Maxillofacial Surgery Clinics of North America*, vol. 23, no. 2, pp. 239–256, 2011.

[5] J. S. Santos, T. D. S. Santos, P. R. S. Martins-Filho, N. von Krockow, P. Weigl, and H. Pablo, "One abutment at one time concept for platform-switched Morse implants: systematic review and meta-analysis," *Brazilian Dental Journal*, vol. 29, no. 1, pp. 7–13, 2018.

[6] B. H. Oliveira and P. Nadanovsky, "Psychometric properties of the Brazilian version of the oral health impact profile-short form," *Community Dentistry and Oral Epidemiology*, vol. 33, no. 4, pp. 307–314, 2005.

[7] G. D. Slade, "Derivation and validation of a short-form oral health impact profile," *Community Dentistry and Oral Epidemiology*, vol. 25, no. 4, pp. 284–290, 1997.

[8] T. Joda and U. Brägger, "Time-efficiency analysis comparing digital and conventional workflows for implant crowns: a prospective clinical crossover trial," *The International Journal of Oral & Maxillofacial Implants*, vol. 30, no. 5, pp. 1047–1053, 2015.

[9] T. K. Divakar, S. Gidean Arularasan, M. Baskaran, I. Packiaraj, and N. Dhineksh Kumar, "Clinical evaluation of placement of implant by flapless technique over conventional flap technique," *Journal of Maxillofacial and Oral Surgery*, vol. 19, no. 1, pp. 74–84, 2020.

[10] R. V. Sunitha and E. Sapthagiri, "Flapless implant surgery: a 2-year follow-up study of 40 implants," *Oral Surgery, Oral Medicine, Oral Pathology and Oral Radiology*, vol. 116, no. 4, pp. e237–e243, 2013.

[11] B. R. Chrcanovic, T. Albrektsson, and A. Wennerberg, "Flapless versus conventional flapped dental implant surgery: a meta-analysis," *PLoS One*, vol. 9, no. 6, 2014.

[12] H. De Bruyn, M. Atashkadeh, J. Cosyn, and T. Van de Velde, "Clinical outcome and bone preservation of single TiUnite™ implants installed with flapless or flap surgery," *Clinical Implant Dentistry and Related Research*, vol. 13, no. 3, pp. 175–183, 2011.

[13] P. F. Allen, "Assessment of oral health related quality of life," *Health and Quality of Life Outcomes*, vol. 1, no. 1, pp. 1–8, 2003.

Immediate Placement and Restoration of a New Tapered Implant System in the Aesthetic Region: A Report of Three Cases

Caroliene M. Meijndert,[1] Gerry M. Raghoebar,[2] Arjan Vissink,[2] and Henny J. A. Meijer[1,2]

[1]*Department of Oral and Maxillofacial Surgery, University of Groningen, University Medical Center Groningen, Groningen, Netherlands*
[2]*Department of Implant Dentistry, Dental School, University of Groningen, University Medical Center Groningen, Groningen, Netherlands*

Correspondence should be addressed to Caroliene M. Meijndert; c.m.meijndert@umcg.nl

Academic Editor: Kevin Seymour

Objective. To assess the clinical, radiographic, aesthetic, and patient-centred outcomes of a new implant system applied for an immediate implant placement and restoration approach in single tooth replacement of anterior maxillary teeth. *Material and Method.* Three cases were treated with a bone level tapered implant. All patients were treated with the same strategy involving flapless extraction and implant placement with simultaneous augmentation. Implants were provisionally restored with a screw-retained restoration at the day of surgery. Definitive restoration was fabricated after 3 months. Follow-up was one year after definitive restoration. *Results.* At the 1-year follow-up, the implants were stable and no complications had occurred. Peri-implant bone levels had increased with a mean value of 0.24 ± 0.30 mm between definitive restoration placement and 1 year of follow-up. Clinical outcome scores showed healthy soft tissues. Mean Pink and White Esthetic scores were rated 7.0 and 7.3, respectively. Mean patient satisfaction had improved from 55.7 (pretreatment) to 90.0 (1-year follow-up) on a 0-100 VAS scale. *Conclusion.* Immediate implant placement and restoration with the new tapered bone level implant system are accompanied by good initial clinical and radiographic results as well as high patient satisfaction.

1. Introduction

Implant placement and restorative procedures have evolved into a procedure that can be performed immediately after tooth extraction. This approach is less time-consuming than the conventional procedure and leads to increasing patient contentment [1]. This is especially beneficial in an aesthetically sensitive area like the anterior maxilla. Studies have shown that this procedure has an outcome comparable to the conventional implant placement and restoration protocols [2, 3].

One of the key conditions for the success of an immediate implant placement and restoration approach is primary stability [4]. Primary stability limits micro movement and allows osteogenic cells to adhere to the implant surface, leading to osseointegration [5, 6]. Factors that influence primary stability are the quality and quantity of bone, surgical techniques, and implant design [7]. If osseointegration is achieved, the next challenge is to maintain stable peri-implant hard and soft tissues. This too has been a topic of research. Amongst others, to reduce peri-implant bone resorption, improvements have been made at the implant-abutment connection by platform switching and by using an internal connection type [8]. An internal conical connection is presumed to be accompanied by less peri-implant bone loss compared to either an external connection or a straight internal connection [9, 10].

A new implant line has recently been presented by Straumann. The bone level implant is equipped with a self-cutting thread design and internal conical implant-abutment connection for high primary stability and minimal bone loss in fresh extraction sockets.

The aim of this case series study is to describe three cases with a failing tooth in the aesthetic region (p1-p1) that were

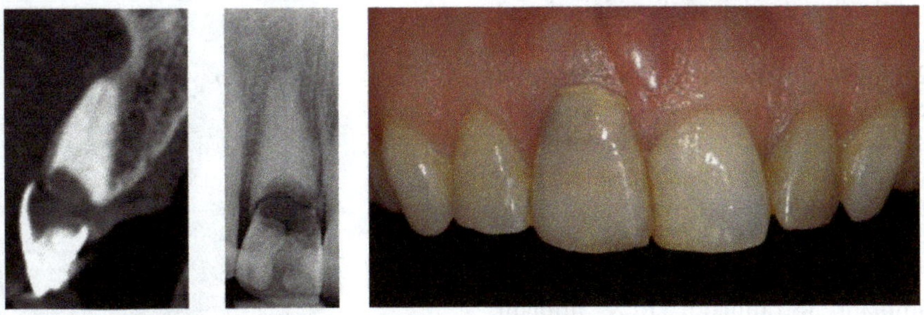

FIGURE 1: Initial situation before treatment of one of the included patients. Note the intact facial bone wall, having at least a thickness of 1 mm in the cervical region.

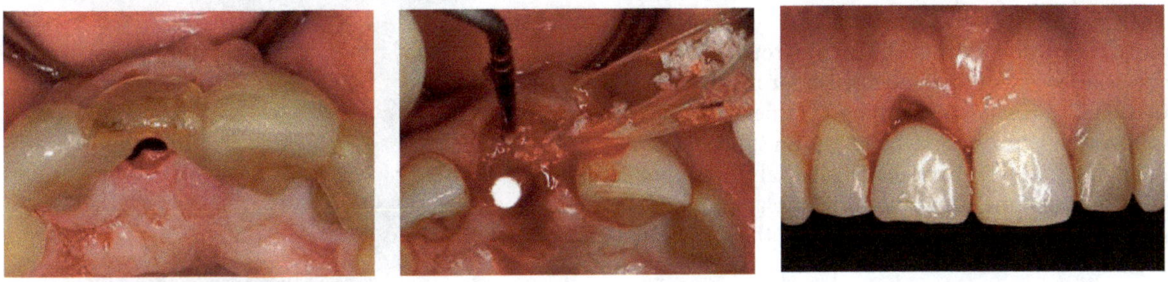

(a) (b) (c)

FIGURE 2: Surgical phase: (a) surgical template in place, (b) bone graft mixture added around the final drill, and (c) restoration at the same day as the implant placement.

treated with this implant system following an immediate implant placement and restoration protocol.

2. Material and Methods

2.1. Study Design. This report describes a prospective case series with a follow-up of one year. Recruitment of patients, implant treatment, and follow-up took place at the Department of Oral and Maxillofacial Surgery of the University Medical Centre Groningen, the Netherlands.

2.2. Patients. Patients were eligible if they met the inclusion criteria: >18year of age, adequate oral hygiene, nonsmoking, no medical and general contraindications for the surgical procedure (ASA score ≥ III [11]), and no periodontal pathology in the remaining dentition, indicated by bleeding on probing combined with pockets ≥ 4 mm. An intraoral radiograph and a cone beam computed tomography (CBCT) were made to determine whether it was likely to expect that the implant would gain sufficient initial stability immediately after tooth removal. Recommendations of Buser et al. [12] were followed concerning immediate implant placement: a fully intact facial bone wall at the extraction site with a thick wall phenotype (>1 mm), a thick gingival phenotype, no acute infection at the extraction site, and sufficient volume of bone apical and palatal of the extraction site to allow implant insertion in a correct 3D position with sufficient primary stability.

Three patients were included: two presented with an irreparable resorption defect in the right central incisor and one patient was referred for a replacement of a fractured left central incisor; (one case is presented to illustrate; see Figure 1). After detailed explanation of the benefits and risks of possible treatment options, the patients chose an implant-supported restoration to replace the failing central incisor. Written informed consents were obtained from the patients before enrolment. All patients were treated following the same immediate placement and restoration protocol as described below.

2.3. After Inclusion. After inclusion, an alginate impression was made and sent to the dental lab where a plaster model was fabricated. An open impression tray was printed based on a scanned version of the plaster cast, and a surgical drilling template was manually produced according to the ideal position of the future crown. The preferred implant position was planned so that the restoration could be screw retained.

2.4. Surgical Procedure. Patients started prophylactic antibiotic treatment one day before the surgery (amoxicillin 500 mg, three times daily for 7 days) and twice a day used a 0.2% chlorhexidine mouth rinse (Corsodyl; GlaxoSmithKline, Utrecht, the Netherlands). After administering local anaesthesia (Ultracaine D-S Forte; Aventis Pharma Deutschland GmbH, Frankfurt am Main, Germany), the periodontal fibers were separated from the tooth after which the affected tooth could be carefully removed without raising a flap. The alveolus was carefully inspected and cleaned of residual granulation tissue. The manufacturer's drilling protocol was followed starting with the needle drill marking the site of implant insertion as dictated by the (semiguided) drilling template (Figure 2(a)). The surgeon ensured that the implant was positioned slightly palatal to the axis of the original root, for sufficient initial stability and ensuring a buccal bone thickness of at least 2 mm in the cervical region. The final implant drill was placed in the osteotomy as a space maintainer during augmentation of the gap between the drill and buccal wall. A 1 : 1 mixture of autologous bone (residual bone chips collected from the burs during osteotomy) and anorganic bovine bone (Geistlich Bio-Oss, Geistlich Pharma AG) was used (Figure 2(b)). Next, the final drill was carefully removed and the implant (Straumann BLX implant, Strauman AG, Basel, Switzerland (Figure 3)) was placed 3 mm apical to the most apical aspect of the prospective clinical crown. The implant was torqued to 45 Ncm. An implant-level open tray impression was made with a vinylpolysiloxane precision impression material (Provil Novo, Medium fast set. Kulzer Mitsui Chemical Group, Germany). The impression was sent to the dental lab for manufacturing the provisional restoration. A healing abutment was placed on the implant. A sterile reabsorbable gelatin sponge haemostat (Cutanplast®, Mascia Brunelli, Milan, Italy) was applied to seal the graft material from the time of placement of the healing abutment until the placement of the provisional restoration.

2.5. Prosthetic Procedure. At the end of the same day, the healing abutment was replaced by the provisional restoration (Figure 2(c)). The provisional consisted of a screw-retained, platform switched titanium stock abutment with an acrylic resin crown. The crown was under-contoured to allow the gingiva to regrow for better aesthetics at final crown stage. The temporary crown was torqued to 25 Ncm and left to heal for 3 months. It was checked that there was no contact with antagonistic teeth during articulation. A CBCT was made to check the implant position (Figure 4(a)).

Two weeks after implant placement and temporary provisionalization, the patients were recalled for checkup (Figure 4(b)). None of the patients reported pain at the time of recall, and only one patient reported having a bruised feeling at the day of implant surgery and one patient reported to have lost a few granulation particles but no major dehiscence was present.

After a 3-month healing period, an open tray implant level impression was made with a polyether precision impression material (Impregum Penta; 3 M ESPE, St. Paul, USA) for the purpose of a definitive restoration. The definitive restoration consisted of a titanium base with zirconium structure and porcelain crown. When the restoration was completed and patients were satisfied, the crown was placed and tightened to 35 Ncm torque and oral hygiene instruction was given. Patients were followed for 12 months after final crown placement (Figures 4(c) and 4(d)).

2.6. Follow-Up. Recall was at 1 month (T_1) and 12 months (T_{12}) after the final restoration was placed. On these follow-up appointments, X-rays were made and clinical variables were measured. Bone level change was measured on a periapical radiograph on the mesial and distal sides of the implant by drawing a line from the implant shoulder to the bone to implant contact point. Change in the midbuccal gingiva level

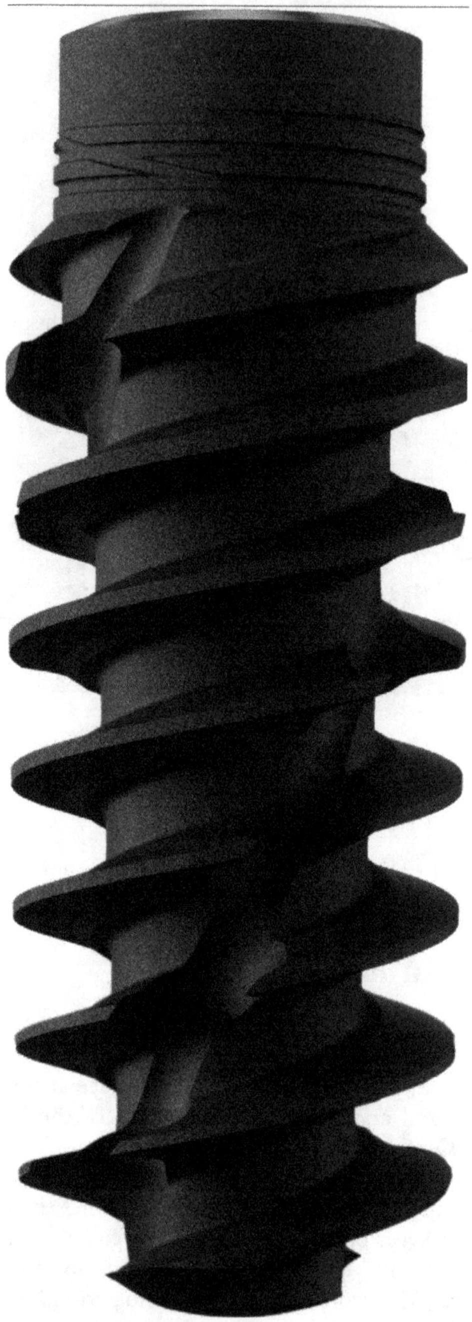

Figure 3: Straumann BLX implant RB. Roxolid® implant material with SLActive® surface. Full tapered core with self-cutting threads, chip flute for redistribution of bone chips, and microthreads on the implant neck to reduce stress at the cortical bone. Conical implant abutment connection (TorcFit™). Courtesy of Straumann AG.

was measured by drawing a (horizontal) line from the top of the midbuccal zenith of both natural lateral incisors and a second (vertical) line was drawn, perpendicular from the horizontal line to the mid buccal zenith of the tooth/implant crown. The length of this vertical line was measured. A periodontal probe was held close to and parallel to the long axis of the implant crown and was used as a calibration [13].

Clinical variables, being the bleeding score (modified Sulcus Bleeding index [14]) and pocket probing depth (using the

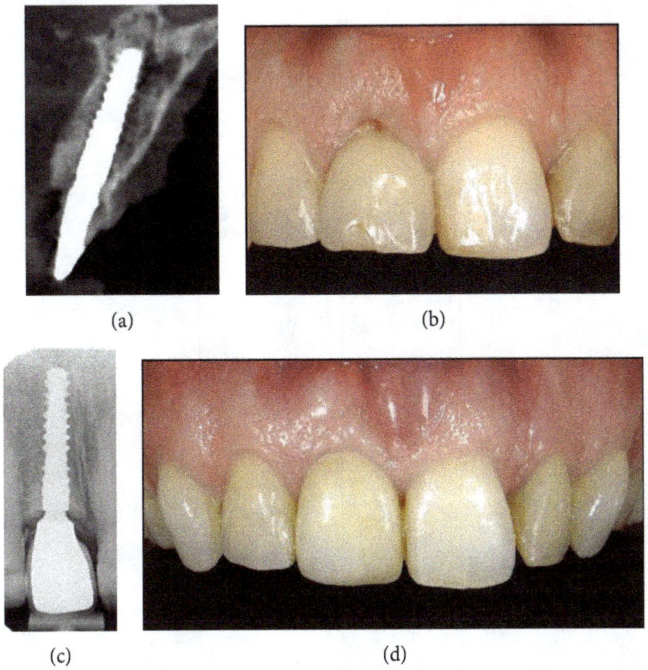

FIGURE 4: (a) Control CBCT at the day of implant placement. (b) Temporary crown 2 weeks after placement. (c, d) Radiographic and clinical images 12 months after definitive crown placement.

Clickprobe with standard pressure of 0.2-0.25 N of KerrHawe Dental Corporation, Bioggio, Switzerland) were scored. Patient satisfaction was scored on a 0-100 mm VAS-scale. Aesthetic outcome was rated on intra-oral photographs using the modified Pink and White Esthetic Score (PES-WES) [15].

3. Results

Results of the outcome measures are depicted in Table 1.

No biological or technical complications had occurred during the whole follow-up time, all implants were stable, and patients were very satisfied with the final result (survival rate 100%).

The peri-implant characteristics of the patient of case 1 started with a gross deviation in midbuccal zenith of 2.24 mm more apical compared to the contralateral incisor. This was improved at the T_{12} measurements, but a slight mismatch of 0.69 mm remained (Figure 5). This did not bother the patient, so no further treatment was initiated. Clinical assessment showed one isolated bleeding on probing at the distobuccal implant site. Pocket probing measured at this site was 3 mm. Radiographs showed high attachment of the bone to the implant up to the implant shoulder.

The peri-implant tissue of patient case 2 showed moderate peri-implant inflammation expressed by a confluent red line on probing, redness, and slight edema of the gingiva sulcus. Pockets were ≤4 mm. Inflammatory signs were also detected at the neighbouring teeth showed by bleeding on probing and slight redness and edema of the sulcular borders and pockets ≤ 3 mm. The patient was pregnant at the time of T_{12} follow-up.

The patient described in case 3 started with no crown to score for PES/WES; therefore, PES/WES was not rated prior to treatment. The patient was very satisfied with aesthetic and functional abilities at the 12-month follow-up. Bleeding on probing was not detected. The periapical radiograph showed good maturation of bone with minimal change in the bone level.

Overall, implant survival rate in the three patients was 100%. The mean bone level increased with 0.24 ± 0.30 mm. The mean PES score improved from score 4.0 at T_{Pre} to 7.0 at T_{12}, WES improved from 3 at T_{Pre} to 7.3 at T_{12}, patient satisfaction improved from 55.7 at T_{Pre} to 90.0 at T_{12} on the VAS scale. No technical or biological complications occurred up to 1-year follow up.

4. Discussion

This case series presents the results of three patients that were treated with the new Straumann BLX tapered bone level implant, immediately after tooth extraction.

After 15 months in function, both patients reported outcome and aesthetic scores were much improved compared to the pretreatment situation. The three patients presented with satisfying hard and soft peri-implant tissues.

Radiographic images 12 months after definitive crown placement (the implants were 15 months in function at this time) show a mean bone level change of $+0.24 \pm 0.30$ mm. de Bruyn et al. reported a bone change of +1.3 mm after 1 year in an immediate implant placement group. They attributed this bone gain to healing of the extraction socket [16]. It is not unlikely that a similar mechanism applies here. The implant is also equipped with features that, in other

Table 1: Clinical, radiographic, and patient-centred outcomes.

	Mesial bone level change (mm) T_1-T_{12}*	Distal bone level change (mm) T_1-T_{12}*	Mean midbuccal gingiva level change (mm) T_{Pre} to T_{12}‡	Mean pockets at T_{12} (mm)	Bleeding score at T_{12}	VAS-score patient satisfaction		PES		WES	
						T_{Pre}	T_{12}	T_{Pre}	T_{12}	T_{Pre}	T_{12}
Case 1	0.00	0.00	+1.74	2.3	1	58	92	4	8	3	7
Case 2	+0.30	0.00	+0.73	3.5	2	56	87	8	8	6	7
Case 3	+0.11	+1.05	+0.32	2.3	0	53	91	na	5	na	8
Mean	0.24 ± 0.15	0.35 ± 0.61	0.93 ± 0.73	2.7	1	55.7	90.0	6.0	7.0	4.5	7.3

T_{Pre} = situation before treatment; T_1 = 1 month after definitive crown placement; T_{12} = 12 months after definitive crown placement; na = not applicable. *Positive value indicates that bone level was increased towards the implant shoulder. Zero indicates bone depicted at or above the implant shoulder at both T_1 and T_{12}. ‡Positive value indicates an incisal displacement of the mid buccal zenith.

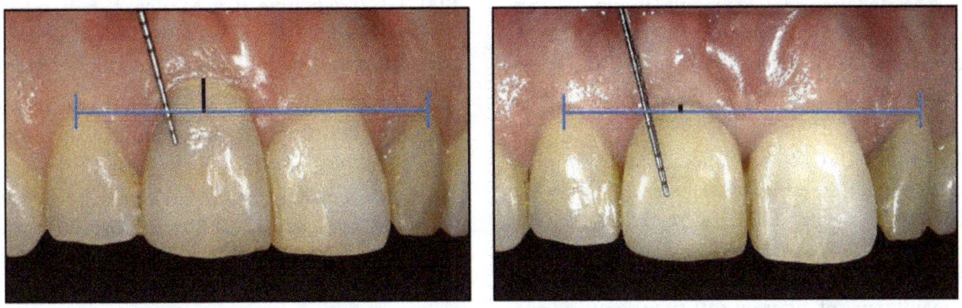

Figure 5: An improvement (1.74 mm) of midbuccal zenith after one year compared to the situation before treatment.

studies, are shown to be favourable in the preservation of cortical bone around the implant, for example, a platform switch [17, 18] and a conical implant-abutment connection [10, 19–21]. There is not much known about the effect of the connection configuration on the aesthetic outcome in the anterior region. Cooper et al. compared three different connection configurations in the anterior region. They found the least bone loss in the conical connection group but found no statistical significant difference in the papilla level change or the PES score. They stated that more research on the effect of implant-abutment interface design is needed [20, 21].

The three studied patients in this report presented with satisfying improvements as expressed in a PES score of 7.0 and patient questionnaire (VAS-scale score of 90.0). This is in line with other studies on immediate placement and provisionalization protocols, where PES scores of 7.5 ± 1.6 [22] and 6.8 ± 1.5 [23] were published on immediate implant placement protocols. All patients reached the threshold of clinical acceptability (score ≥ 6) [15].

One patient was pregnant at the final follow-up and showed signs of inflammation around the implant and other teeth. There is a connection between increased plasma levels during pregnancy and gum disease [24]. Because the same inflammatory signs were present at the neighbouring teeth, it can be assumed that the marginal peri-implant soft tissues are affected due to the pregnancy hormones.

The initial results of this implant are favourable. However, this is a report of three patients followed for a short period of time. Studies with larger population and a longer follow-up are needed to view the stability of the facial hard and soft tissues in the long-term, as various studies have shown that hard and soft tissue alterations can be observed after many years in function [25–27].

5. Conclusion

Within the limitations of this study, it can be concluded that immediate implant placement and provisionalization using this implant have the potential to result in favourable clinical, radiographic, aesthetic, and patient satisfaction outcomes.

References

[1] V. Joshi and S. Gupta, "Immediate implant placement in anterior aesthetic region and assessment using cone-beam computed tomography scan technology," *Journal of International Oral Health*, vol. 7, no. 2, pp. 99–102, 2015.

[2] M. Esposito, G. Zucchelli, G. Cannizzaro et al., "Immediate, immediate-delayed (6 weeks) and delayed (4 months) post-extractive single implants: 1-year post-loading data from a randomised controlled trial," *European Journal of Oral Implantology*, vol. 10, no. 1, pp. 11–26, 2017.

[3] K. W. Slagter, L. den Hartog, N. A. Bakker, A. Vissink, H. J. A. Meijer, and G. M. Raghoebar, "Immediate placement of dental implants in the esthetic zone: a systematic review and pooled analysis," *Journal of Periodontology*, vol. 85, no. 7, pp. e241–e250, 2014.

[4] P. Papaspyridakos, C. J. Chen, S. K. Chuang, and H. P. Weber, "Implant loading protocols for edentulous patients with fixed prostheses: a systematic review and meta-analysis," *International Journal of Oral and Maxillofacial Implants*, vol. 29, Supplement, pp. 256–270, 2014.

[5] D. Rodrigo, L. Aracil, C. Martin, and M. Sanz, "Diagnosis of implant stability and its impact on implant survival: a prospective case series study," *Clinical Oral Implants Research*, vol. 21, no. 3, pp. 255–261, 2010.

[6] R. Smeets, B. Stadlinger, F. Schwarz et al., "Impact of Dental Implant Surface Modifications on Osseointegration," *BioMedical Research International*, vol. 2016, article 6285620, pp. 1–16, 2016.

[7] A. Gill and P. L. Rao, "Primary stability: the password of implant integration," *Journal of Dental Implants*, vol. 2, no. 2, p. 103, 2012.

[8] A. Pozzi, M. Tallarico, and P. K. Moy, "Three-year post-loading results of a randomised, controlled, split-mouth trial comparing implants with different prosthetic interfaces and design in partially posterior edentulous mandibles," *European Journal of Oral Implantology*, vol. 7, no. 1, pp. 47–61, 2014.

[9] T. Koutouzis, "Implant-abutment connection as contributing factor to peri-implant diseases," *Periodontology 2000*, vol. 81, no. 1, pp. 152–166, 2019.

[10] R. Caricasulo, L. Malchiodi, P. Ghensi, G. Fantozzi, and A. Cucchi, "The influence of implant-abutment connection to peri-implant bone loss: a systematic review and meta-analysis," *Clinical Implant Dentistry and Related Research*, vol. 20, no. 4, pp. 653–664, 2018.

[11] E. C. Smeets, K. J. M. de Jong, and L. Abraham-Inpijn, "Detecting the Medically Compromised Patient in Dentistry by Means of the Medical Risk-Related History: A Survey of 29,424 Dental Patients in the Netherlands," *Preventive Medicine*, vol. 27, no. 4, pp. 530–535, 1998.

[12] D. Buser, V. Chappuis, U. C. Belser, and S. Chen, "Implant placement post extraction in esthetic single tooth sites: when immediate, when early, when late?," *Periodontology 2000*, vol. 73, no. 1, pp. 84–102, 2017.

[13] E. G. Zuiderveld, H. J. A. Meijer, A. Vissink, and G. M. Raghoebar, "The influence of different soft-tissue grafting procedures at single implant placement on esthetics: a randomized controlled trial," *Journal of Periodontology*, vol. 89, no. 8, pp. 903–914, 2018.

[14] A. Mombelli, M. A. C. Oosten, E. Schürch, and N. P. Lang, "The microbiota associated with successful or failing osseointegrated titanium implants," *Oral Microbiology and Immunology*, vol. 2, no. 4, pp. 145–151, 1987.

[15] U. C. Belser, L. Grütter, F. Vailati, M. M. Bornstein, H.-P. Weber, and D. Buser, "Outcome evaluation of early placed maxillary anterior single-tooth implants using objective esthetic criteria: a cross-sectional, retrospective study in 45 patients with a 2- to 4-year follow-up using pink and white esthetic scores," *Journal of Periodontology*, vol. 80, no. 1, pp. 140–151, 2009.

[16] H. De Bruyn, F. Raes, L. F. Cooper et al., "Three-years clinical outcome of immediate provisionalization of single Osseospeed(™) implants in extraction sockets and healed ridges," *Clinical Oral Implants Research*, vol. 24, no. 2, pp. 217–223, 2013.

[17] Y. T. Hsu, G. H. Lin, and H. L. Wang, "Effects of platform-switching on peri-implant soft and hard tissue outcomes: a systematic review and meta-analysis," *International Journal of Oral and Maxillofacial Implants*, vol. 32, no. 1, pp. e9–e24, 2017.

[18] F. P. Strietzel, K. Neumann, and M. Hertel, "Impact of platform switching on marginal peri-implant bone-level changes. A systematic review and meta-analysis," *Clinical Oral Implants Research*, vol. 26, no. 3, pp. 342–358, 2015.

[19] S. K. Mishra, R. Chowdhary, and S. Kumari, "Microleakage at the different implant abutment Interface: A Systematic review," *Journal of Clinical and Diagnostic Research*, vol. 11, no. 6, pp. ZE10–ZE15, 2017.

[20] L. Cooper, G. Reside, C. Stanford et al., "Three-year prospective randomized comparative assessment of anterior maxillary single implants with different abutment interfaces," *International Journal of Oral and Maxillofacial Implants*, vol. 34, no. 1, pp. 150–158, 2019.

[21] C. A. Barwacz, C. M. Stanford, U. A. Diehl et al., "Electronic assessment of peri-implant mucosal esthetics around three implant-abutment configurations: a randomized clinical trial," *Clinical Oral Implants Research*, vol. 27, no. 6, pp. 707–715, 2016.

[22] H. J. A. Meijer, K. W. Slagter, A. Vissink, and G. M. Raghoebar, "Buccal bone thickness at dental implants in the maxillary anterior region with large bony defects at time of immediate implant placement: a 1-year cohort study," *Clinical Implant Dentistry and Related Research*, vol. 21, no. 1, pp. 73–79, 2018.

[23] E. G. Zuiderveld, H. J. A. Meijer, L. den Hartog, A. Vissink, and G. M. Raghoebar, "Effect of connective tissue grafting on peri-implant tissue in single immediate implant sites: a RCT," *Journal of Clinical Periodontology*, vol. 45, no. 2, pp. 253–264, 2018.

[24] I. L. C. Chapple, B. L. Mealey, T. E. Van Dyke et al., "Periodontal health and gingival diseases and conditions on an intact and a reduced periodontium: consensus report of workgroup 1 of the 2017 World Workshop on the Classification of Periodontal and Peri-Implant Diseases and Conditions," *Journal of Periodontology*, vol. 89, pp. S74–S84, 2018.

[25] J. Cosyn, A. Eghbali, A. Hermans, S. Vervaeke, H. De Bruyn, and R. Cleymaet, "A 5-year prospective study on single immediate implants in the aesthetic zone," *Journal of Clinical Periodontology*, vol. 43, no. 8, pp. 702–709, 2016.

[26] J. Y. Kan, K. Rungcharassaeng, J. L. Lozada, and G. Zimmerman, "Facial gingival tissue stability following immediate placement and provisionalization of maxillary anterior single implants: a 2- to 8-year follow-up," *International Journal of Oral and Maxillofacial Implants*, vol. 26, no. 1, pp. 179–187, 2011.

[27] S. Raes, A. Eghbali, V. Chappuis, F. Raes, H. De Bruyn, and J. Cosyn, "A long-term prospective cohort study on immediately restored single tooth implants inserted in extraction sockets and healed ridges: CBCT analyses, soft tissue alterations, aesthetic ratings, and patient-reported outcomes," *Clinical Implant and Dentistry Related Research*, vol. 20, no. 4, pp. 522–530, 2018.

Distraction Osteogenesis of Severely Resorbed Mandible

Salah Sakka, Ali Al Rafedah, Nasser Alqhtani, and Adel Alenazi

Department of Oral and Maxillofacial Surgery and Diagnostic Sciences, Prince Sattam Bin Abdulaziz University, Al-Kharj, KSA, Saudi Arabia

Correspondence should be addressed to Salah Sakka; s.sakka@psau.edu.sa

Academic Editor: Asja Celebic

Edentulous patients require an adequate rehabilitation so that the alveolar ridge in the interforaminal region be restored for subsequent implant-supported overdentures. The ultimate goal of distraction is to reconstruct the alveolar ridge to a suitable height and width compatible with Atwood class 2 in an appropriate direction allowing the sagittal interalveolar relation to be normally restored. *Methods.* A 65-year-old man presented with a grade 4 Mandibular atrophy as per Atwood classification which resulted in unsatisfactory treatment with full dentures. Endo-Distractor Krenkel® device was used for anterior mandibular vertical distraction osteogenesis. Four mandibular implants (ITI Straumann, Basel, Switzerland) measuring diameter $\varnothing = 4.1$ mm and length $L = 16$ mm were inserted after the required retention period. Standardized prosthetic treatment was completed with titanium bar retained over dentures. *Results.* A distraction of 11 mm was achieved within 18 days followed by a retention period of 4 months. No signs of infection nor distractor anchorage loosening were detected, and minimal lingual tilting has occurred. *Conclusion.* Distraction is possible on severely atrophic mandibles. The quality of bone reconstruction is satisfactory for both functional and esthetic results.

1. Introduction

Severely resorbed mandibular alveolar ridges are always being a genuine challenge for dentists to attain an adequate oral rehabilitation. Dental implant surgery techniques have been successfully used for the treatment of such dilemma of severe atrophy [1]. However, serious complications were also associated with such treatment approach [2, 3].

In 1992, the concept of distraction osteogenesis was pioneered in oral and maxillofacial surgery for lengthening of the human mandible by gradual distraction [4]. Several clinical cases were then reported [5–7]. Many of the related devices are bulky and anchored by two miniplates which require removal in a second procedure.

In 2009, the Endo-Distractor Krenkel® was presented [8]. The screw of this simple device is anchored in the center of the bony arch and the osteotomized alveolar segment. It gently separates the bony segments gradually to a carefully chosen distance in the decided direction.

In this paper, we present a case of an elderly male patient with severe mandibular alveolar ridge. The Endo-Distractor Krenkel® was used for bone regeneration in order to support a subsequent implant placement.

2. Case Description

A 65-year-old man of nonsignificant medical history presented with a chief complaint of unsatisfactory conventional treatment with full dentures, resulting in severe atrophy of the alveolar ridge. Class 4 Mandibular atrophy was graded according to Atwood classification [9] using preoperative lateral transcranial X-rays. The patient was evaluated clinically and by orthopantomography and cephalograms after the distraction and before placing the implants.

Surgery was done under general anesthesia because of the danger of bleeding in the floor of the mouth. A fully vascularized osteotomy surface is an essential precondition for an optimal distraction osteogenesis, and that was achieved by supraperiosteal dissection of the osteotomy segment. The dissection of the soft tissues was a modified Edlan-Mejchar technique [10]. The only difference was in creating a superior pedicle periosteal flap for coverage of the osteotomy gap (Figures 1(a) and 1(b)).

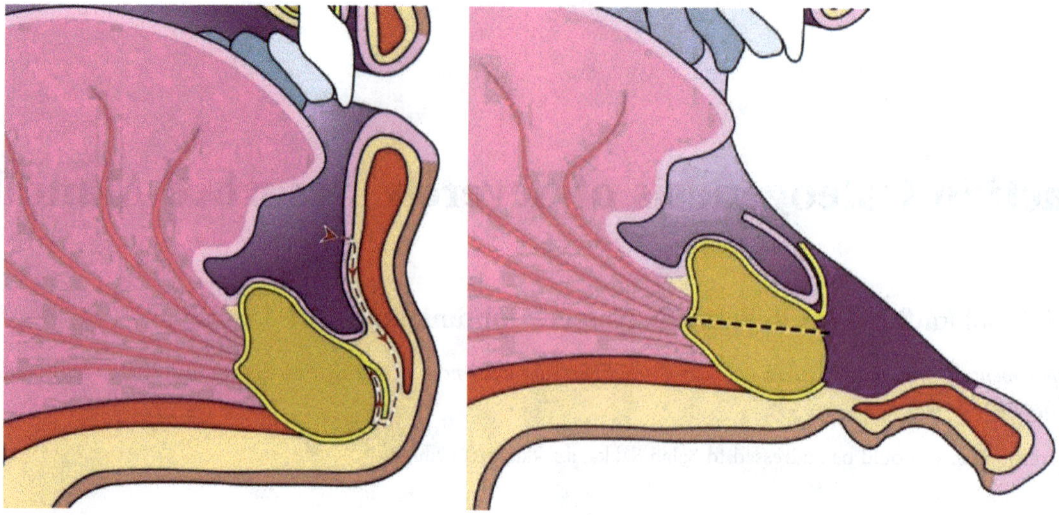

(a) (b)

FIGURE 1: Schematic drawing showing (a) soft tissue preparation technique and (b) deflected tissues after dissection and the osteotomy line.

The next would be the identification of the mental nerves for the lateral extension of the osteotomy. A bone height of 8 mm should be available to obtain segments of 4 mm each. Then, the osteotomy was performed parallel to the lower edge of the mandible (mandibular plane) using a W&H surgical microsaw-blade shape handpiece. According to the planned direction, a tap hole (Ø = 2.0 mm) was prepared in the body of the basal segment for the right-hand threaded distraction screw. In the osteotomy segment, a larger tap hole (Ø = 3.2 mm) was prepared for the left-hand threaded hollow screw. The distraction screw protrudes through the tap hole of the hollow screw 5 mm above the alveolar crest for the use of the screwdriver. The threaded distraction screw was covered by the threaded hollow screw, which is permanently anchored in the marginal bone segment (Figure 2).

The right-hand thread of the distraction screw and the left-hand thread of the hollow implant guarantee the stable fixation of the hollow implant when gradually unscrewing the threaded screw during distraction. The primary osteotomy gap of 3 mm would help in the initial thickness of callus formation.

After surgery, the Endo-Distraction Implant Krenkel® was safeguarded and blocked with a cover screw during the first retention time (Figure 3(a)). The resultant callus formation would predispose for the anticipated distraction osteogenesis.

The distraction period would start postoperatively after the first retention time for 7 days. The ends of the threaded screw are square headed, and each thread has a lead of 1 mm for one full turn.

The patient or one of his relatives did the distraction, exactly as instructed by the surgeon, on an "at home" basis with weekly controls.

The number and the amount of the daily extension movements was increased according to the thickness and stretchability of the newly formed distraction callus. The initial start was for 0.25 mm once a day for the first 8 days which allowed a "soft start." This was necessary for a safe osteogenesis without creating fresh bleedings within the osteotomy gap bearing in mind that the daily distraction distance should not exceed more than one tenth of the momentary distraction gap. The twist movements would be increased up to 2×0.25 mm a day for the next 6 days followed by a period of 3×0.25 mm for 4 days. Thus, a distraction of 11 mm was achieved within 18 days. At the end of the distraction period, the Endo-Distraction Implant Krenkel® is again safeguarded and blocked by the cover screw for the second retention period of 4 months (Figure 3(b)).

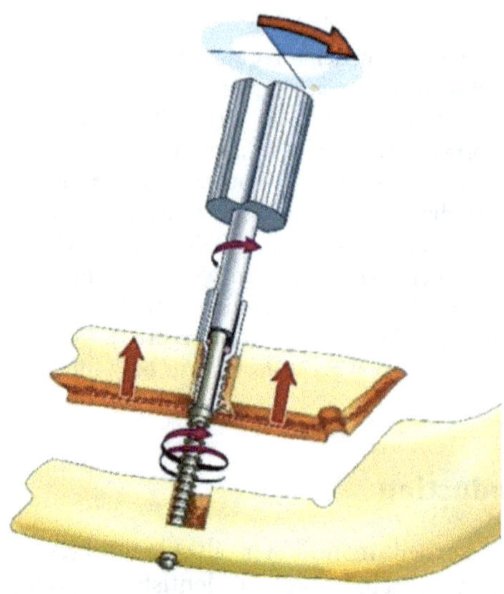

FIGURE 2: Schematic drawing and split image of the Endo-Distraction Implant Krenkel® and its biomechanical function.

No signs of infection nor distractor anchorage loosening were detected, and minimal lingual tilting has occurred. The amount of tilting was assessed by lateral transcranial radiographs with the distraction screw postoperatively and at the end of the retention period.

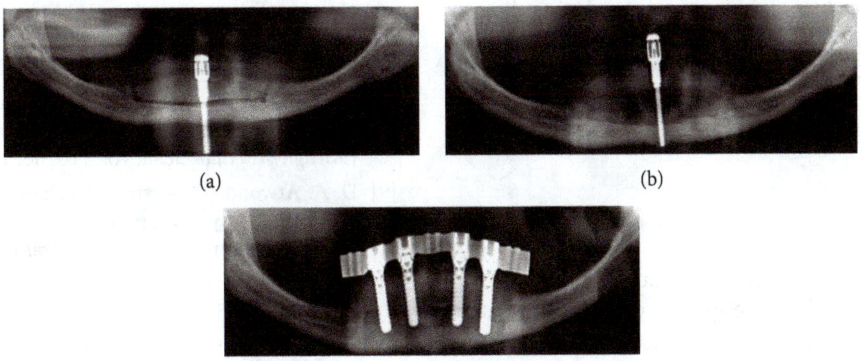

(a) (b) (c)

FIGURE 3: Orthopantomography follow-up. (a) X-ray performed after the placement of the Endo-Distraction device with an initial gap between the osteotomized segments. (b) X-ray showing bone formation after 6 months of retention period. (c) Posttreatment X-ray with fully functional implants connected by a bar.

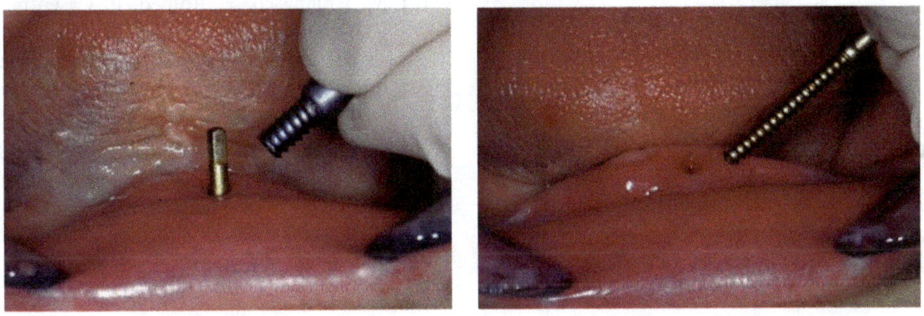

(a) (b)

FIGURE 4: (a) Simple removal of the left-hand threaded hollow screw. (b) Easy removal of the right-handed distraction screw leaving a tiny hole in the mucosa, which subsequently healed.

Perfect preoperative oral hygiene and oral mouth rinsing with chlorhexidine as well as treating with systemic antibiotics for three days are mandatory to prevent the infection.

The device was then retrieved and easily unscrewed as the screws were not firmly osseointegrated (Figures 4(a) and 4(b)).

The patient was scheduled for insertion of 4 mandibular implants (ITI Straumann, Basel, Switzerland) measuring diameter $Ø = 4.1$ mm and length $L = 16$ mm.

Standardized prosthetic treatment was performed with titanium bar retained over dentures. Additional 10-15 mm distal extensions lead the force distributed to the interforaminal implants, protecting the highly atrophic molar region (Figure 3(c)).

3. Discussion

The most important indication for this technique of distraction osteogenesis is a mandible with severe Atwood class 4 to 6 atrophy [11]. It primarily aims to rebuild the alveolar ridge to an adequate height and width consistent with Atwood class 2 in an appropriate direction to restore the sagittal interalveolar relation to normal.

The vertical bone gain obtained by distraction may reach 15 mm in a more "physiological" way than the vertical guided bone regeneration (GBR), without the need for bone grafting, and features less morbidity [12].

Vertical alveolar distraction osteogenesis is not an uncomplicated procedure, and complications can range from fractures of basal bone, fracture of transport segment, breakage of distractor, and lingual displacement of the distracted segment [13]. Conventional distraction devices require secondary surgery for the removal of plates, with repeated dissection of the mental muscles which may jeopardize the esthetic outcome. On the other hand, no need for secondary surgery for removal of the Endo-Distractor device used since the threaded distraction screw and the threaded hollow screw are visible in the oral cavity and the retrieval instruments can be easily used. Lingual tilting of the proximal bone segment is a related common complication of the conventional devices that requires secondary bone grafting before implant placement [14]. In contrast, lingual tilting of the distraction device used in this clinical report was negligible. Moreover, temporary dentures are no longer recommended during the retention time to prevent overloading the system that may induce anchorage loosening of the distraction device [8].

Special attention should be paid to blood supply, especially in the proximal segment, to prevent necrosis and infection. Terminal branches of the sublingual arteries should also be preserved to avoid hemorrhage during dissection and implant placement in the interforaminal region [15]. No other postoperative complications were observed like anchorage loosening of the distractor device, osteomyelitis, mandibular fracture, and implant failure.

4. Conclusion

The results show that alveolar distraction is possible on severely atrophic mandibles. The quality of bone generated was satisfactory for both functional and esthetic results. Surgical difficulty was lesser than with conventional distraction techniques, and the rate of complications was minimal.

Consent

Written informed consent was obtained from the patient for publication of this case report and accompanying images.

Acknowledgments

The authors would like to thank the Prince Sattam bin Abdulaziz University and the deanship of scientific research for their continuous support.

References

[1] M. Cuesta Gil, T. Bucci, B. Duarte Ruiz, and F. Riba García, "Reconstruction of the severely atrophic mandible using autologous calvarial bone graft: an inverted sandwich graft technique and dental rehabilitation with fixed implant-supported prostheses," *Journal of Craniomaxillofacial Surgery*, vol. 38, no. 5, pp. 379–384, 2010.

[2] B. R. Chrcanovic and A. L. Custódio, "Mandibular fractures associated with endosteal implants," *Oral and Maxillofacial Surgery*, vol. 13, no. 4, pp. 231–238, 2009.

[3] M. Almasri and M. El-Hakim, "Fracture of the anterior segment of the atrophic mandible related to dental implants," *International Journal of Oral and Maxillofacial Surgery*, vol. 41, no. 5, pp. 646–649, 2012.

[4] J. G. McCarthy, J. Schreiber, N. Karp, C. H. Thorne, and B. H. Grayson, "Lengthening the human mandible by gradual distraction," *Plastic and Reconstructive Surgery*, vol. 89, no. 1, pp. 1–8, 1992.

[5] A. García-García, M. Peñarrocha-Diago, M. Somoza-Martín, P. Gándara-Vila, and F. Camacho, "Modified LEAD system distractor to prevent tilting during alveolar distraction in the mandibular symphyseal region," *British Journal of Oral and Maxillofacial Surgery*, vol. 46, no. 2, pp. 141–143, 2008.

[6] F. B. Perdijk, G. J. Meijer, C. Krenkel, and R. Koole, "The use of intra-osseous versus extra-osseous distraction devices in atrophic mandibles," *International Journal of Oral and Maxillofacial Surgery*, vol. 41, no. 4, pp. 521–526, 2012.

[7] K. A. Kumar, A. K. Masrom, K. Patil, R. Kunusoth, F. Begum, and V. Venkatesh, "Evaluation of vertical bone gain following alveolar distraction osteogenesis in the anterior edentulous mandible: a clinical study," *Journal of Maxillofacial and Oral Surgery*, vol. 13, no. 4, pp. 539–545, 2014.

[8] C. Krenkel and I. Grunert, "The endo-distractor for preimplant mandibular regeneration," *Revue de Stomatologie et de Chirugie Maxillo-facial*, vol. 110, no. 1, pp. 17–26, 2009.

[9] D. A. Atwood, "Postextraction changes in the adult mandible as illustrated by microradiographs of midsagittal sections and serial cephalometric roentgenograms," *Journal of Prosthetic Dentistry*, vol. 13, no. 5, pp. 810–824, 1963.

[10] A. Edlan and B. Mejchar, "Plastic surgery of the vestibulum in periodontal therapy," *International Dentistry Journal*, vol. 13, pp. 593–596, 1963.

[11] G. M. Raghoebar, R. S. Liem, and A. Vissink, "Vertical distraction of the severely resorbed edentulous mandible. A clinical, histological and electron microscopic study of 10 treated cases," *Clinical Oral Implants Research*, vol. 13, pp. 558–565, 2002.

[12] M. Chiapasco, E. Romeo, P. Casentini, and L. Rimondini, "Alveolar distraction osteogenesis vs. vertical-guided bone regeneration for the correction of vertically deficient edentulous ridges: a 1-3 year prospective study on humans," *Clinical Oral Implants Research*, vol. 15, pp. 82–95, 2004.

[13] T. Günbay, B. O. Koyuncu, M. C. Akay, A. Sipahi, and U. Tekin, "Results and complications of alveolar distraction osteogenesis to enhance vertical bone height," *Oral Surgery Oral Medicine Oral Patholology Oral Radiology and Endodontology*, vol. 105, no. 5, pp. e7–13, 2008.

[14] P. Schleier, C. Wolf, H. Siebert et al., "Treatment options in distraction osteogenesis therapy using a new bidirectional distractor system," *International Journal of Oral and Maxillofacial Implants*, vol. 3, pp. 408–416, 2007.

[15] S. Sakka and C. Krenkel, "Hemorrhage secondary to interforaminal implant surgery: anatomical considerations and report of a case," *Journal of Oral Implantology*, vol. 39, no. 5, pp. 603–607, 2013.

24

The Socket-Shield Technique: Digital Planning, Guided Surgery and Immediate Implant Loading—2-Year Follow-Up

Sušić Mato,[1] Smojver Igor,[2] Stojić Luka,[3] Katalinić Ivan,[2] Gerbl Draženа,[4] and Vuletić Marko[1]

[1]*School of Dental Medicine, Department of Oral Surgery, Zagreb, Croatia*
[2]*St. Catherine Specialty Hospital, Zagreb, Croatia*
[3]*Private Dental Office, Zagreb, Croatia*
[4]*Department of Anaesthesiology & Critical Care, University Hospital Centre Zagreb, Zagreb, Croatia*

Correspondence should be addressed to Smojver Igor; ismojver@gmail.com

Academic Editor: Gianrico Spagnuolo

Anterior aesthetic zone implant placement and tooth restoration can be a quite challenging procedure. Modern technology offers new tools that can help maximize results in both aesthetic and functional ways. The socket-shield technique, as described by Hürzeler et al., boosted with the 3D diagnostics, digital planning, and 3D printing, could provide a valuable alternative to traditional approaches. This case report describes a clinical workflow for an efficient anterior implant-prosthetic restoration.

1. Introduction

Restoring lost frontal tooth can be a complex challenge for every clinician. After the tooth extraction, alveolar bone and adjacent soft tissues start immediate adaptation and remodelation. The labial bone of the upper anterior teeth resorbs relatively fast due to the loss of blood supply from the cancellous bone [1, 2]. This chain of events can impair final aesthetic results of the implant-supported restoration in terms of unpredictable long-term soft and hard tissue margins in regard to the dental crown and the implant neck. Salama et al. [3] demonstrated retaining a tooth root is potentially an effective method of soft and hard tissue preservation. Following this finding, Parlar et al. [4] placed an implant into a previously prepared intra-root space without actually extracting the root itself. Unfortunately, the approach failed due to the lack of osseointegration and connective tissue grown into the space between the implant and the root wall. Hürzeler et al. [5] introduced the socket-shield technique in order to overcome previously described problems. Gluckman et al. [6] further refined the treatment and proposed vertical root sectioning along with mesio-distal cutting into oral and vestibular portions. Probably the main challenge with this relatively new technique is an accurate tooth fragment preparation. A full-thickness flap approach would be useful to gain visual control over the preparation but is not recommended in order to help prevent bone resorption emerging from surgical trauma and temporary loss of blood supply [7]. As previously stated, precision is of paramount importance; proper and precise root segment preparation and implant placement dictate the outcome of the treatment [8]. Digital planning and surgical guides could assist overcoming this issue. With the help of digital technology, one can plan the final crown in advance, prepare temporary crown that can be attached immediately post-operative, and 3D print surgical template to ensure precise implant placement.

This clinical report presents the variation of the socket-shield protocol described by Zhang et al. [9], combining the use of digital planning, surgical guide, and free-hand preparation.

2. Case Report

A 47-year-old patient was referred to our clinic because of a horizontal fracture of the root of tooth #11 without other

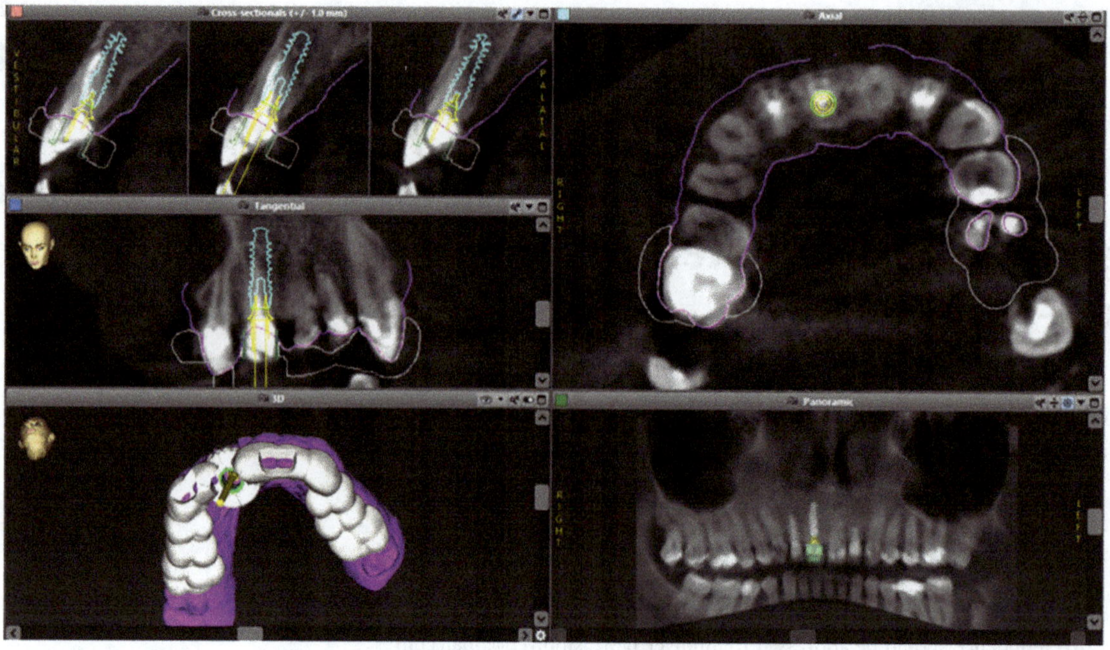

Figure 1: The virtual planning in the specialist software.

medical problems and diseases. In addition to the above, he also wanted to solve the aesthetics of the remaining front upper teeth that had old metal-ceramic crowns (teeth #12, #21, and #22). After the clinical examination and analysis of the cone-beam computed tomography (CBCT) image, an unfavorable horizontal fracture of tooth #11 was confirmed. Two options for prosthetic rehabilitation were offered: (1) a fixed ceramic bridge on the remaining teeth and (2) an implant in position #11 with new individual crowns on the remaining front teeth (#13, #12, #21, #22, and #23). The patient insisted on individual crowns with an implant at position #11. As it was an aesthetic zone, we decided on a socket-shield procedure due to the favorable fracture line and in order to maintain the morphology of the soft tissues in a minimally invasive way. Considering the sensitivity of adequate prosthetic implant positioning in the aesthetic zone and the consequent impact on long-term aesthetic stability, we insisted on a guided surgical implantation procedure. In this way, we used the benefits of both the socket-shield technique in terms of preserving the soft tissue architecture and the guided surgery for prosthetic positioning of the implant and immediate temporary restoration.

2.1. Digital Implant Procedure Planning. In order to properly prepare for implant placement procedure, the coDiagnostiX® (Dental Wings Inc., Montreal, QC, Canada) digital planning software was used (Figure 1). In this software, the CBCT scan exported in DICOM format (Orthophos SL, Densply Sirona, Bensheim, Germany) was overlapped with the .STL file obtained from patient intraoral scanning with the 3Shape TRIOS 3 scanner (3Shape, Copenhagen, Denmark; Figures 2 and 3).

After digital merging of DICOM and .STL files, tooth #11 was virtually extracted, and the implant was positioned bearing in mind the final position of the new crown as well as the root fragment that is to remain inside the alveola after the *in vivo* extraction. Surgical stent adjusted for Straumann BLX SLActive RB implant 4.0 length 14 mm (Straumann Group, Basel, Switzerland) was 3D printed following the virtual design (Figure 4).

2.2. Dental Laboratory Phase. The future implant position has been digitally planned as follows: virtual model export option together with the "Scanbody" implant position has been selected in the CoDiagnostiX planning software (Straumann CARES RB/WB Mono Scanbody, Straumann Group). The (CAM) computer-aided manufacturing design software (3Shape Dental Designer) has been used for temporary crow design. Working model with prepared space for RB Repositionable Implant Analog has been designed with the 3Shape Model Bilder software. The model has been printed with Straumann® P20+ printer using P Pro Master Model Grey/P Pro Gingiva Mask resin (Straumann Group). The temporary crown (Telio CAD LT, Ivoclar Vivadent, Schaan, Liechtenstein) has been made utilising computer-aided design(CAD)/CAM technology. The crown has been cemented on the implant abutment (RB Variobase®, Straumann Group, for Crown AS) with the self-adhesive composite cement (Multilink® Hybrid Abutment, Ivoclar Vivadent). Surgical guide has been 3D printed (Straumann® P20+, Straumann Group) in Pro Surgical Guide resin (Rapid Shape, Heimsheim, Germany).

2.3. Surgical and Restorative Phase. After the application of local anaesthesia (4% articaine with epinephrine 1 : 200,000; 1.8 mL), according to the Zuhr/Hürzeler protocol [5], the fractured clinical crown of the tooth was removed, and the coronal buccal root segment was separated from the rest of the root using a Lindemann surgery bur (NTI, Kahla,

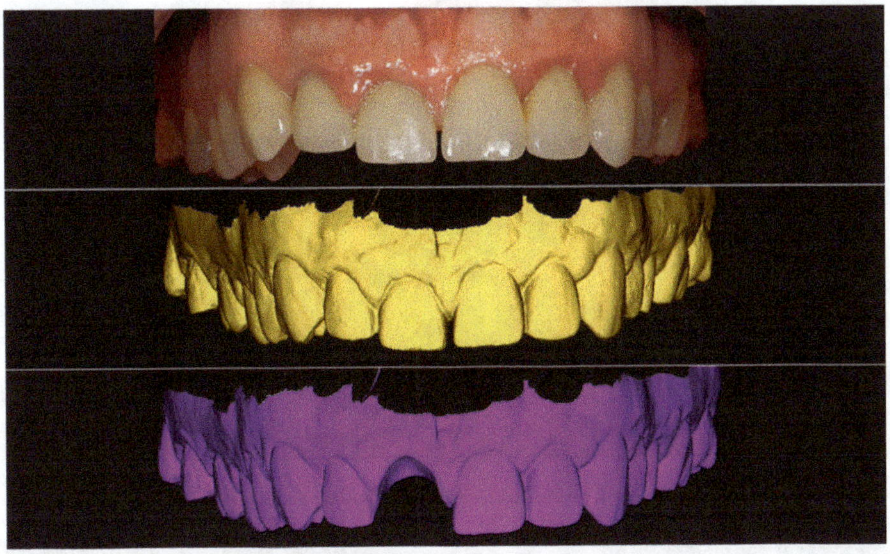

Figure 2: The planning phases overlapped: intraoral starting point—.STL scan of starting position—tooth #11 virtual extraction.

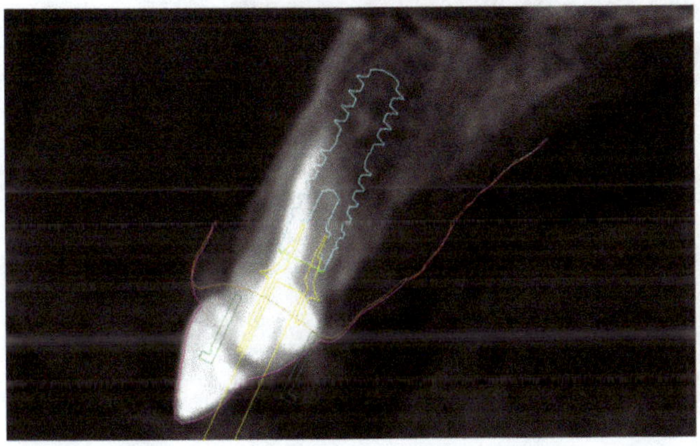

Figure 3: Virtual implant placement planning—superimposition of future implant and the root.

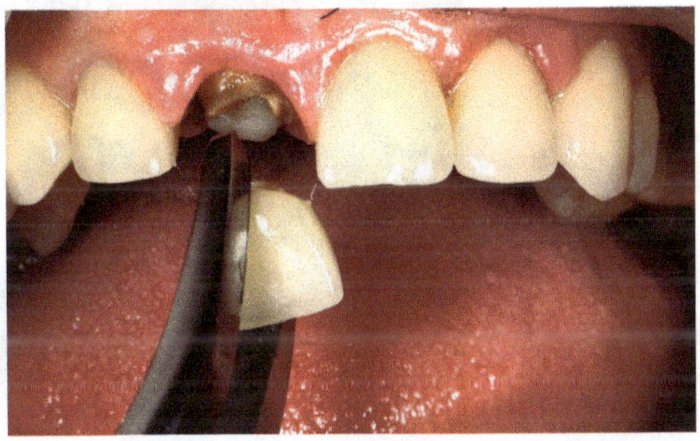

Figure 5: The old crown removal and root preparation/sectioning.

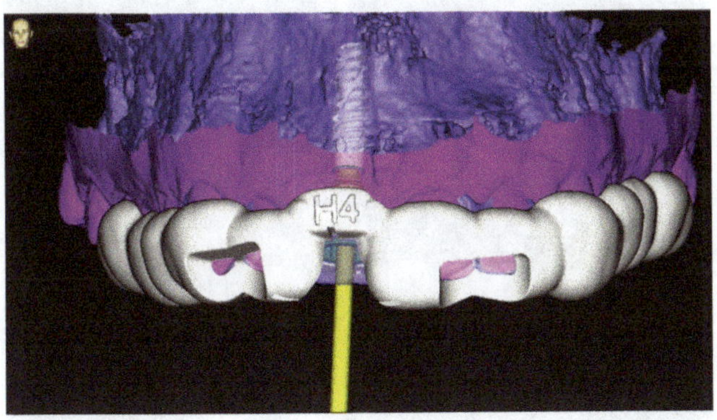

Figure 4: Surgical implant stent digital planning.

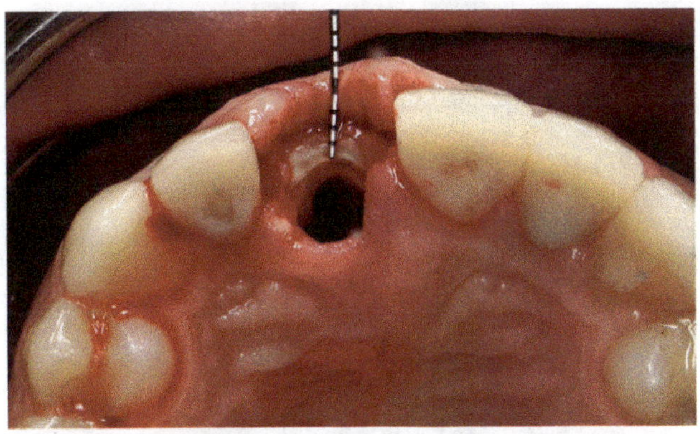

Figure 6: The buccal root "shield" in place after sectioning.

Germany) with the visual aid of light and magnification loupes (Figure 5).

The remaining pieces of the root were removed using a periotome (Carl Martin, Solingen, Germany), without placing excessive stress on the buccal tissues. This resulted in a part of the former root in the area of the buccal bony socket, which was thinned out to a thickness of 2 mm using a round diamond bur (NTI) under sterile saline cooling (Figure 6). Then, implant bed preparation was performed with surgical guide according to the manufacturer's guidelines for BLX full guided surgery (Figures 7 and 8). Before the implant was inserted, a buccal root was smeared with Emdogain gel

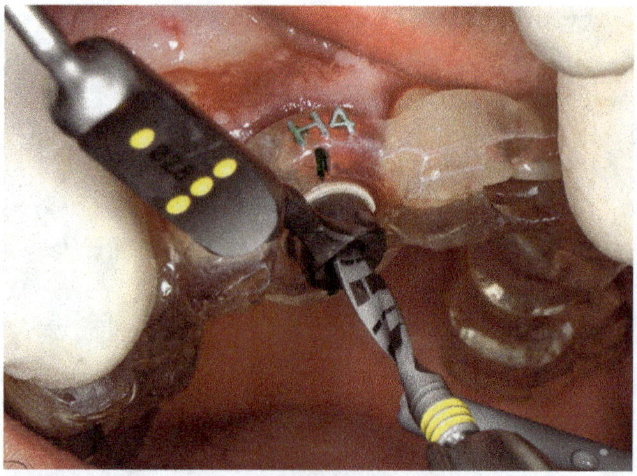

FIGURE 7: The surgical stent-drill guide fixed in place.

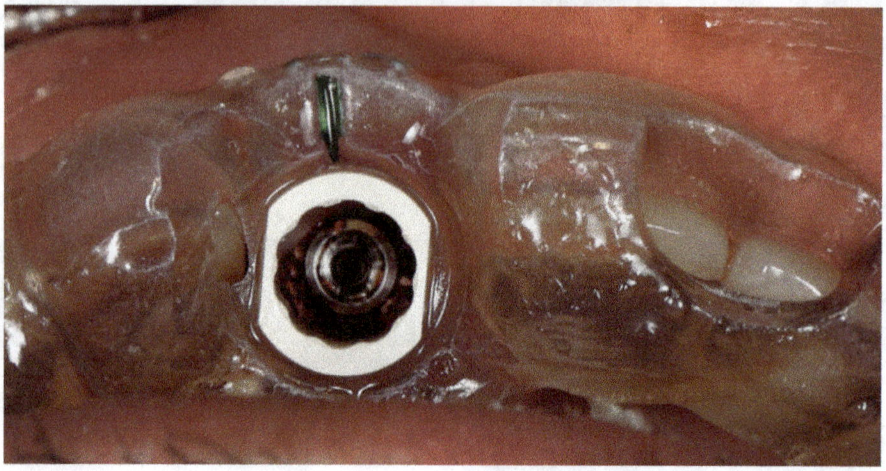

FIGURE 8: The occlusal view through stent.

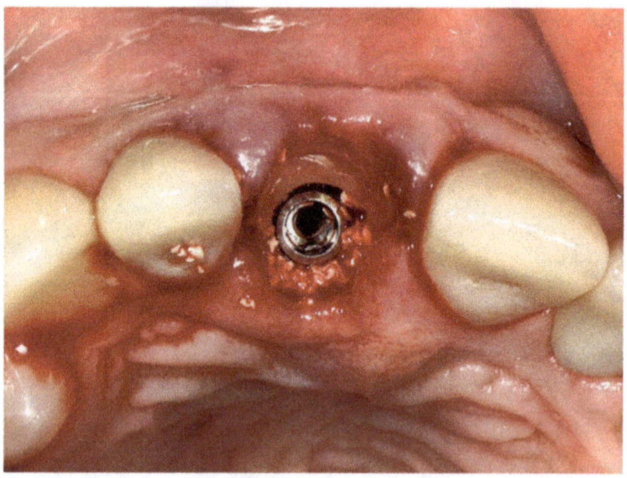

FIGURE 9: The implant in place—socket shield can be observed buccally along with some xenograft material.

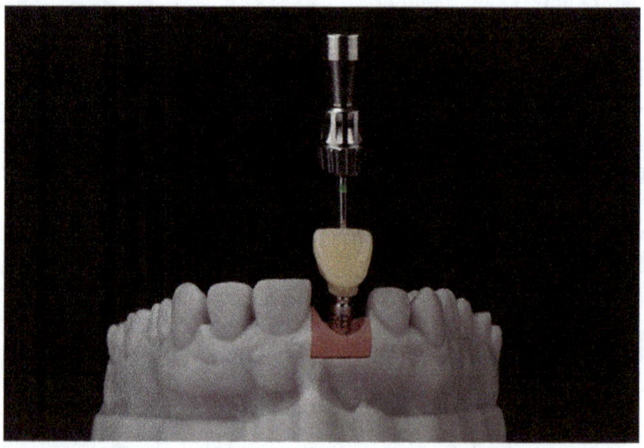

FIGURE 10: The temporary crown on the 3D printed lab model.

(Straumann Group) to prevent epithelial proliferation and bacterial colonization [5, 10], and a microgap was filled with xenograft bone substitute (Straumann Xenograft 0.5 g, Straumann Group; Figure 9).

Temporary crown was fitted, and mesial papilla was repositioned with 5-0 monofilament suture (Prolene, Ethicon, Johnson & Johnson, Somerville, NJ, USA; Figures 10 and 11). Antibiotic therapy (amoxicillin and clavulanic acid) was prescribed for 7 days after surgery for all patients.

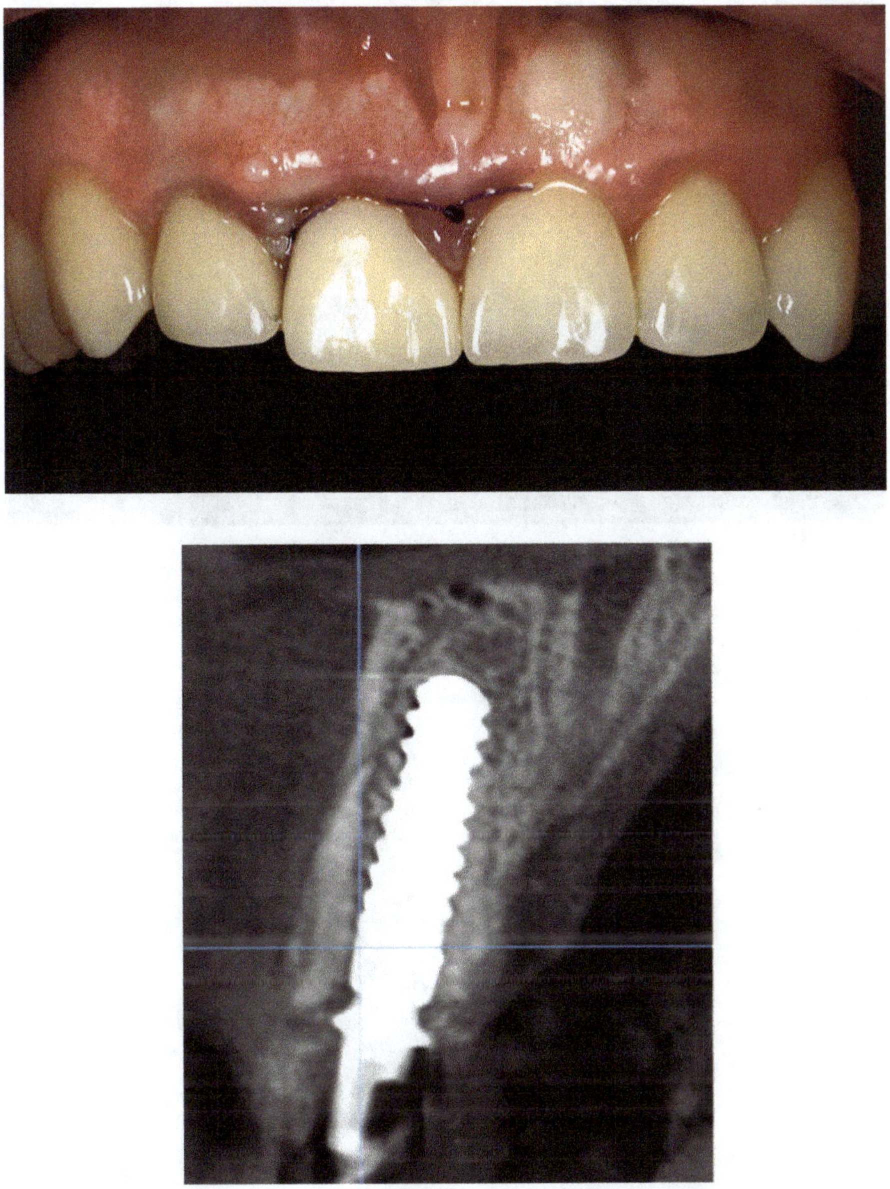

FIGURE 11: Immediate post-operative with fitted immediate crown and CBCT.

After 6 months, teeth #23, #22, #21, #12, and #23 were prepared and crowned, first with temporary crowns (Protemp 4, 3M, Neuss, Germany) and then with lithium disilicate crowns (IPS e.max ceram, Ivoclar Vivadent). The definitive permanent screw-retained hybrid zirconia ceramic crown was made (Zolid Zirconia block—Amann Girrbach, cladding ceramics Celtra Ceram, Dentsply Sirona, Charlotte, NC, USA). Crown has been cemented on the implant abutment (RB Variobase® for Crown AS) with the self-adhesive composite cement (Multilink® Hybrid Abutment, Ivoclar Vivadent; Figures 12 and 13).

3. Discussion

The potential for reducing or avoiding buccal bone loss after the tooth loss has been recorded when opting for conservation of a buccal root portion followed by an immediate implant insertion or so called socket-shield protocol [5]. Preserved root portion retains its periodontal ligament and supra-periosteal attachment, which stabilizes neighboring soft and hard tissues and prevents them from receding [5]. This approach, being a part of a concept called "partial extraction therapies," challenges the well-established "extract and augment" approach [11]. Although it seems quite promising, some complications may emerge during socket-shield protocol. They are mainly connected with improper management of the root fragment and unprecise implant placement. For instance, if there are pulp tissue remnants, an inflammation can occur. If the root fragment is too thin, socket-shield could fracture. In addition, the large contact surface between an implant and a root can cause root fragment migration and lower rate of osseointegration (connective tissue ingrowth) [12]. Free-hand preparation of the root fragment followed by implantation requires rather skilled clinician and good

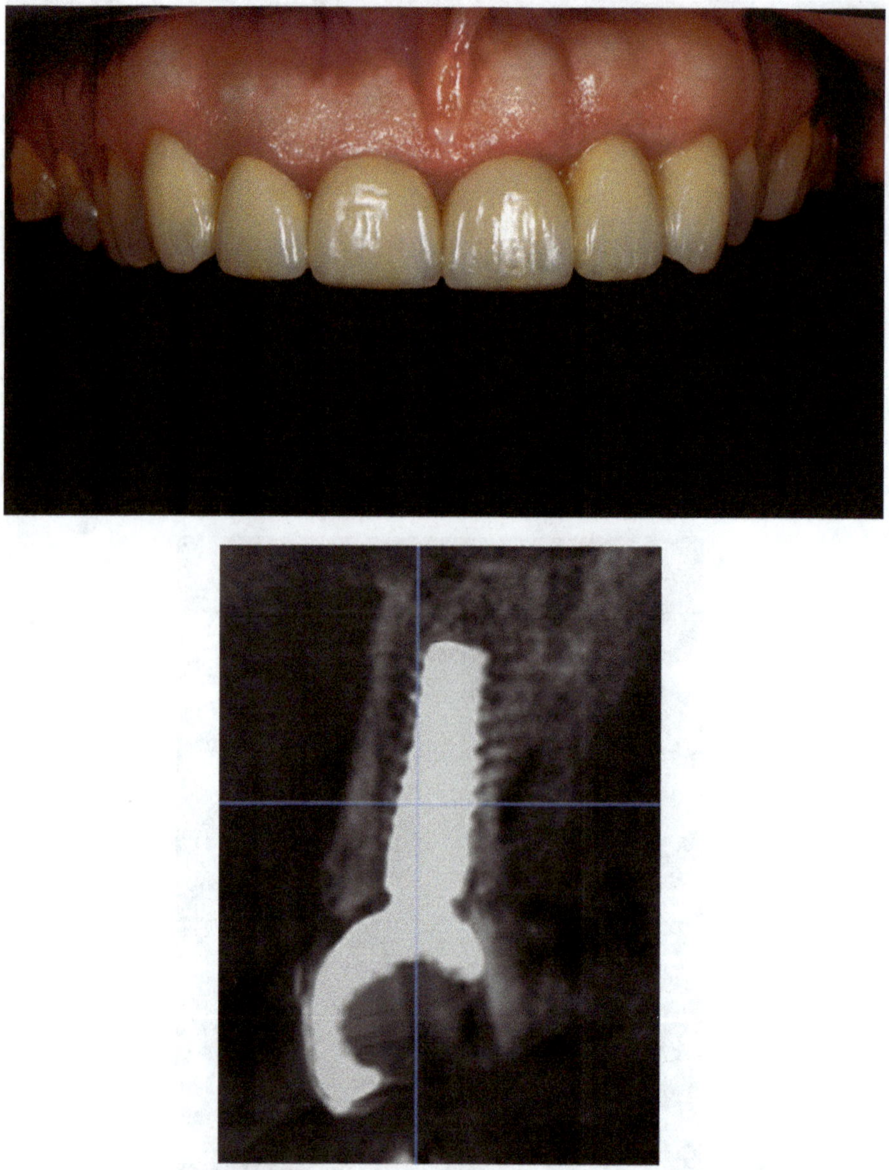

FIGURE 12: The final restoration in place with control CBCT after 2 years post-operative.

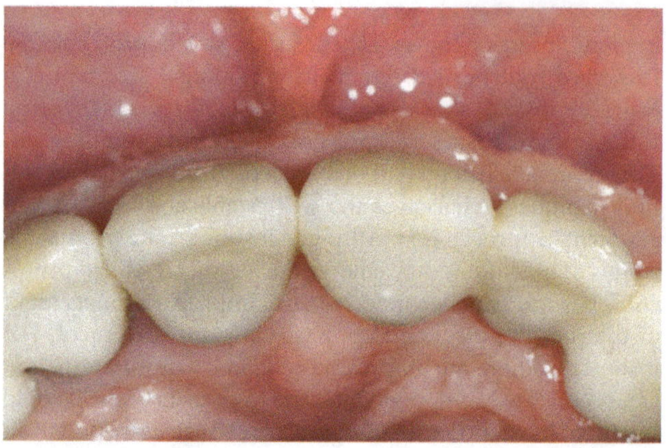

FIGURE 13: The occlusal view on the tooth #11 and the soft tissue adaptation to the final restoration.

pre-operative preparation, also keeping final restoration in mind. The 3D printed surgical guide based on 3D planning is a tool that can help in both properly preparing remaining root fragment and assist with precise implant insertion. In contrast to Zhang et al. [9] clinical case report, we did not use two guides: one for the root fragment preparation and other for implantation. Instead, we have used only one template, which is for an implant placement. In the current case, it was more convenient for the surgeon to adequately prepare the root segment free-handed, due to the need for crown lengthening procedure. In order to shape final aesthetics of the future crown and adjust it to the adjacent tooth, the edge of the bone (the anterior socket wall) was reduced by 1 mm. Thus, the edge of the root fragment was also reduced by 1 mm. Sharp new drills, as proposed by Zhang et al. [9], have been used to minimize the damaging potential on the shield and adjacent tissues. We have chosen Straumann BLX SLActive® (Straumann Group) implant for this specific case. The hydrophilic nano-structured implant surface should increase chances for successful osseointegration as this type of surface supports potent fibrin network formation and mineralization [13].

The implant crown shape, size, and position were also planned prior the treatment, which enabled us to provide the patient with the aesthetic temporary restoration immediately after the implantation. This detail improves predictability of the adjacent soft tissue remodelation. Finally, this modified socket-shield protocol allowed us to achieve predictable and stable results: good osseointegration, proper function, and satisfying aesthetics.

4. Conclusion

The modified socket-shield technique shown in this case, using both free-hand preparation of the field of interest along with the guided implantation based on previous 3D analysis and planning, showed satisfying results in both functional and aesthetic aspects without facing serious complications during or after the treatment.

References

[1] D. E. Cutright, "The proliferation of blood vessels in gingival wounds," *Journal of Periodontology*, vol. 40, no. 3, pp. 137–141, 1969.

[2] B. Le, A. Borzabadi-Farahani, and B. Nielsen, "Treatment of labial soft tissue recession around dental implants in the esthetic zone using guided bone regeneration with mineralized allograft: a retrospective clinical case series," *Journal of Oral and Maxillofacial Surgery*, vol. 74, no. 8, pp. 1552–1561, 2016.

[3] M. Salama, T. Ishikawa, H. Salama, A. Funato, and D. Garber, "Advantages of the root submergence technique for pontic site development in esthetic implant therapy," *The International Journal of Periodontics & Restorative Dentistry*, vol. 27, no. 6, pp. 521–527, 2007.

[4] A. Parlar, D. D. Bosshardt, B. Unsal, D. Cetiner, C. Haytac, and N. P. Lang, "New formation of periodontal tissues around titanium implants in a novel dentin chamber model," *Clinical Oral Implants Research*, vol. 16, pp. 259–267, 2010.

[5] M. B. Hürzeler, O. Zuhr, P. Schupbach, S. F. Rebele, N. Emmanouilidis, and S. Fickl, "The socket-shield technique: a proof-of-principle report," *Journal of Clinical Periodontology*, vol. 37, no. 9, pp. 855–862, 2010.

[6] H. Gluckman, M. Salama, and T. J. Du, "A retrospective evaluation of 128 socketshield cases in the esthetic zone and posterior sites: partial extraction therapy with up to 4 years follow-up," *Clinical Implant Dentistry and Related Research*, vol. 20, pp. 122–129, 2017.

[7] H. Gluckman, K. Nagy, and J. Du Toit, "Prosthetic management of implants placed with the socket-shield technique," *The Journal of Prosthetic Dentistry*, vol. 121, no. 4, pp. 581–585, 2019.

[8] M. Glocker, T. Attin, and P. R. Schmidlin, "Ridge preservation with modified "socket-shield" technique: a methodological case series," *Dental Journal*, vol. 2, no. 1, pp. 11–21, 2014.

[9] X. Zhang, J. Wang, Q. Wan, and L. Li, "Guided residual root preparation for socket-shield procedures: a clinical report," *The Journal of Prosthetic Dentistry*, vol. 124, no. 6, pp. 625–631, 2020.

[10] D. Bäumer, O. Zuhr, S. Rebele, D. Schneider, P. Schupbach, and M. Hürzeler, "The socket-shield technique: first histological, clinical, and volumetrical observations after separation of the buccal tooth segment—a pilot study," *Clinical Implant Dentistry and Related Research*, vol. 17, no. 1, pp. 71–82, 2015.

[11] H. Gluckman, M. Salama, and J. Du Toit, "Partial extraction therapies (PET) part 1: maintaining alveolar ridge contour at pontic and immediate implant sites," *The International Journal of Periodontics & Restorative Dentistry*, vol. 36, no. 5, pp. 681–687, 2016.

[12] C. W. Schwimer, H. Gluckman, M. Salama, K. Nagy, and J. Du Toit, "The socket-shield technique at molar sites: a proof-of-principle technique report," *The Journal of Prosthetic Dentistry*, vol. 121, no. 2, pp. 229–233, 2019.

[13] E. Müller, M. Rottmar, S. Guimond et al. The interplay of surface chemistry and (nano-)topography defines the osseointegrative potential of Roxolid® dental implant surfaces, eCM Meeting Abstracts 2017, Collection 3; SSB+RM (p. 31).

25

Clinical Versatility of the Facility-Equator Implant System as Mandibular Overdenture Retainers

Anna Paula da Rosa Possebon,[1] **Alessandra Julie Schuster**,[2] **Amália Machado Bielemann**,[2] **Ana Paula Pinto Martins**,[1] **Samille Biasi Miranda**,[3] **Otacílio Luiz Chagas-Júnior**,[4] **Luciana de Rezende Pinto**,[2] **and Fernanda Faot**[2]

[1]*Graduate Program in Dentistry, School of Dentistry, Federal University of Pelotas, RS, Brazil*
[2]*Department of Restorative Dentistry, School of Dentistry, Federal University of Pelotas, RS, Brazil*
[3]*School of Dentistry, Federal University of Pelotas, RS, Brazil*
[4]*Department of Oral and Maxillofacial Surgery and Maxillofacial Prosthodontics, School of Dentistry, Federal University of Pelotas, RS, Brazil*

Correspondence should be addressed to Fernanda Faot; fernanda.faot@gmail.com

Academic Editor: Mine D ndar

The use of mandibular overdentures (MO) for the rehabilitation of totally edentulous individuals with limited bone availability is widespread and has proven clinical success. Narrow diameter implants (NDI) are available on the market as MO retainers to solve problems related to limited bone availability and bone thickness, providing a low-cost, minimally invasive treatment option. This technique evolved over the years, and changes frequently involved the number of implants used as MO retainers, as the adoption of a smaller number of implants can generate biomechanical disadvantages, contributing to the increased stress in peri-implant tissues, which may accelerate marginal bone loss (MBL), in addition to reducing masticatory capacity and satisfaction with rehabilitation. Some studies pointed out that the use of 3 or more implants as MO retainers improves the biomechanics. Thus, the objective of this study was to report 3 different clinical cases where 3 or more NDI were adopted to retain mandibular overdentures in association with diverse loading protocols: (i) 3 implants adopting conventional loading, (ii) 4 implants using progressive loading, and (iii) 4 implants with hybrid loading. The case with 4 implants and progressive loading showed a slight worsening of masticatory function at 1 year, in addition to a more pronounced MBL compared to other cases, but with improvements in satisfaction and oral health-related quality of life. Thus, NDI can be used as MO retainers with predictability and clinical success, using different numbers of implants and loading protocols.

1. Introduction

Complete denture wearers often report complaints related to lack of stability and retention, especially of the mandibular prostheses [1]. These complaints are mainly related to bone availability and residual ridge morphology, which are dependent on the severity of bone resorption and the time of edentulism [1]. These factors result in difficulties using mainly the mandibular prosthesis that directly affect quality of life and contribute to maintaining an impaired or deficient chewing pattern [2, 3].

According to the McGill consensus, mandibular overdentures (MO) retained by 2 implants should be the minimum treatment offered to this profile of patients, due to the benefits that this type of rehabilitation promotes, such as increased bite force, decreased discomfort during function, improvements in masticatory function, and neuromuscular control, thus ensuring greater quality of life and patient satisfaction [4]. Several MO retention systems are available and differ mainly in terms of whether or not they use implant splinting. Currently, nonsplinted systems are used more frequently, both in cases of conventional and immediate

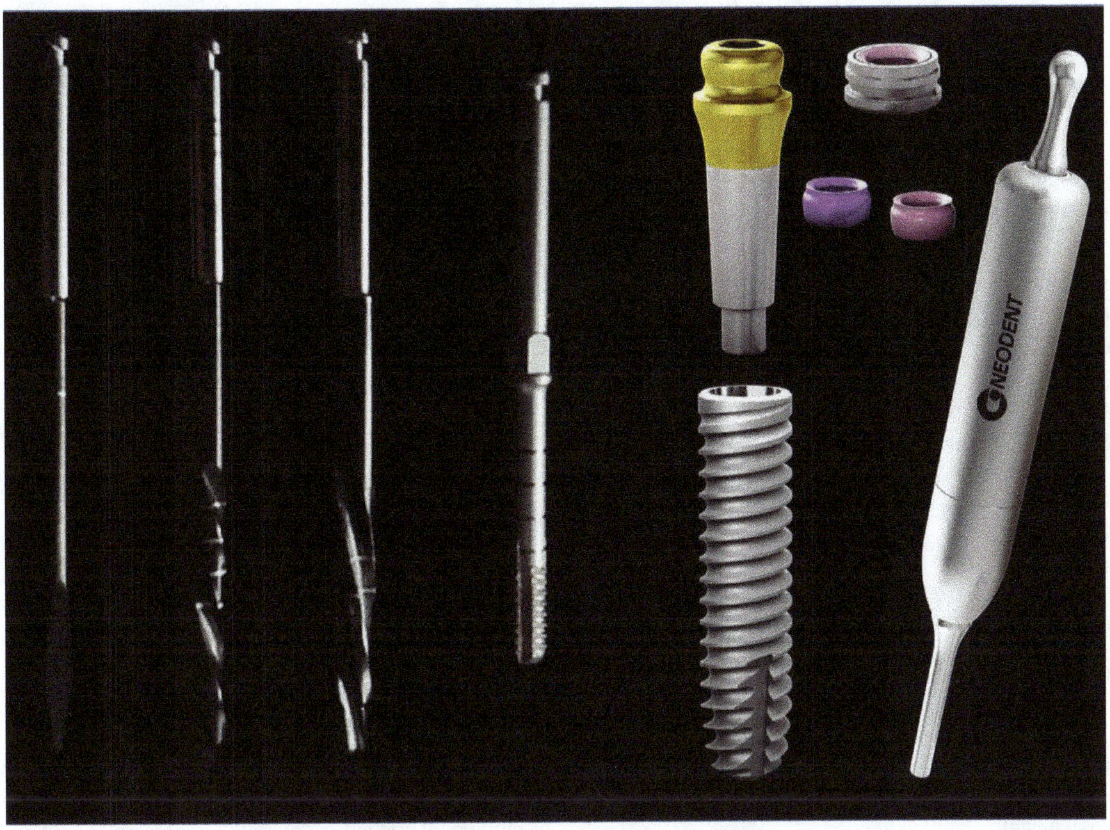

FIGURE 1: The Facility-Equator system. Sequence of drills used for installing the narrow diameter implant (Facility Initial Drill, Facility Twist Drill 2.0, Facility Drill 10, Facility); Facility implant (Ø 2.9 mm × 10,12,14 mm); Facility-Equator attachment, Equator O-ring with Cylinder, Equator O-ring (pink: less retention; purple: more retention), and Facility Abutment Placement Aid.

loading, ensuring treatment with high predictability and safety, in addition to easy handling by the patient and simplified maintenance routine [5, 6].

Narrow diameter implants (NDI) have become an alternative rehabilitation for patients with limited bone availability, especially for elderly patients, guaranteeing the rehabilitation of edentulous patients with residual ridge atrophy, who often could not undergo an extensive surgical procedure with prolonged healing time [7]. The Facility-Equator NDI implant system is available on the market since 2013 and consists of a small diameter implant (2.9 mm) with a 5° Morse cone connection based on frictional retention. Its prosthetic system uses a screwless button-type fitting system that is installed with the help of a hammer (Facility Equator attachment; transmucosal heights range from 1.5 to 4.5 mm) [8]. Previous studies that investigated the predictability and success of the Facility-Equator system [3, 8–11] show that the use of 2 implants leads to excellent clinical and functional performance for the rehabilitation of totally edentulous individuals. However, younger edentulous patients using MO retained by only 2 implants still complain about retention in the posterior region. In this sense, some studies show that the use of 3 or more implants as MO retainers would improve the biomechanics, since MO retained by 2 implants can still present the tendency to move in the anteroposterior direction. Thus, the use of a 3rd or 4th implant would guarantee greater retention and stability, in addition to reducing anteroposterior movement [12–14].

Thus, the objective of this study was to explore the effect of using different numbers of NDI (Facility-Equator system) to retain MO combined with various loading protocols in a series of clinical cases describing the predictability of this system by monitoring clinical, functional, and patient-centered outcomes after 1 year of use. The following combinations of implant numbers and type of occlusal loading were adopted in these 3 clinical cases: (i) 3 NDI with conventional loading, (ii) 4 NDI with progressive loading, and (iii) 4 NDI with hybrid loading.

2. Clinical Case Reports

First, all individuals that agreed to participate in this study were asked to sign an informed consent form. This case series reportfollowed the CARE Guidelines [15]. In all clinical cases, the individuals were nonsmokers, did not have systemic diseases, and were totally edentulous in the upper arch. In the mandible, 1 participant used complete dentures and 2 used removable partial dentures. All patients showed clinically limited bone thickness with Class IV mandibular ridge resorption according to Cawood and Howell's descriptive classification and experienced persistent lack of retention and stability of their mandibular prostheses [16], in addition

TABLE 1: Sociodemographic, clinical, radiographic, and financial data.

Case	1	2	3
Gender	Masculine	Feminine	Feminine
Age	68	59	50
Ethnicity	White	White	White
Profession	Retired (merchant)	Housewife	Guard
Marital status	Married	Widow	Married
Time since mandibular edentulism	1	0	0
Time since maxillary edentulism	5	2	4
Distance between foramens	61.9	52.2	43.6
Cawood & Howell atrophy (anterior height/posterior height)	Nonatrophic (32.5 mm/29.9 mm)	Nonatrophic (25.5 mm/21.3 mm)	Nonatrophic (25.0 mm/19.1 mm)
Wical atrophy (mental foramen evaluation)	Atrophic	Atrophic	Atrophic
Kapur atrophy (clinical evaluation)	Nonatrophic	Atrophic	Atrophic
Main complaint for MO option	Lack of retention and stability of the lower prosthesis	Dissatisfaction with the appearance of the teeth and lack of retention of the lower prosthesis	Dissatisfaction due to pain and discomfort caused by lower prosthesis
Comorbidity	Alcoholic for 20 years and smoker for 9 years	—	Arterial hypertension
Transmucosal height	3.5 mm—left and midline; 2.5—right	2.5 mm—right and left	4.5 mm—right and left
Materials used	3 implants + 3 healing caps + 3 Equator	4 implants + 4 healing caps + 4 Equator	4 implants + 2 healing caps + 4 Equator
Minimum cost (BRL)	720.00	960.00	920.00

to discomfort, pain, and poor masticatory efficiency that led them to stop using their removable mandibular prostheses.

MO retained by NDI (Facility-Equator) was indicated for all patients; 3 or 4 implants were installed between the mental foramen, depending on the patients' preference, desired degree of retention, financial situation, and bone availability. The implant insertion torque determined the type of loading used in the 3 cases: (i) immediate loading was used when the implant insertion torque was ≥32 N, (ii) conventional loading when the insertion torque was <32 N, and (iii) hybrid loading was applied in cases where 4 implants were used and where at least 2 implants achieved the minimum insertion torque required for immediate loading, and the remaining cases were loaded 3 months after surgery. In all cases, implant installation followed the bone drilling protocol recommended by the manufacturer (Figure 1), adopting a minimally invasive technique with a soft tissue flap restricted to the implant area. The procedure was performed by an experienced surgeon (OLCJ). Equator-type attachment was installed with a hammer (Facility Abutment Placement Aid) designed for insertion of prosthetic components through impact (Figure 1). Postsurgical instructions included the use of medication ((i) antibiotic: amoxicillin 875 mg, 1 tablet every 12 hours for 7 days; for those allergic to penicillin, azithromycin 500 mg, 1 tablet every 24 hours for 5 days; (ii) anti-inflammatory: nimesulide 100 mg, 1 tablet every 12 hours for 4 days; (iii) analgesic: dipyrone 500 mg, 2 tablets every 6 hours in case of pain or fever; for those allergic to dipyrone, paracetamol 750 mg, 1 tablet every 6 hours in case of pain or fever). The patients were recommended to eat cold and pasty food in the first 48 hours and to rest and avoid intense physical exercise, spitting, sucking, and exposure to hot sun during the first 48 hours. The sutures were removed 10 days after surgery. Table 1 lists the clinical information and characteristics of all patients in this case series.

2.1. Case 1. The patient presented an ovoid mandibular ridge with a rounded asymmetric residual ridge and a medium muscle insertion. In this case, 3 implants were installed because the patient is younger and requested a higher degree of retention. The patient was unsatisfied with his prosthetic experience after extraction of the lower teeth, as he was unable to adapt to the immediate mandibular total prosthesis in the short period of edentulism (3 months). Conventional loading was applied since no implant achieved the minimum insertion torque of 32 N during installation. Figure 2 shows the radiographic exams performed prior to surgery and those made in the immediate postoperative period and after 1 year (Figures 2(a)–2(c)). Figures 2(d)–2(f) illustrate the adaptation of peri-implant tissues around the healing caps immediately after replacement by Equatorattachments after 3 months of osseointegration. Figure 3 shows the capture

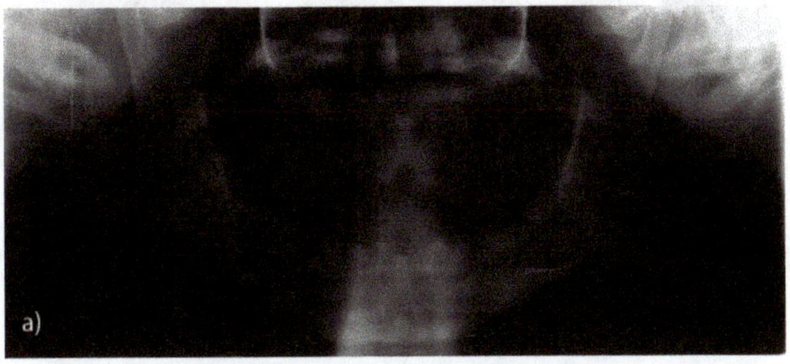

(a)

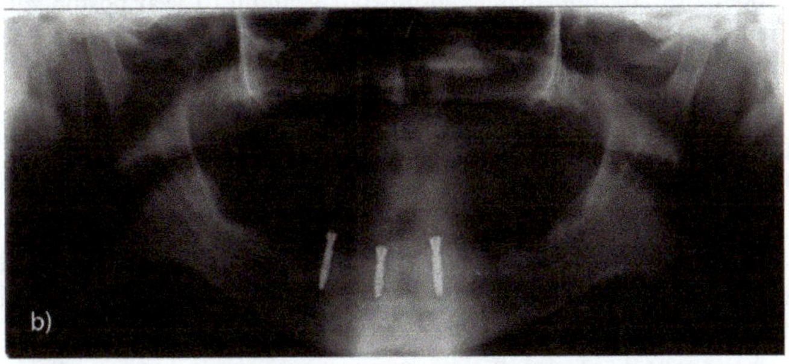

(b)

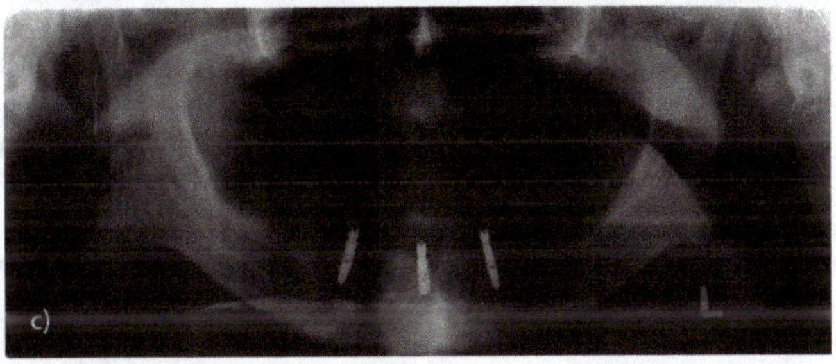

(c)

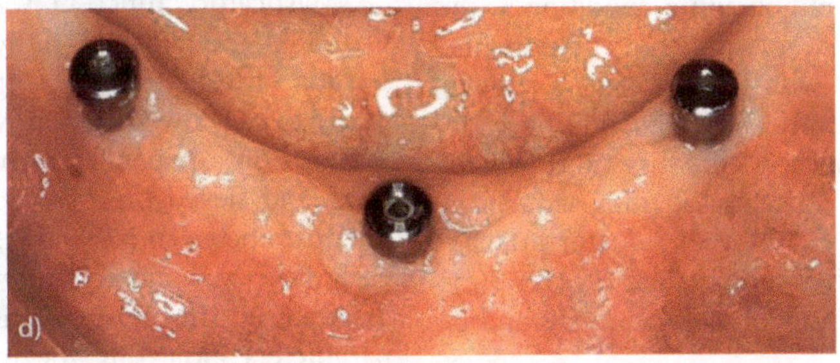

(d)

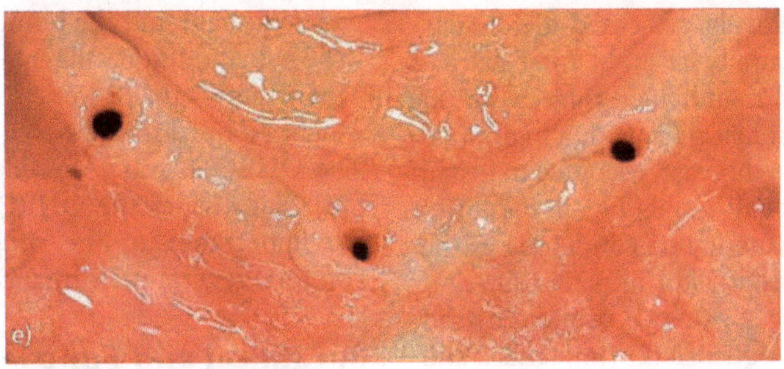

(e)

FIGURE 2: Continued.

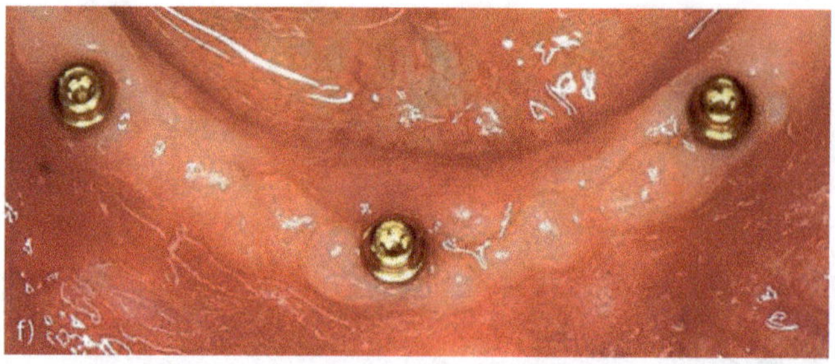

(f)

Figure 2: Panoramic X-rays: (a) preoperative, (b) immediately postoperative, and (c) 1 year postoperative; (d) peri-implant healing after 3 months; (e) tissue condition after removal of the healing caps; (f) installation of prosthetic attachment and adaptation of peri-implant tissues around the Equator attachment.

sequence of each O-ring with cylinder for the loading phaseseparately.

2.2. Case 2. Patient 2 preoperatively presented a Kennedy Class I modification I type mandibular arch. After extraction, the patient had an ovoid mandibular ridge with an asymmetric, rounded residual ridge with a high muscle insertion close to the ridge. In this case, we opted to install 4 implants due to the patient's young age and request for high retention. However, because the patient's lower teeth were extracted at the time of surgery, adequate bone beds for all 4 implants were initially unavailable, so we opted to install implants 2 and 4 first, followed by installation of implants 1 and 3 after 2 months. The type of loading was conventional and progressive. Neither the first 2 implants (implants 2 and 4) nor the last 2 (implants 1 and 3) reached a minimum torque of 32 N, and all implants were thus loaded conventionally after 3 months of osseointegration. Figure 4(a) shows the preoperative radiographic exams; the radiographic condition with installation of implants 2 and 4 with the components installed and implants 1 and 3 with healing caps is shown in Figure 4(b). Figure 4(c) illustrates the final condition after loading all implants. Figure 4(d) shows the surgical timeline. Figure 5 summarizes the clinical occlusal loading sequence: Figures 5(a) and 5(b) show the capture of Equator attachments 2 and 4 three months after surgery, and Figures 5(c) and 5(d) show the capture of Equator attachemnts 1 and 3 three months after surgery 2.

2.3. Case 3. Patient 3 preoperatively presented a Kennedy Class I, modification II type mandibular arch. After extraction, the patient had an ovoid mandibular ridge, with an asymmetric, knife edge-type residual ridge with a high muscle insertion close to the ridge. In this case, we opted to install 4 implants immediately after dental extractions in the lower arch. The bone availability and bone bed conditions at the time of surgery permitted to install all 4 implants simultaneously. However, unlike in case 2, patient 3 received hybrid loading: two implants reached torque > 32 N (implants 2 and 4) and received immediate occlusal loading, while the other two (implants 1 and 3) did not reach the minimum torque and received conventional loading. At the time of surgery, 4 Equatorattachments were installed but only two were immediately loaded. Figure 6(a) shows the preoperative radiographic exams (Figure 6(a1)) and those made in the immediate postoperative period (Figure 6(a2)). Figure 6(b) illustrates the adopted occlusal loading scheme: immediate loading for implants 2 and 4 (Figures 6(b1) and 6(b2)) and conventional loading for implants 1 and 3 (Figures 6(b3) and 6(b4)).

2.4. Monitoring of Clinical and Patient-Centered Variables. Assessments of the masticatory function and oral health-related quality of life (OHRQoL) were carried out before installation and after 1 year of MO use. All individuals had high expectations for the treatment and reported complaints related to masticatory function and showed dissatisfaction with their own oral health and quality of life. Peri-implant health and marginal bone loss (MBL) around the implants was monitored to verify the presence of differences in these outcomes in cases with different numbers of installed implants.

Masticatory function was assessed via the swallowing threshold test wherein individuals chewed a standardized portion of test food (3.7 g Optocal cubes) until they felt the desire to swallow [17]. Afterwards, the chewed material was expelled on a paper filter, dried at room temperature for 7 days, and sieved on a shaker with a sieve stack with sieve apertures between 5.6 and 0.5 mm. The material retained in each sieve was subsequently weighed, and the values were inserted in the Rosin-Rammler equation to calculate 2 parameters indicating the minimum opening of the sieve through which at least 50% of the chewed material would pass (ST_X50) and the homogeneity of the chewed particles (STB). In addition, the masticatory efficiency parameters ME5.6 and ME2.8 were calculated as the percentage of weight retained in the sieves with 5.6 and 2.8 mm apertures. The OHRQoL was assessed using the DIDL questionnaire [18] that divides the OHRQoL into 5 domains relating to the appearance of the prosthesis, pain during use, oral comfort, general performance, and eating and chewing.

3. Clinical and Functional Results after the MO Loading

All patients showed signs of healthy peri-implant conditions during healing and postloading. The patient in case 2 showed the greatest peri-implant bone loss (Table 2). The ST_X50

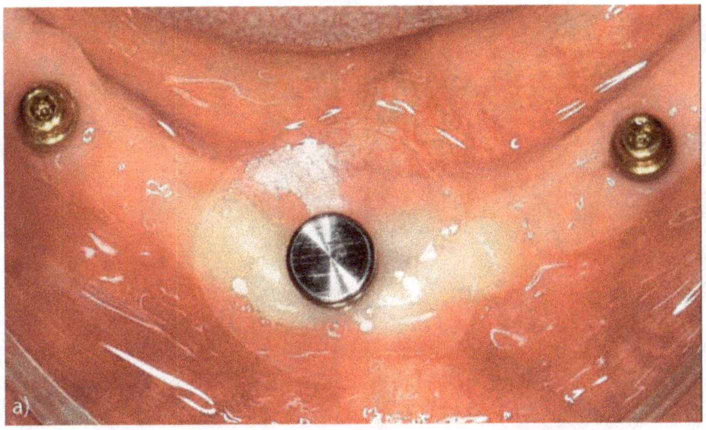

(a)

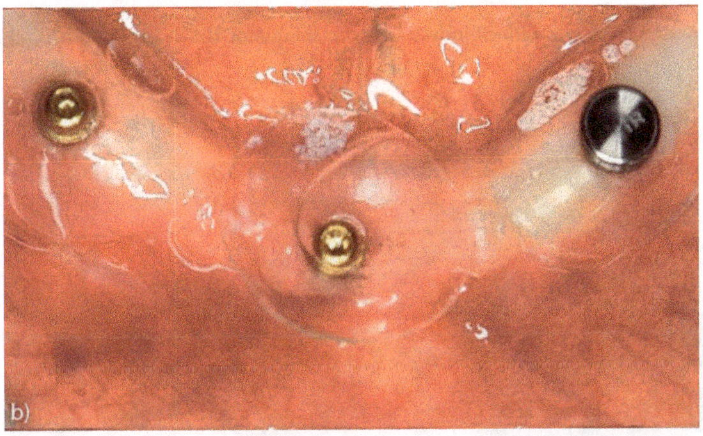

(b)

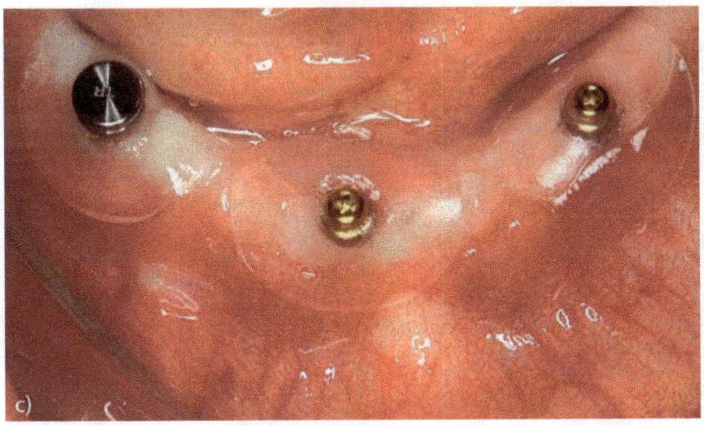

(c)

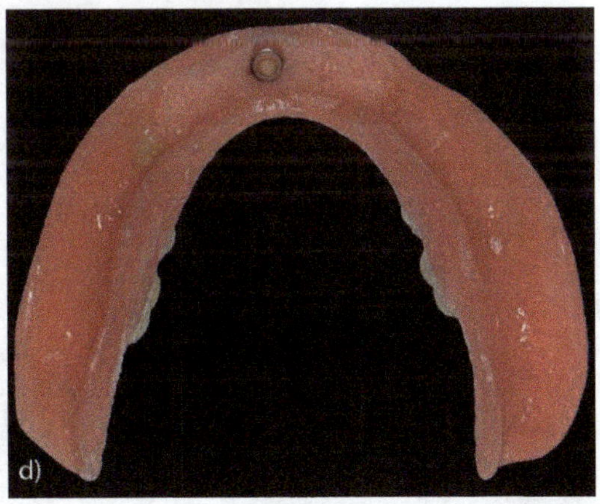

(d)

FIGURE 3: Continued.

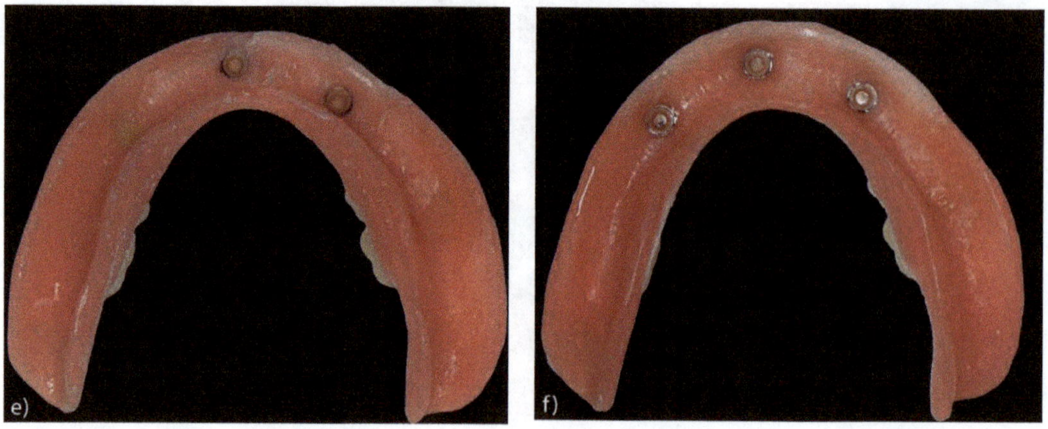

(e) (f)

Figure 3: (a–c) Capture sequence for the O-rings with cylinders; (d) central Equator attachment capture; (e) left Equator attachment; (f) right Equator attachment capture.

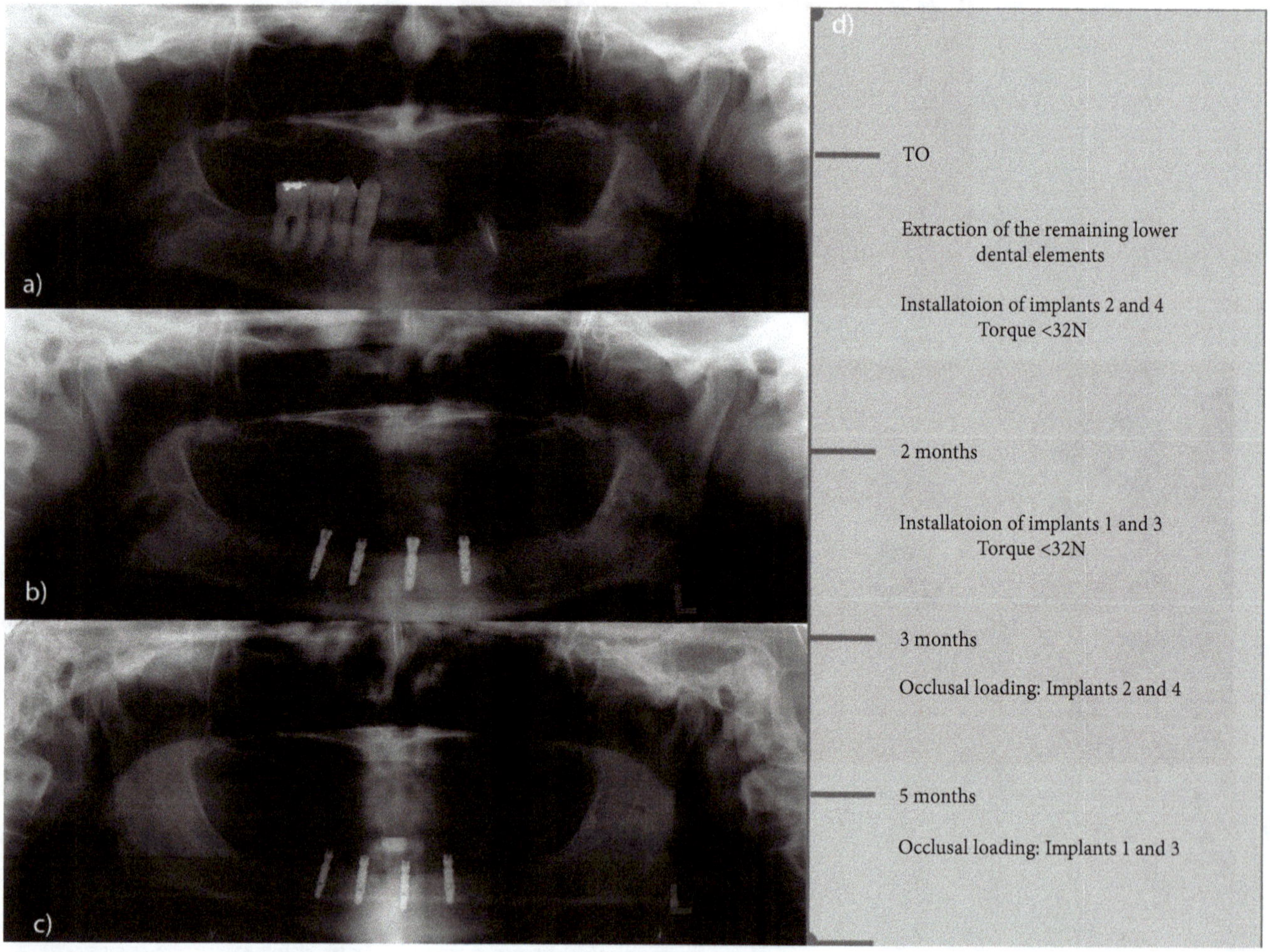

Figure 4: (a) Preoperative panoramic X-rays; (b) panoramic X-rays with installation of implants 2 and 4 (components installed) and implants 1 and 3 (healing caps); (c) final condition after loading all implants; (d) surgical timeline.

values for 2 out of 3 patients decreased, indicating that food trituration improved after 1 year of MO use regardless of the number of implants installed as retainers. The trituration capacity of patient 2 deteriorated slightly (ST_X50 + 4.30%) as well as the homogeneous particle size distributions after 1 year of MO use, as indicated by an increase of 33.82% in

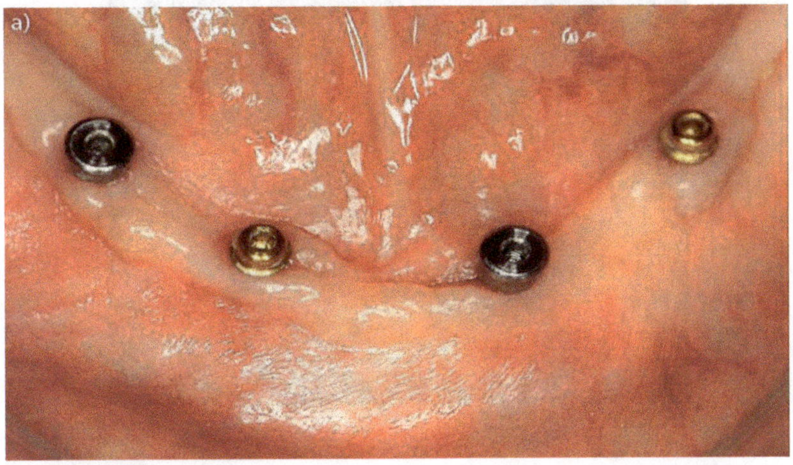

(a)

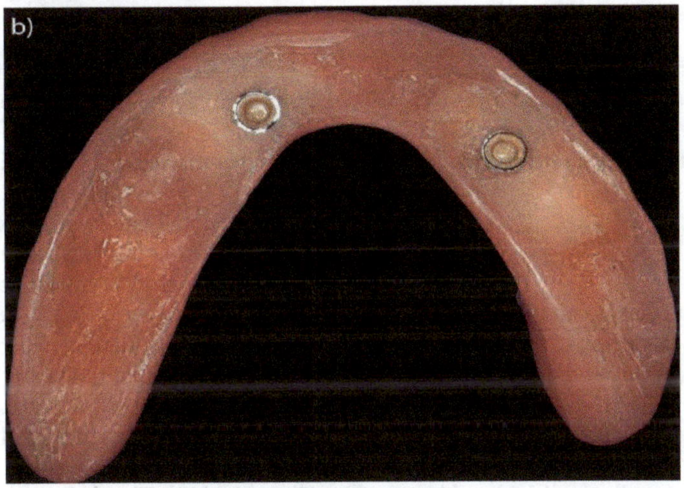

(b)

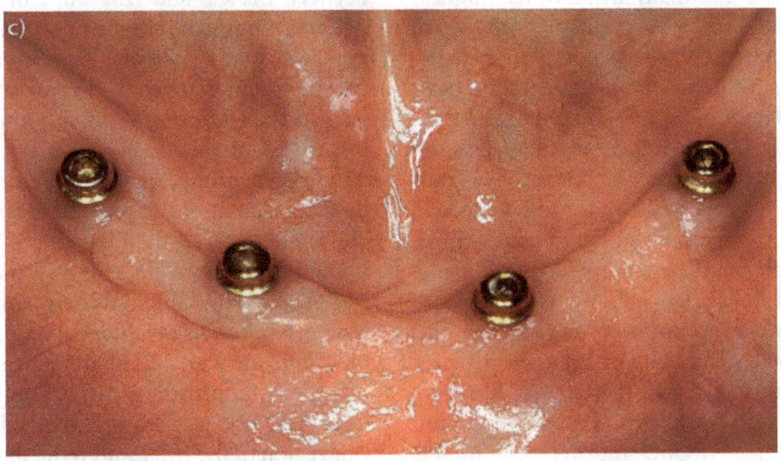

(c)

Figure 5: Continued.

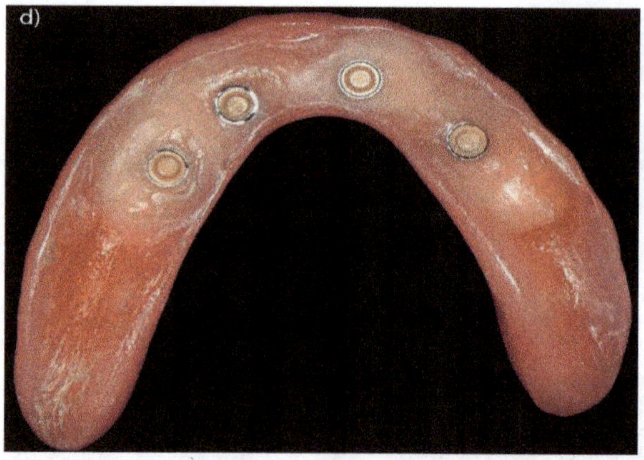

(d)

Figure 5: Clinical occlusal loading sequence: (a) occlusal view of Equator attachments connected to implants 2 and 4 and healing caps connected to implants 1 and 3; (b) base of the prosthesis after capturing the O-rings of implants 2 and 4; (c) occlusal view after installation of the Equator attachments connected to implants 1 and 3; (d) prosthesis base after capturing.

STB (Figure 7(a)). The masticatory efficiency measured by ME5.6 improved in all cases, with the exception of case 3 (Figure 7(b)). All cases reported self-perceived OHRQoL improvements in the oral comfort and eating and chewing domain (Figure 7(c)).

4. Discussion

Treatment with dental implants has become an integral part of modern dentistry, even in challenging situations, such as completely edentulous elderly patients with systemic impairments, long periods of edentulism, mandibular bone atrophy, and/or poor-quality bone. The specialized literature shows that MO use for rehabilitation of totally edentulous individuals with low bone availability is well established and has satisfactory success and survival rates alongside a major positive impact on patients' quality of life [10, 19, 20]. MO treatment benefits from fast, low-cost minimally invasive techniques, and these have been undergoing innovations over the years [4]. Narrow diameter implant (NDI) systems designed for rehabilitation of patients with low bone availability have recently been studied to determine short- and long-term predictability and the maintenance regime required. A systematic review [7] showed that NDI have a 98% survival rate and a 96% success rate in up to 4 years, indicating that NDI are a safe treatment option with excellent long-term predictability and are thus a viable option to improve retention and stability of complete dentures [21].

Studies of this research group that investigated the Facility-Equator NDI system have observed that patients show a fast and significant increase in masticatory function 30 days after installation of 2 implant-retained MO; after three months, there is an OHRQoL improvement in the functional, oral comfort, and psychosocial domains [10, 11]. We also investigated the influence of anteroposterior discrepancies on the masticatory function and found that only Class II patients still had masticatory difficulties after 1 year of MO use [3]. While bone remodeling values of -0.06 ± 0.64 mm indicate that MBL 1 year after implant placement was similar to the MBL immediately after implant placement, dislodgements of the prosthetic and surgical components were the most common prosthetic complications [8]. In addition, monitoring clinical peri-implant health-related parameters, smoking habit, and time since edentulism in patients rehabilitated with this NDI system is important, as they can predict implant success rates [22].

The biological performance of the Facility-Equator system in the early and late osseointegration period was also evaluated according to conventional loading (CL) and immediate loading (IL) [23]. During the initial 3-month period, IL implants were associated with a smaller and thus more favorable probing depth than CL implants, while inflammatory markers such as TNF-α and IL-1β were more stable in the CC group [23]. The drilling depth remained lower in the IL group until 1 year after loading, and no significant differences in MBL, masticatory function, and OHRQoL were found between the CL and IL groups in this period. However, IL patients require more time to acquire similar chewing performance than CL patients. The survival rates and number of prosthetic intercurrences were also similar in both groups: 90% in the CL group (2 losses) and 85% in the IL group (3 losses); 33 prosthetic events occurred in the CL group and 23 in the IL group, mainly Equator dislodgements, followed by replacement of the prosthetic abutment [24].

There is currently a tendency to increase the number of implants used to retain MO, as some studies have shown that MO retained by 2 implants between the mental foramen have biomechanical disadvantages compared to MO retained by 3 or 4 implants, as 2 implants permit anteroposterior movements of the prosthesis, increasing the tension around the implants [13], accelerating MBL and bone loss in the posterior region of the ridge and reducing the masticatory capacity and satisfaction with the rehabilitation [12, 13, 25]. However, individual results can deviate strongly from such general tendencies. Cases 1 and 3 all show marked improvements in both food trituration and food homogenization and in the percentage of retention in the 5.6 and 2.8 mm sieves. Meanwhile, case 2 with MO retained by 4 progressively loaded

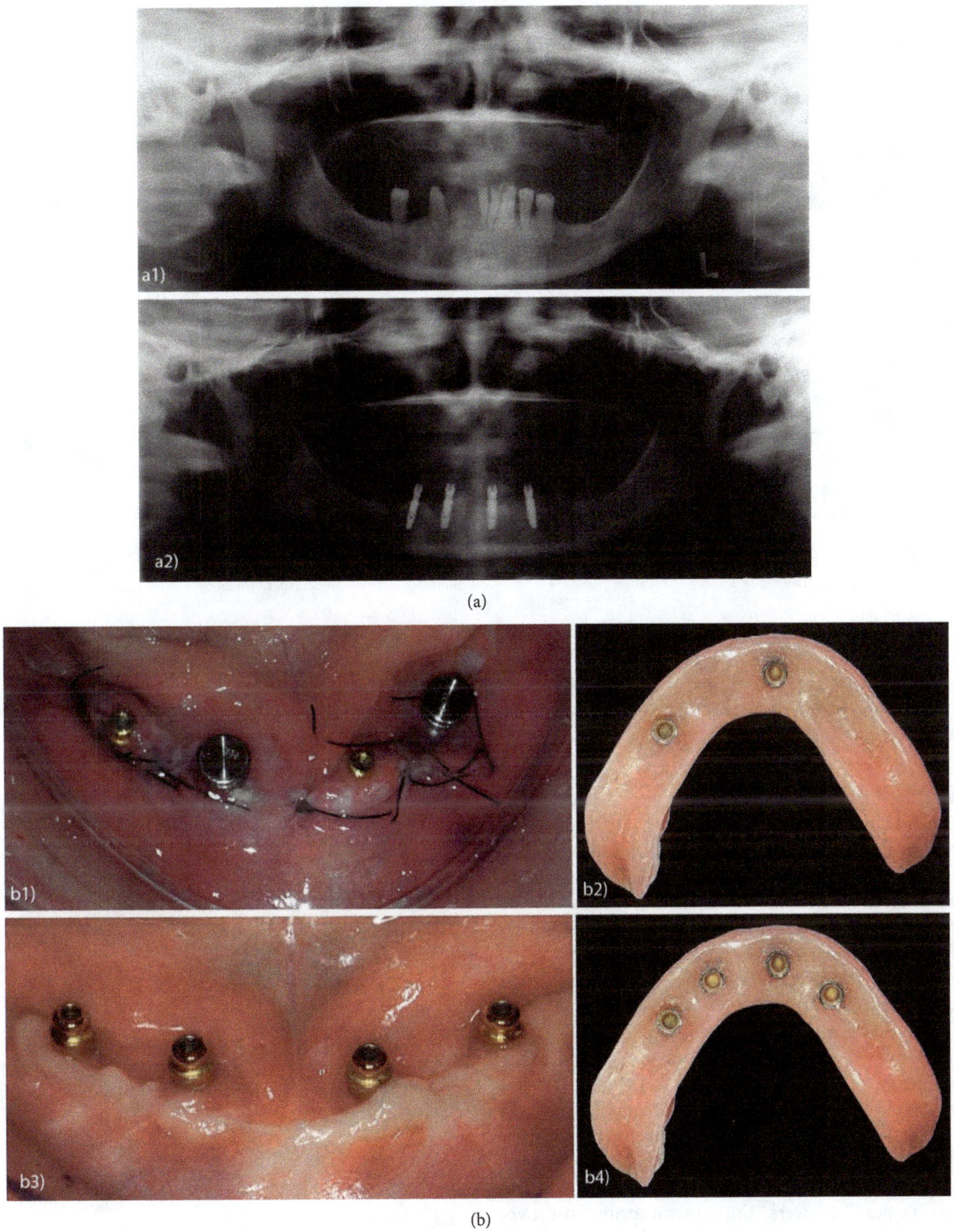

FIGURE 6: : (a) Panoramic X-rays: (a1) preoperative and (a2) immediate postoperative; (b) hybrid occlusal loading: (b1) occlusal view of the O-rings with cylinders in position for capture; (b2) view of the prosthesis base after capturing the O-rings with cylinders of implants 2 and 4; (b3) occlusal view of the attachments prior to capturing implants 1 and 3; (b4) view of the prosthesis base after final capturing.

implants experienced a slight deterioration (by 4.30%) for the ST X50 and 33.82% for the STB and 84.51% in ME2.8. In addition, there was a more marked MBL in all implants in case 2, although this patient reported improvements in satisfaction and OHRQoL. The observed MBL in case 2 is unexpected since several studies [13, 14, 26] demonstrate that a greater number of implants guarantees lower tensions in the bone tissue around the implants and consequently less peri-implant bone loss is expected. A finite element study [13] showed that a greater number of implants result in more bone deformation around these implants, resulting in greater tension in the cortical bone around them, presenting greater

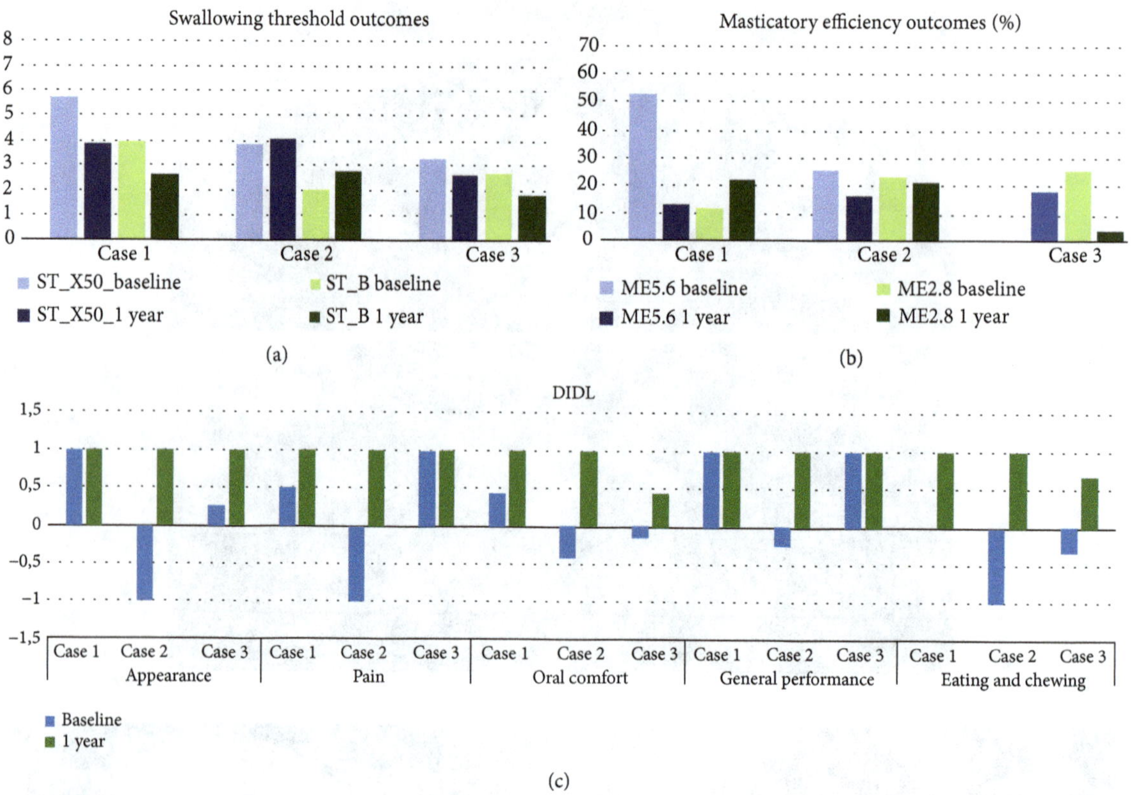

FIGURE 7: (a) Swallowing threshold outcomes (in mm). (b) Masticatory efficiency outcomes (in %). (c) Oral health-related quality of life outcomes (DIDL questionnaire scores; higher is better).

MBL, while the masticatory force mostly affects the mucosa in cases with a lower number of implants. Such a process could account for the observed MBL in case 2. The lack of improvement in masticatory function in case 2 could be attributed to faster chewing by this patient, enabled by the greater retention and stability. Indeed, van der Bilt [27] has shown that a smaller number of cycles and time can directly interfere with the grinding of food (ST_X50), as individuals tend to chew less often and want to swallow the food faster. In addition, subjects with good masticatory function do not always swallow food after a smaller number of cycles, as the ST is partly influenced by the physiology of the individuals (masticatory muscles) and by the social context [27]. When chewing faster, with fewer cycles and due to the masticatory musculature being used only for this purpose and no longer to stabilize the prosthesis in the mouth, individuals perceive themselves as good chewers, thus guaranteeing improvements in the mastication and oral comfort domains, regardless of the number of implants.

It is clear that MO retained by 3 or 4 NDI loaded with conventional, immediate, progressive, and hybrid loading protocols can promote improvements in masticatory function, OHRQoL, and MBL of totally edentulous patients with limited bone availability. However, since a longitudinal clinical study [28] demonstrated that MO retained by three implants have similar survival rates as those retained by four implants and because our case report illustrates that using 4 implants can lead to suboptimal results in some cases, we emphasize that using 2 and 3 implants appears to reduce retention and stability problems of complete dentures sufficiently in many cases [9–12], while avoiding overtreatment and reducing financial costs for the patient, thus constituting treatment options with better cost-effectiveness.

TABLE 2: Marginal bone loss by case, number of implants (I), and type of loading. Abbreviations: IL: immediate loading; CL: conventional loading; HL: hybrid loading.

		Baseline	1 year
Case 1-3I CL	I2	0.00	0.00
	I1	-0.12	1.13
	I2	0.00	1.70
	I3	0.00	1.57
Case 2-4I CL	I1	0.00	-0.62
	I2	0.00	-0.74
	I3	0.00	-0.45
	I4	0.00	-1.94
Case 3-4I HL	I1	0.00	0.00
	I2	0.00	-0.30
	I3	0.00	0.00
	I4	0.00	0.00

The strengths of these approaches include the predictability of the treatment using narrow diameter implants that is attributed to (i) detailed case planning that took into account the clinical conditions along with the patient's preference and expectations and (ii) consistent clinical, functional, and OHRQoL improvements, regardless of the number of implants. We emphasize that MO retained by a smaller number of implants can fulfill their role adequately, with positive bone tissue, chewing, and quality of life responses, as in our case with 3 NDI. Therefore, this option can be strongly indicated for individuals with low bone availability and a reduced budget. The limitations for the proposed approaches are (i) the financial aspect: both the initial costs and the maintenance costs scale with the number of implants (e.g., O-rings require replacement annually) and (ii) with progressive aging and cognitive and motor decline, the increased retention of MO promoted by the greater number of implants can result in difficulties removing them; conversion to retention by 2 implants is recommended in these cases.

Finally, narrow diameter implants can be successfully used as MO retainers in diverse clinical scenarios where mandibular ridge atrophy is present. The available treatment options in these cases include the use of 3 or 4 implants and adopting conventional, conventional progressive, or hybrid loading, illustrating the versatility of the available clinical options. We recommend clinicians to analyze each case individually, taking into account the clinical conditions and the patient's preferences, together with the literature recommendations. Furthermore, we suggest that MO retained by 3 NDI can be indicated in the clinical routine as an optimal option when the patients wish increased retention and stability at a lower budget.

Acknowledgments

The authors thank Neodent's Research Support Program for supplying the dental implants and attachments used in the study. This study was conducted in a Graduate Program supported by CAPES, Brazil. Finance Code: 001.

References

[1] R. M. Marcello-Machado, A. M. Bielemann, G. G. Nascimento, L. R. Pinto, A. A. del Bel Cury, and F. Faot, "Masticatory function parameters in patients with varying degree of mandibular bone resorption," *Journal of Prosthodontic Research*, vol. 61, no. 3, pp. 315–323, 2017.

[2] A. J. Schuster, R. M. Marcello-Machado, A. M. Bielemann, L. R. Pinto, and F. Faot, "Is predicting masticatory function based on mandibular bone atrophy as defined by clinical and radiographic parameters possible? A clinical study," *The Journal of Prosthetic Dentistry*, vol. 121, no. 3, pp. 432–439, 2019.

[3] A. P. da Rosa Possebon, R. M. Marcello-Machado, A. M. Bielemann, A. J. Schuster, L. de Rezende Pinto, and F. Faot, "Masticatory function of conventional complete denture wearers changing to 2-implant retained mandibular overdentures: clinical factor influences after 1 year of function," *Journal of Prosthodontic Research*, vol. 62, no. 4, pp. 479–484, 2018.

[4] J. M. Thomason, S. A. M. Kelly, A. Bendkowski, and J. S. Ellis, "Two implant retained overdentures - a review of the literature supporting the McGill and York consensus statements," *Journal of Dentistry*, vol. 40, no. 1, pp. 22–34, 2012.

[5] A. Kutkut, M. Rezk, D. Zephyr, D. Dawson, R. Frazer, and M. al-Sabbagh, "Immediate loading of unsplinted implant retained mandibular overdenture: a randomized controlled clinical study," *The Journal of Oral Implantology*, vol. 45, no. 5, pp. 378–389, 2019.

[6] A. Y. Alqutaibi and A. F. Kaddah, "Attachments used with implant supported overdenture," *International Dental & Medical Journal of Advanced Research - VOLUME 2015*, vol. 2, no. 1, pp. 1–5, 2016.

[7] R. M. Marcello-Machado, F. Faot, A. J. Schuster, G. G. Nascimento, and A. A. del Bel Cury, "Mini-implants and narrow diameter implants as mandibular overdenture retainers: a systematic review and meta-analysis of clinical and radiographic outcomes," *Journal of Oral Rehabilitation*, vol. 45, no. 2, pp. 161–183, 2018.

[8] R. M. Marcello-Machado, F. Faot, A. J. Schuster, A. M. Bielemann, O. L. Chagas Júnior, and A. A. del Bel Cury, "One-year clinical outcomes of locking taper Equator attachments retaining mandibular overdentures to narrow diameter implants," *Clinical Implant Dentistry and Related Research*, vol. 20, no. 4, pp. 483–492, 2018.

[9] A. P. D. R. Possebon, A. J. Schuster, A. M. Bielemann, B. L. Porto, N. Boscato, and F. Faot, "Evaluation of Bite Force and Masticatory Performance: Complete Denture vs Mandibular Overdenture Users," *Brazilian Dental Journal*, vol. 31, no. 4, pp. 399–403, 2020.

[10] R. M. Marcello-Machado, F. Faot, A. J. Schuster, A. M. Bielemann, G. G. Nascimento, and A. A. del Bel Cury, "How fast can treatment with overdentures improve the masticatory function and OHRQoL of atrophic edentulous patients? A 1-year longitudinal clinical study," *Clinical Oral Implants Research*, vol. 29, no. 2, pp. 215–226, 2018.

[11] A. J. Schuster, R. M. Marcello-Machado, A. M. Bielemann et al., "Short-term quality of life change perceived by patients after transition to mandibular overdentures," *Brazilian Oral Research*, vol. 31, 2017.

[12] E. Emami, R. F. de Souza, J. Bernier, P. Rompré, and J. S. Feine, "Patient perceptions of the mandibular three-implant overdenture: a practice-based study," *Clinical Oral Implants Research*, vol. 26, no. 6, pp. 639–643, 2015.

[13] J. Liu, S. Pan, J. Dong, Z. Mo, Y. Fan, and H. Feng, "Influence of implant number on the biomechanical behaviour of mandibular implant-retained/supported overdentures: a three-dimensional finite element analysis," *Journal of Dentistry*, vol. 41, no. 3, pp. 241–249, 2013.

[14] Misch, *Contemporary Implant Dentistry*, Elsevier Health Sciences, St. Loius, MIssouri, 2007.

[15] J. J. Gagnier, the CARE Group, G. Kienle et al., "The CARE guidelines: consensus-based clinical case reporting guideline development," *Journal of Medical Case Reports*, vol. 7, no. 1, 2013.

[16] J. I. Cawood and R. A. Howell, "A classification of the edentulous jaws," *International Journal of Oral and Maxillofacial Surgery*, vol. 17, no. 4, pp. 232–236, 1988.

[17] F. A. Fontijn-Tekamp, A. van der Bilt, J. H. Abbink, and F. Bosman, "Swallowing threshold and masticatory performance in dentate adults," *Physiology & Behavior*, vol. 83, no. 3, pp. 431–436, 2004.

[18] M. K. Al-Omiri, O. A. Hammad, E. Lynch, P. J. Lamey, and T. J. Clifford, "Impacts of implant treatment on daily living,"

The International Journal of Oral & Maxillofacial Implants, vol. 26, no. 4, pp. 877–886, 2011.

[19] R. Doornewaard, M. Glibert, C. Matthys, S. Vervaeke, E. Bronkhorst, and H. de Bruyn, "Improvement of quality of life with implant-supported mandibular overdentures and the effect of implant type and surgical procedure on bone and soft tissue stability: a three-year prospective split-mouth trial," *Journal of Clinical Medicine*, vol. 8, no. 6, p. 773, 2019.

[20] M. Tallarico, L. Ortensi, M. Martinolli et al., "Multicenter retrospective analysis of implant overdentures delivered with different design and attachment systems: results between one and 17 years of follow-up," *Dental Journal*, vol. 6, no. 4, p. 71, 2018.

[21] R. A. Bulard and J. B. Vance, "Multi-clinic evaluation using mini-dental implants for long-term denture stabilization: a preliminary biometric evaluation," *The Compendium of Continuing Education in Dentistry*, vol. 26, pp. 892–897, 2005.

[22] R. R. Marcello-Machado, F. Faot, A. J. Schuster, A. M. Bielemann, G. G. Nascimento, and A. A. Del Bel Cury, "Mapping of inflammatory biomarkers in the peri-implant crevicular fluid before and after the occlusal loading of narrow diameter implants," *Clinical Oral Investigations*, vol. 24, no. 3, pp. 1311–1320, 2020.

[23] A. M. Bielemann, R. M. Marcello-Machado, A. J. Schuster, O. L. Chagas Júnior, A. A. del Bel Cury, and F. Faot, "Healing differences in narrow diameter implants submitted to immediate and conventional loading in mandibular overdentures: a randomized clinical trial," *Journal of Periodontal Research*, vol. 54, no. 3, pp. 241–250, 2018.

[24] A. J. Schuster, R. M. Marcello-Machado, A. M. Bielemann, A. P. da Rosa Possebon, O. L. Chagas Júnior, and F. Faot, "Immediate vs conventional loading of Facility-Equator system in mandibular overdenture wearers: 1-year RCT with clinical, biological, and functional evaluation," *Clinical Implant Dentistry and Related Research*, vol. 22, no. 3, pp. 270–280, 2020.

[25] S. Bhat, R. Chowdhary, and S. Mahoorkar, "Comparison of masticatory efficiency, patient satisfaction for single, two, and three implants supported overdenture in the same patient: a pilot study," *The Journal of Indian Prosthodontic Society*, vol. 16, no. 2, pp. 182–186, 2016.

[26] R. Mericske-Stern, "Clinical evaluation of overdenture restorations supported by osseointegrated titanium implants: a retrospective study," *The International Journal of Oral & Maxillofacial Implants*, vol. 5, no. 4, pp. 375–383, 1990.

[27] A. van der Bilt, "Assessment of mastication with implications for oral rehabilitation: a review," *Journal of Oral Rehabilitation*, vol. 38, no. 10, pp. 754–780, 2011.

[28] J. Balaguer, J. Ata-Ali, D. Peñarrocha-Oltra, B. García, and M. Peñarrocha-Diago, "Long-term survival rates of implants supporting overdentures," *The Journal of Oral Implantology*, vol. 41, no. 2, pp. 173–177, 2015.

26

Flapless Cone Beam Computed Tomography-Guided Implant Surgery with Contextual Transcrestal Sinus Lift Augmentation using New Bone Compactor Tools

Ferdinando Attanasio,[1] Sergio Bortolini,[2] Daniele Carbone,[3] and Andrea Pacifici[3]

[1]*Department of Health Sciences, Magna Graecia, University of Catanzaro, Catanzaro, Italy*
[2]*CHIMOMO, Università di Modena e Reggio Emilia, Largo del Pozzo 71, 41125 Modena, Italy*
[3]*Department of Oral and Maxillo-Facial Science, Sapienza University of Rome, Rome 00100, Italy*

Correspondence should be addressed to Andrea Pacifici; andrea.pacifici@uniroma1.it

Academic Editor: Jamil Awad Shibli

In the present paper, the authors present a case report of premolar edentulism in the upper jaw treated through a guided flapless oral implant surgery with contextual crestal sinus lift, performed with a system of manual screw-tapered bone expanders (B&B Dental, San Benedetto, BO, Italy). The surgery was planned by means of dedicated software, through which the data obtained from the CBCT and from intraoral scanner impression were matched, with consequent production of a surgical template. The proposed surgical procedure is minimally invasive, very simple, and fast and ensures good comfort for the patient by avoiding the elevation of mucoperiosteal flaps and uncomfortable malleting maneuvers. In addition, the presented method shows a good degree of correspondence between the ideal position of the implant in the planning phase and the actual one detectable after the surgery.

1. Introduction

A tooth lost in the posterior areas of the upper jaws besides leaving a chewing deficit can also lead to a slow but inexorable expansion of the maxillary sinus in the side affected by edentulism [1, 2]. The pneumatization of the maxillary sinus therefore brings about a lessening of the available surgical space for the implant insertion without recurring to any bone augmentation procedure [3]. International reports in various studies [4, 5] have underlined the anatomical limits that allow the surgeon to obtain a better prognosis for the prosthetic rehabilitation on implants in posterior edentulous areas of the upper jaw [6]. In particular, a residual ridge lesser than 5 mm in height requires a surgical approach through the elevation of a lateral window, while a residual ridge greater than 5 mm in height can be approached through a transcrestal elevation procedure with excellent success rates [7]. Several different techniques have been proposed by various authors for transcrestal sinus elevation surgery: from the osteotomy proposed by Summers [8, 9] to the more recent fluid dynamic technique [10] or the use of a compactor/expander or even the use of dedicated implants which allow the insertion of the fixture and the contextual elevation of the sinus membrane [11–13].

In this case report, the authors propose a computer-guided surgery procedure consisting in crestal maxillary sinus lift performed with bone expanders (B&B Dental, San Benedetto, BO, Italy) and contextual oral implant insertion. Through the exposed technique, instead of penetrating the bone tissue with osteotomes by percussion in the apical direction (for example, the Summers type), we have the insertion of a series of compactors with a gradually increasing diameter, which allow the safe fracture of the maxillary sinus floor resulting in a totally atraumatic and painless procedure for the patient. This protocol allows raising the height of the ridge by even 3-4 mm in the antral direction. Moreover, the preparation of the implant site through the use of the compactors allows increasing the density of the bone in the implant site in order to obtain higher insertion torque and gain a greater primary stability of the fixture compared to traditional implant site preparation drills or to percussion osteotomies of Summers [14]. In order to obtain even greater bone volume around the apical zone of the implant, it is possible to insert an autogenous bone graft or bone substitute [15]. This maneuver must be performed with accuracy and precision in order to avoid the laceration of the Schneiderian membrane [16].

2. Case Presentation

A healthy 34-year-old woman presented to our observation requesting clinical evaluation of her upper left maxilla and implant prosthetic treatment of second left upper premolar edentulism (Figures 1(a)–1(c)). The missing tooth was extracted several years before due to a history of dentoalveolar infections. The patient reported no smoking or significant illness while referring good oral hygiene habits.

As a predictable, significative vertical ridge defect was present, probably due to both bone resorption and maxillary sinus expansion, which made the anatomical site seriously compromised and inadequate for implant-supported rehabilitation. In fact, the radiographic examination clearly displayed that the bone height in this area was not sufficient for standard length implant placement (5 mm bone height) while the horizontal bone thickness appeared to be sufficient (Figure 2).

The treatment plan included the immediate placement of one fixture with a contextual transcrestal sinus lift procedure to ideally restore the shape, function, and esthetics of the alveolar defect. In order to minimize the trauma as much as possible, avoiding flaps from opening and increasing the bone volume only for the necessary portion, we decided to perform the preparation of the implant site and the positioning of the implant through static computer-aided implant surgery.

In order to proceed with the computer-assisted implant surgery, a CBCT (Pax i-3d Green, Vatech, Yongin, Korea) of the affected area was preliminarily performed. Furthermore, a digital acquisition of the dental arch's surface profile was performed through an intraoral scanner (CEREC Omnicam v4.5.1; Dentsply Sirona), and the obtained .stl file has been extracted. The two files have been imported into dedicated software (B&B Dental Guide System, B&B Dental San Benedetto, BO, Italy) so as to allow the digital superimposition of the .stl file containing all the data of soft tissue and teeth and the .dcm file that brings along the bone and internal anatomical structures' information in order to allow the correct digital positioning of the proper size and kind implant for the structure of the upper jaw. The .dcm and .stl file matching was performed to overlap the obtained information and clearly display the patient's situation in a very detailed manner. By the idea that the patient is semiedentulous, the acquisition of the CBCT was made without the use a radiographic template with radiopaque markers, as the B&B Dental Guide System software allows the overlapping of the impression made by Omnicam v4.5.1 (Dentsply Sirona) directly with the .dicom file by recognizing some anatomical portions of the residual teeth.

Surgeons evaluated the obtainable volumes through the sinus lifting procedure and then digitally positioned an implant of 4Ø× 8 mm length (Duravit 3P, B&B Dental, San Benedetto, BO, Italy), suitable with the anatomical structure and in a prosthetically guided positioning to obtain screw-retained rehabilitation.

In order to precisely determine the depth of the osteotomy, it is necessary to use cross-sectional images of the elevation site and measure the distance between the top of the bony crest and the maxillary sinus floor along with the implant axis on the three-dimensional model (Figures 3(a)–3(d)).

As a result of the evaluations made through the software, it was possible to perform an accurate digital implant positioning and to design a template and export the resulting .stl file. This file can be sent to any laboratory for printing; in our case, we relied on B&B Dental guided surgery and printing service to receive both a printed model and the finished surgical template.

The surgical template is printed in acrylic material and contains hexagonal polyether ether ketone (PEEK) sleeves (4.2Ø× 5 mm height) in correspondence with the planned implants' position and with their own inclination. The internal diameter of the sleeves perfectly fit the neck of all the instruments inside the dedicated guided surgery kit (B&B Dental guided surgery kit, B&B Dental, San Benedetto, BO, Italy) in order to accurately direct the instrument to prepare the planned osteotomy. All the drills' necks are 9 mm long while the cutting edges have variable sizes according to the producer's implant sizes.

The chosen material for the sleeves allows lower dimensional tolerance, thus improving the accuracy of the sleeve instrument fitting in order to guarantee higher precision in terms of directing the drill while avoiding any temperature rising.

Before starting the procedure, the surgical template is checked for proper seating and secured in place with a tooth support (Figure 4(a)), thus ensuring the greatest possible precision [17, 18].

The stabilization of the surgical template is a key point to reproduce the virtual surgery in the mouth of the patient with high accuracy [19]. The loss of accuracy may result from movements of the surgical guide during implant preparation or from the so-called "intrinsic" error of the template [20].

The patient was premedicated with amoxicillin+clavulanic acid (2 g) 1 hour before surgery, and then, 875 mg of amoxicillin and 125 mg of clavulanic acid were administered twice per day for 1 week following the surgery.

The patient rinsed with a 0.20% chlorhexidine gluconate solution (Curasept, Curaden HealthCare, Italy) for 1 minute; then, the skin surrounding the surgical site was disinfected. The patient presented a thick biotype. Under local anesthesia (2% lidocaine with 1 : 80,000 epinephrine), an operculectomy was performed with the use of a rotating circular tissue punch mounted on a handpiece, after which a pilot drill was used to cut the cortical bone and assess the tissue consistency (Figures 4(b) and 4(c)).

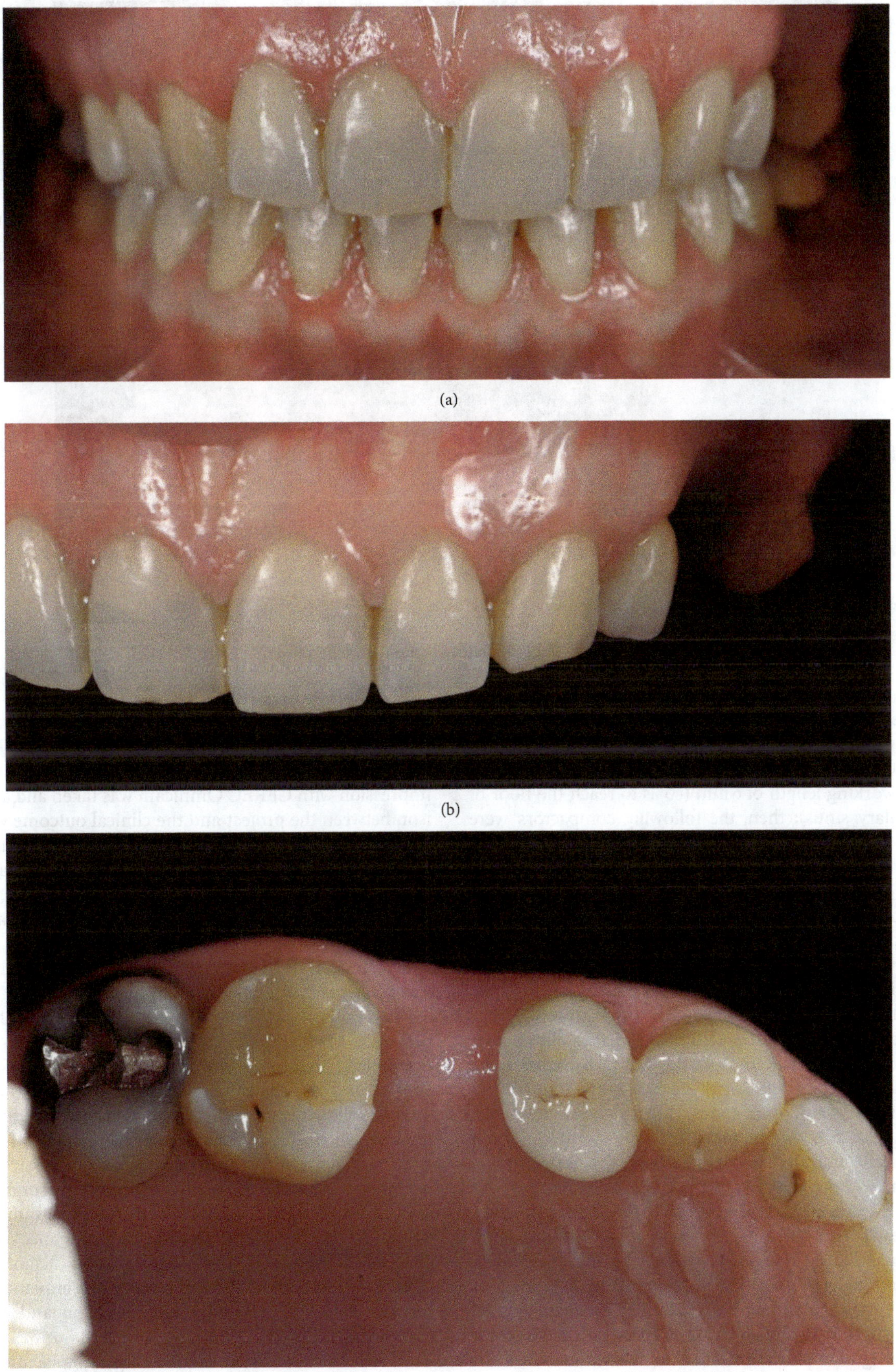

FIGURE 1: (a) Intraoral preoperatory frontal view. (b) Intraoral preoperatory frontal view. (c) Intraoral preoperatory occlusal view.

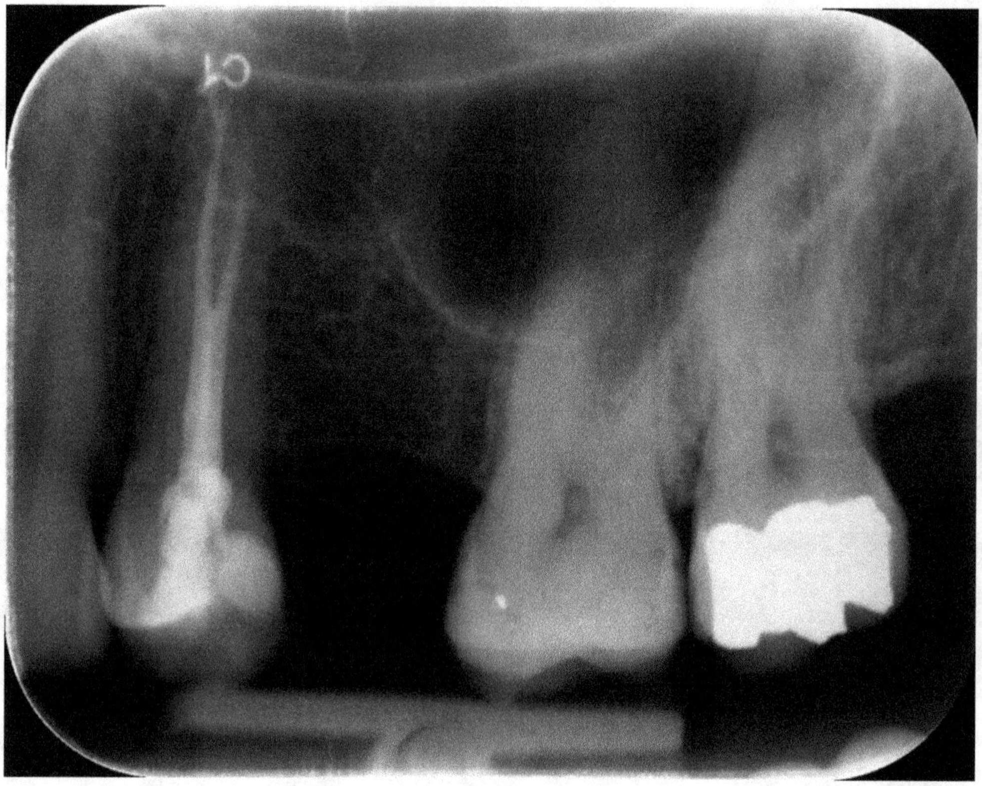

Figure 2: Preoperatory endoral radiography.

Subsequently, bone compactors with a convex apex of increasing diameter and length were inserted with a clockwise rotation. We started with a 2.2 mm in diameter compactor for a working length of 6 mm (so as to reach the floor of the maxillary sinus); then, the following compactors were 3.0, 3.5, and 4.0 mm in diameter and have been used in sequence up to a length of 10 mm (Figures 5(a)–5(c)).

Once the osteotomy for the preparation of the implant site was finished, the patient performed the Valsalva maneuver, which showed the absence of perforations of the sinus membrane. The implant site was filled with inorganic bovine bone-derived mineral (ABBM) (Bio-Oss, Geistlich Pharma, Wolhusen, Switzerland) (Figure 5(d)).

The convex rounded tip of the compactors allows performing compressions and expansions of the alveolar bone by pushing and compacting it at the ends of the implant site (both vertically and horizontally). This allows not only fracturing the floor of the maxillary sinus completely and atraumatically but also, above all, lifting the Schneiderian membrane without the need to use other instruments.

At this point, using the mounter from the surgical kit, a soft thread 4Ø× 8 mm long implant was placed (Figure 5(e)). The mounter has the function of guiding the final insertion of the implant in terms of angle, height, and orientation. This component has a landmark hexagon whose faces are aligned with those of the implant's hexagonal connections. The faces of the hexagon must be matched to the direction of the sleeve inside the surgical guide that has been planned to allow the correct positioning of the prosthetic abutment (Figure 5(f)).

The precision of the final implant position was monitored through an endoral X-ray (Figure 6(a)).

Before the end of the surgical procedures, an optical impression with CEREC Omnicam was taken and a comparison between the project and the clinical outcome was made through a digital superimposition. This showed that, despite the contextual positioning of the implant and the transcrestal sinus elevation, there were 1.88 mm of deviation on the position of the apex, 0.96 mm of deviation at the head of the implant, and an angle deviation of 4.73°.

At the end of the surgery, a transmucosal healing screw was placed and no sutures had to be inserted.

In addition to the pre- and postoperative antibiotics described above, an anti-inflammatory medication (ibuprofen 600 mg) has been administered immediately after the surgery and was thereafter prescribed three times a day for 1 week following surgery. 0.20% chlorhexidine digluconate mouthwash rinses were prescribed twice daily for ten days, starting 24 hours after the surgery. It was not possible to carry out radiographic control 4.5 months after the surgery due to the patient's pregnancy. Before proceeding with the impressions for the prosthetic restoration, resonance frequency analysis (Osstell ISQ™ device, Integration Diagnostics AB, Göteborg, Sweden) of the osteointegrated implant was performed: values of 81 in the B/L direction and 80 in the M/D were recorded.

About 5 months after the surgery, a screw-retained implant-supported metal porcelain crown was applied; all the laboratory steps followed a completely digital workflow. Intraoral examination showed healthy a peri-implant

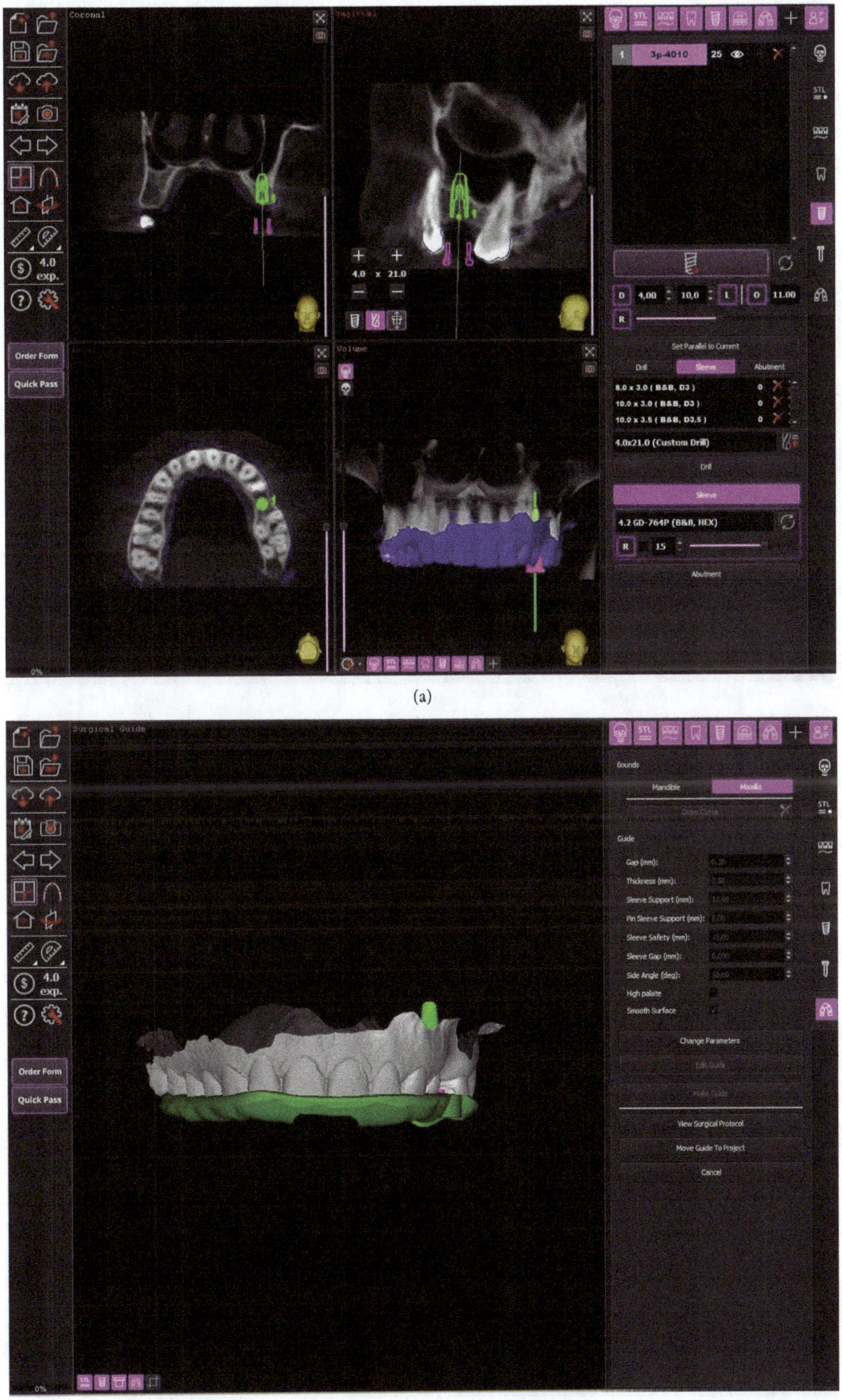

(a)

(b)

FIGURE 3: Continued.

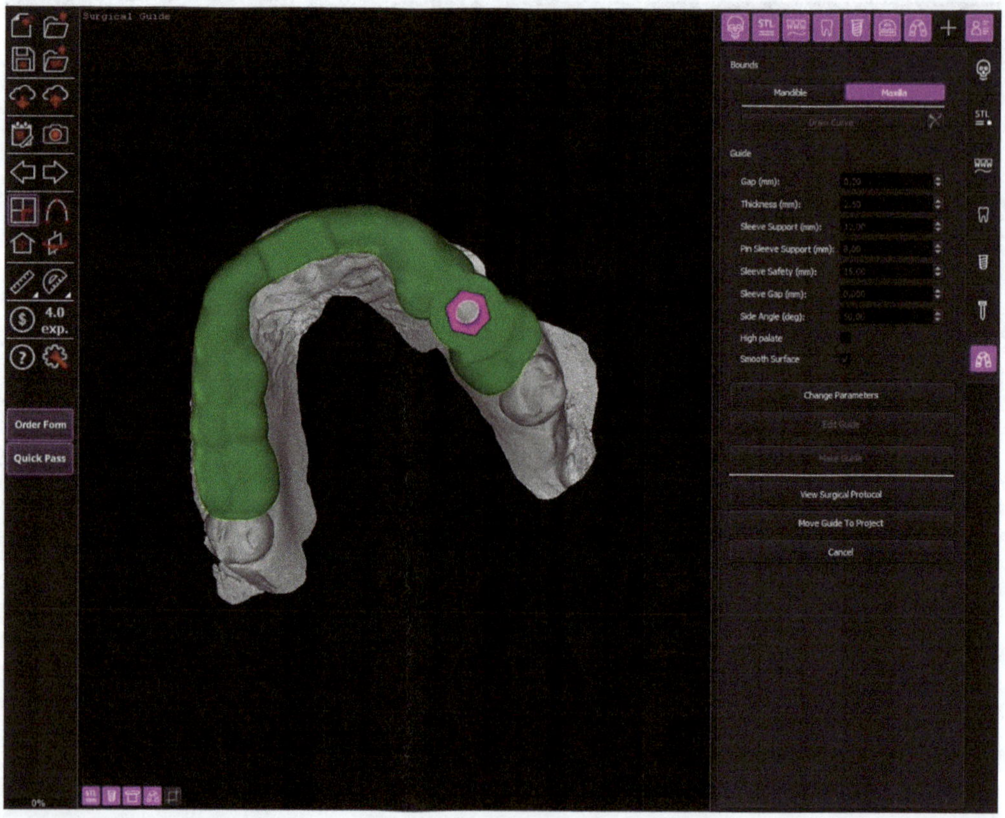

(c)

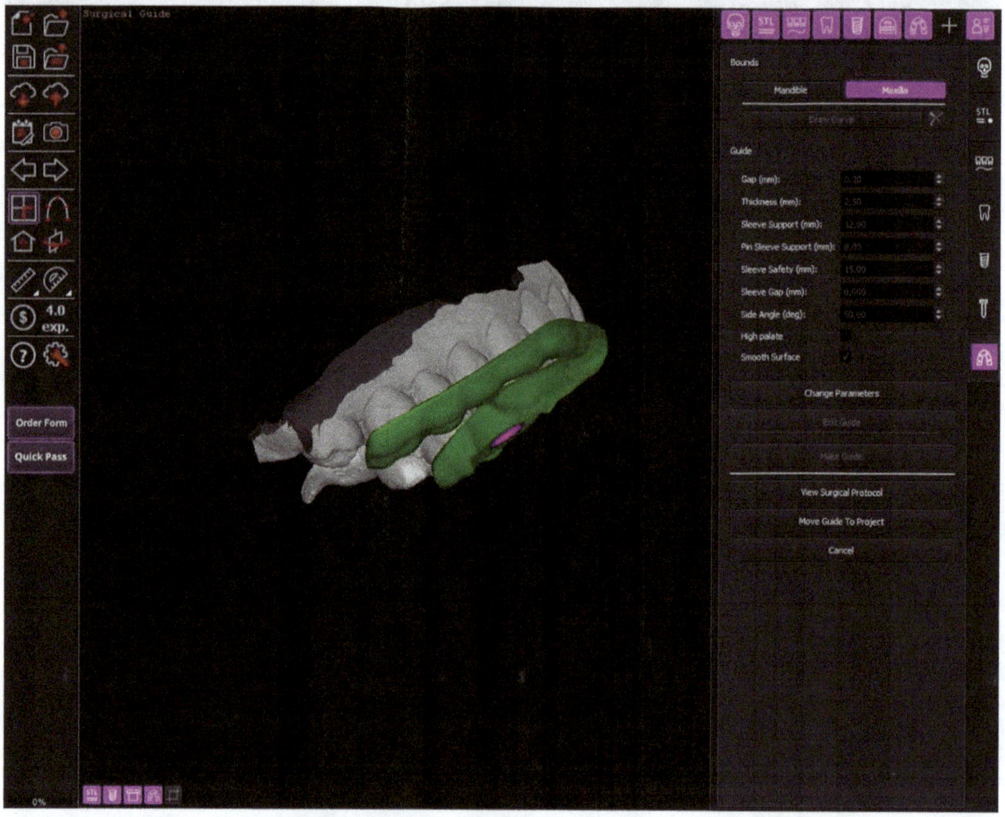

(d)

FIGURE 3: (a) Software evaluation and digital planning of the surgical procedure. (b–d) Digital modeling of the surgical template.

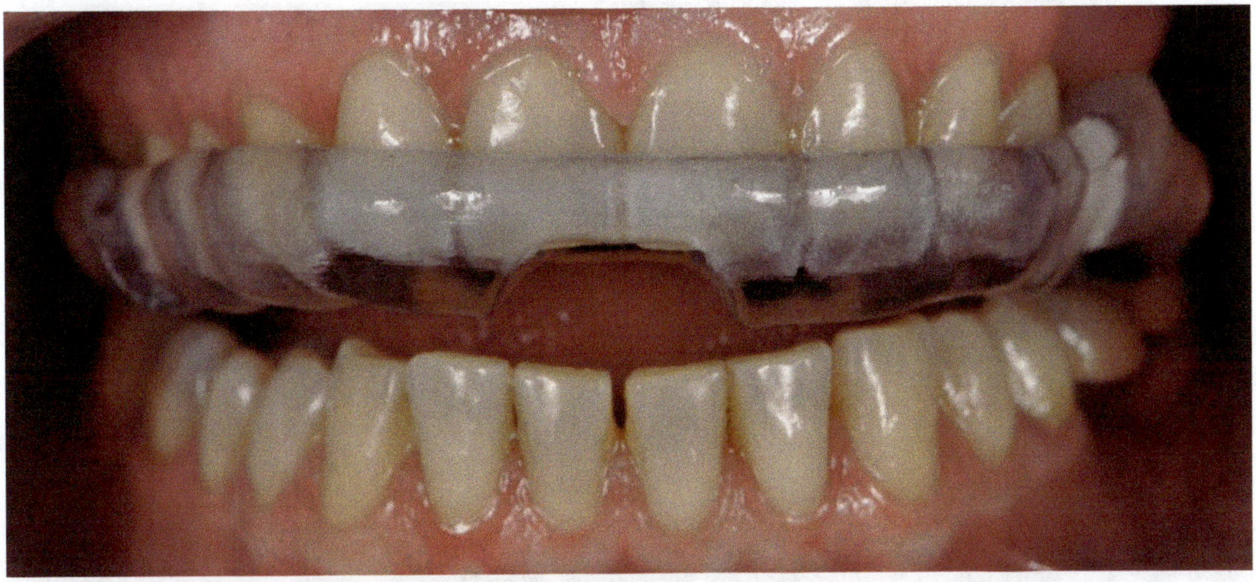

(a)

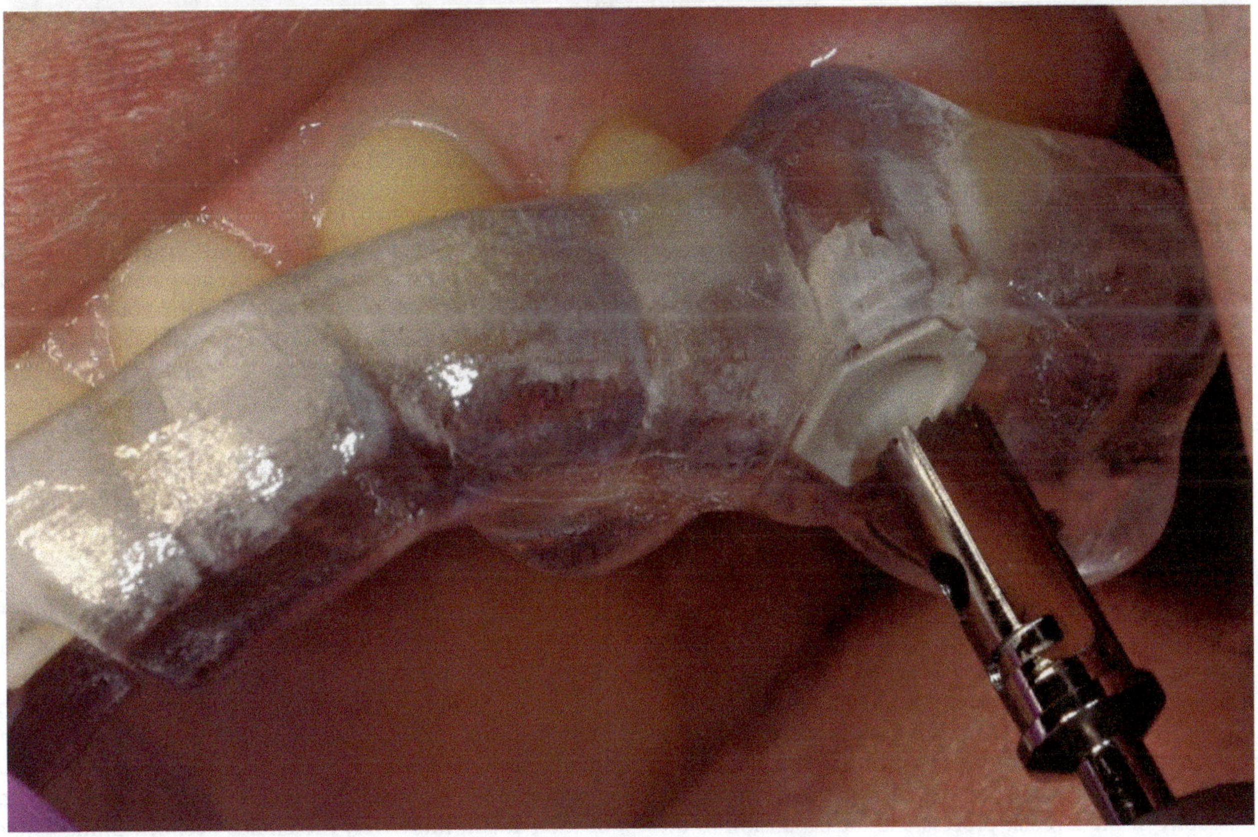

(b)

FIGURE 4: Continued.

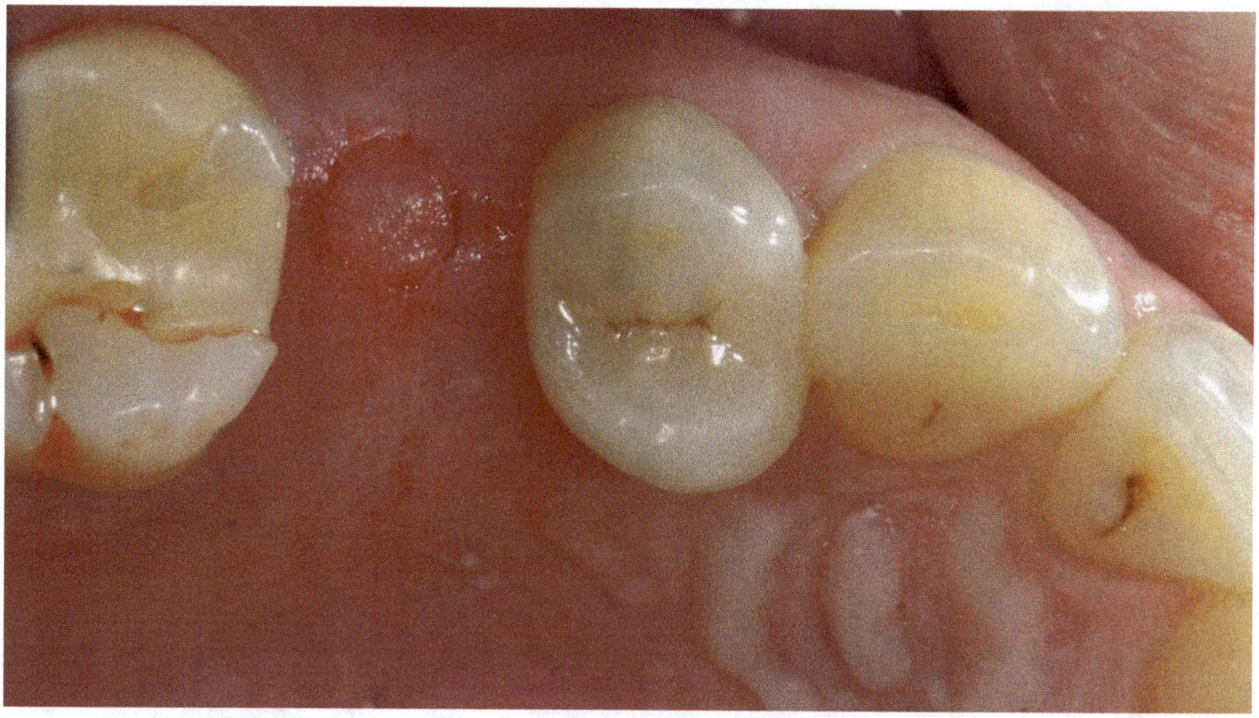

(c)

FIGURE 4: (a) Template positioning before the surgery. (b) Rotating circular tissue punch. (c) Operculectomy through the gingiva.

mucosa without suppuration, swelling, or erythema close to the implant site. The patient did not complain of foreign body sensation, pain, or dysesthesia.

Endoral radiographies performed immediately after the end of the procedure and after 9 months (4 months after the implant underwent prosthetic loading) showed good osseointegration of the fixture and the absence of pathological signs (Figure 6(b)).

3. Discussion

The rehabilitation of partial or total edentulous patients using implant prosthesis techniques has become a routine practice with reliable long-term success rates [21, 22]; however, local conditions of the alveolar edentulous ridge can seriously disadvantage implant positioning. In particular, the posterior edentulous jaw bone has often represented a challenge for oral surgeons because of the insufficient bone volume, as a consequence of crestal resorption caused by the atrophy of the alveolar process and the expansion of the maxillary sinus. Moreover, the quality of the residual bone can further reduce the primary stability of implants [23].

Procedures for sinus floor elevation have become an argument of great interest since the introduction of the technique by Tatum in 1976 [24, 25]. The first publication dates back to 1980, in an article by Boyne [26].

The traditional technique for the maxillary sinus floor augmentation foresees the opening of a lateral window, the elevation and medialization of the membrane with rounded off instruments, the grafting of particulate material, and the use of a membrane to cover the access window.

Historically, the maxillary sinus lift surgery that was performed in the early 80s involved hospitalization of the patient. During the procedure, an autologous bone graft was used in block or in the form of particulates, with simultaneous or deferred placement of endoosseous implants [26–28]. This technique was also widely used in the 90s [29–31]. The autologous block grafts within the preimplant regenerative oral surgery showed several critical issues including reduced survival rate and postoperative discomforts [27].

To get around these problems, researchers studied the use of heterologous bone graft substitutes [32, 33]. Moreover, research into the guided bone regeneration brought about the introduction of membranes to cover the lateral access window [34, 35].

The technique of maxillary sinus floor elevation and bone grafting through lateral window osteotomy is commonly performed, nowadays, with foreseeable results in an outpatient setting, avoiding in this way the hospitalization of the patient; moreover, the choice between immediate or deferred implant insertions depends on the capacity of the surgeon to obtain a good primary stability [36, 37]. According to the revision of Wallace and Froum [38], once the primary stability has been reached, the difference in the survival rates between the implants positioned contextually or after the graft is unimportant.

The maxillary sinus floor elevation technique through a lateral access window is usually used when the height of the residual bone is inferior to 4-5 mm.

In 1994, Nedir et al. [7] introduced a sinus floor augmentation technique through a transcrestal access; from that

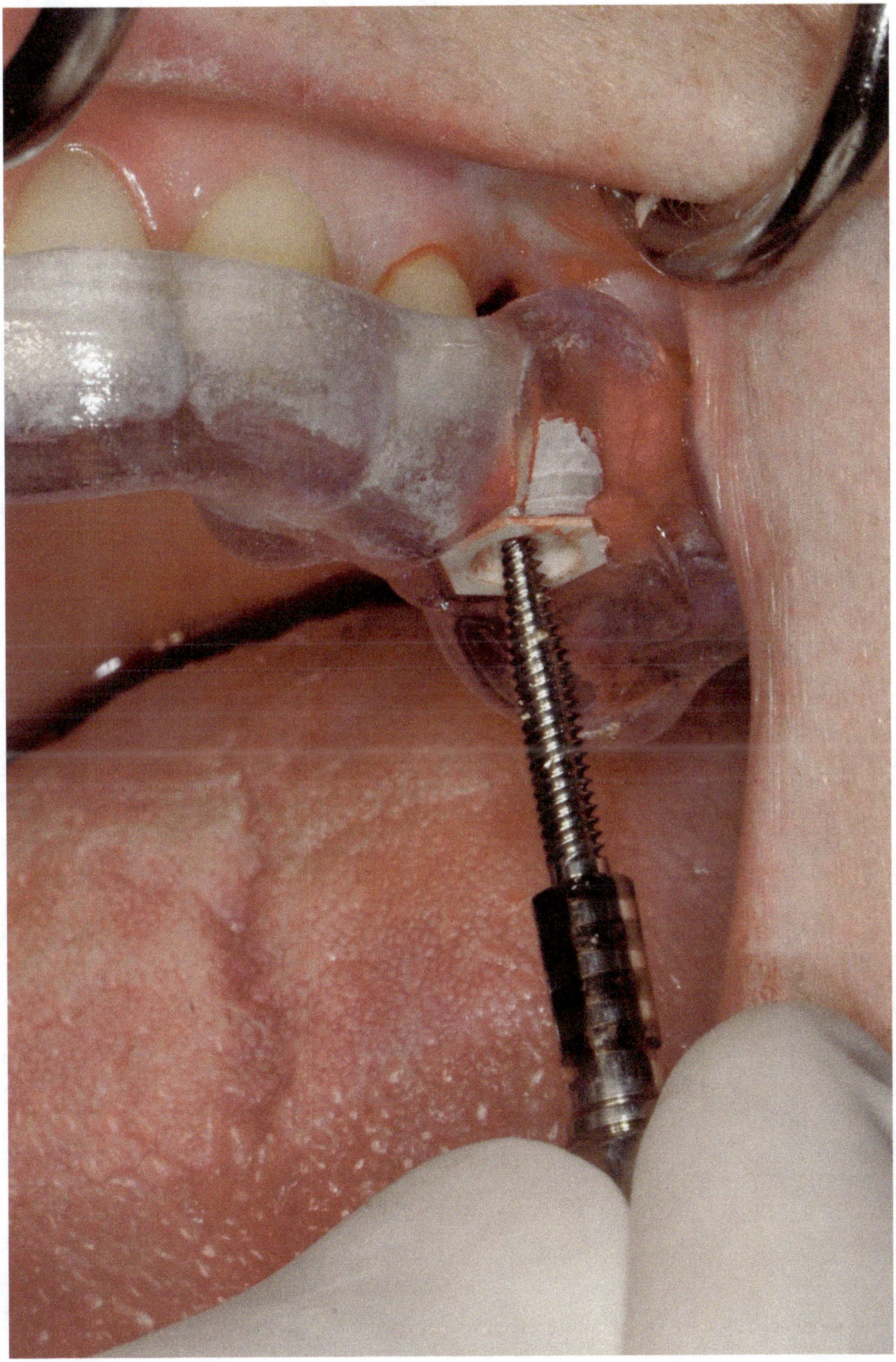

(a)

FIGURE 5: Continued.

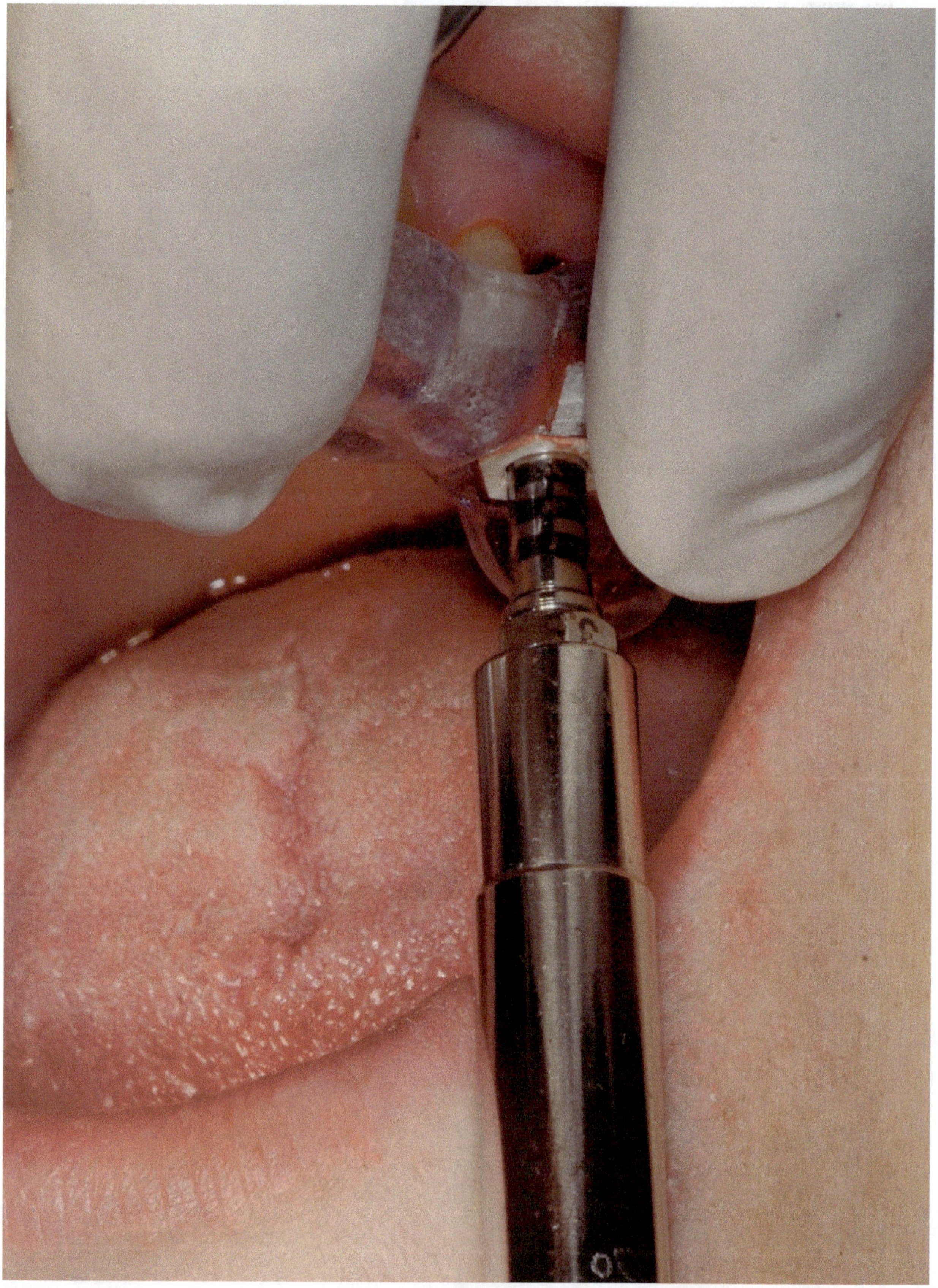

(b)

Figure 5: Continued.

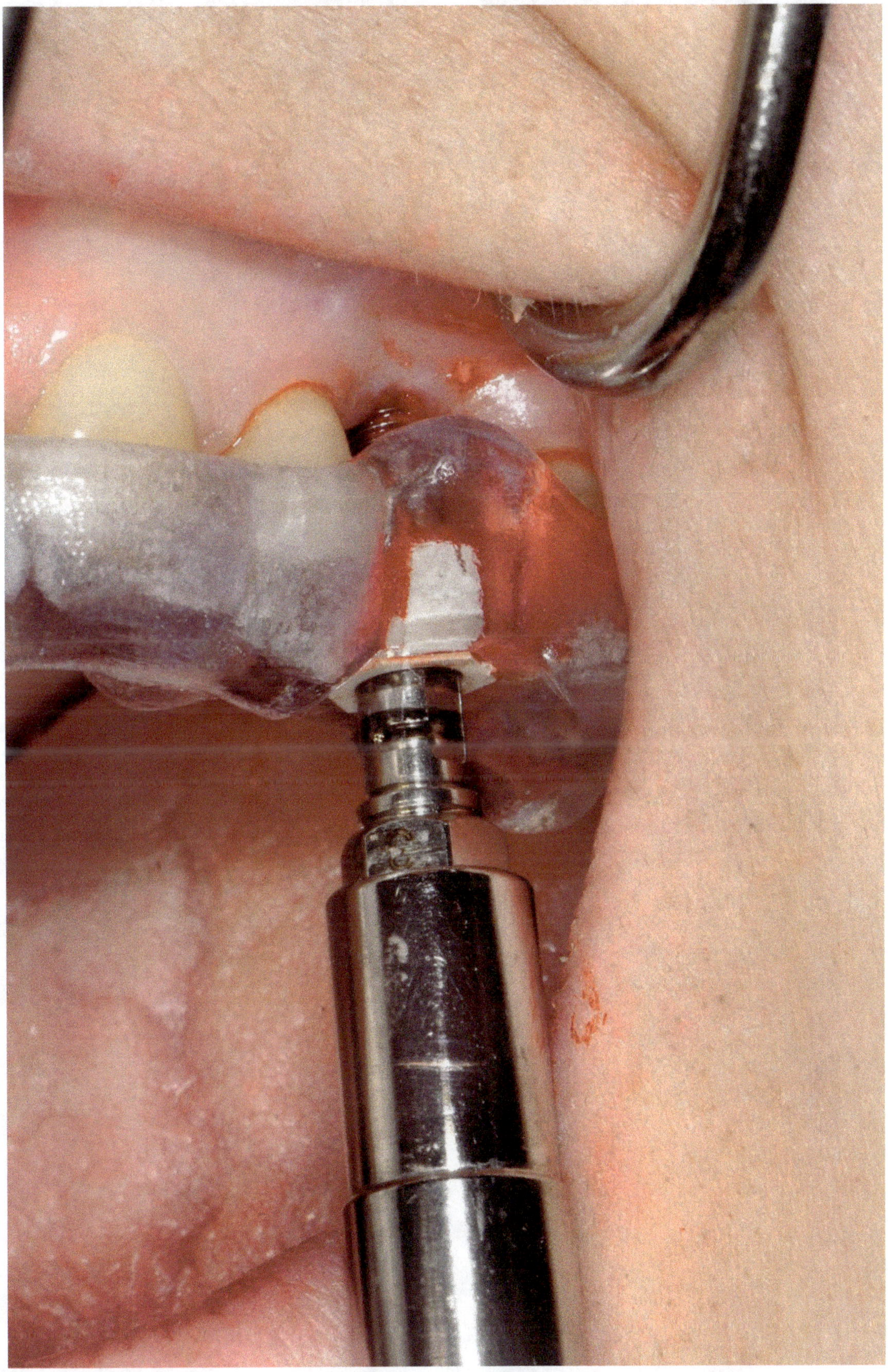

(c)

FIGURE 5: Continued.

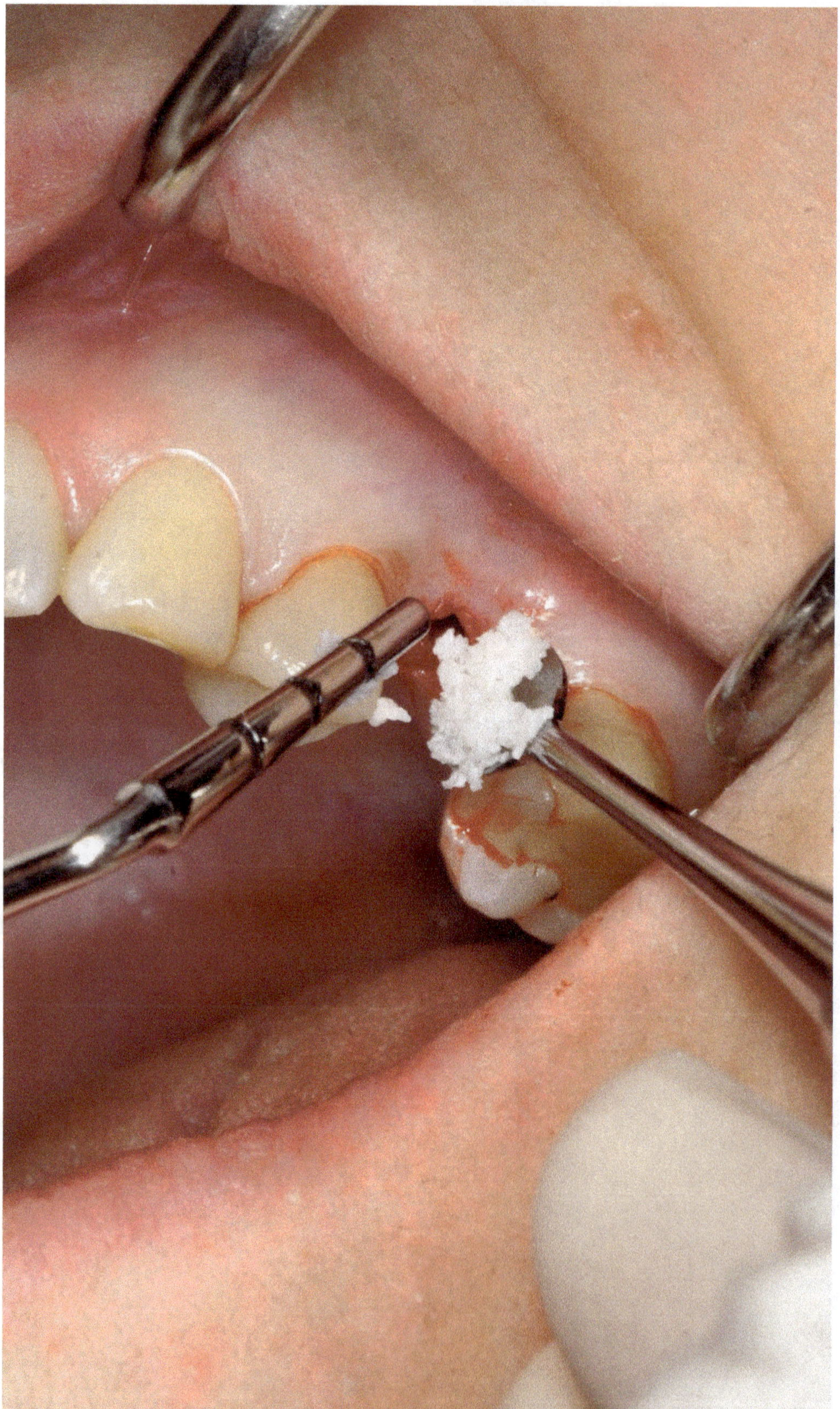

(d)

Figure 5: Continued.

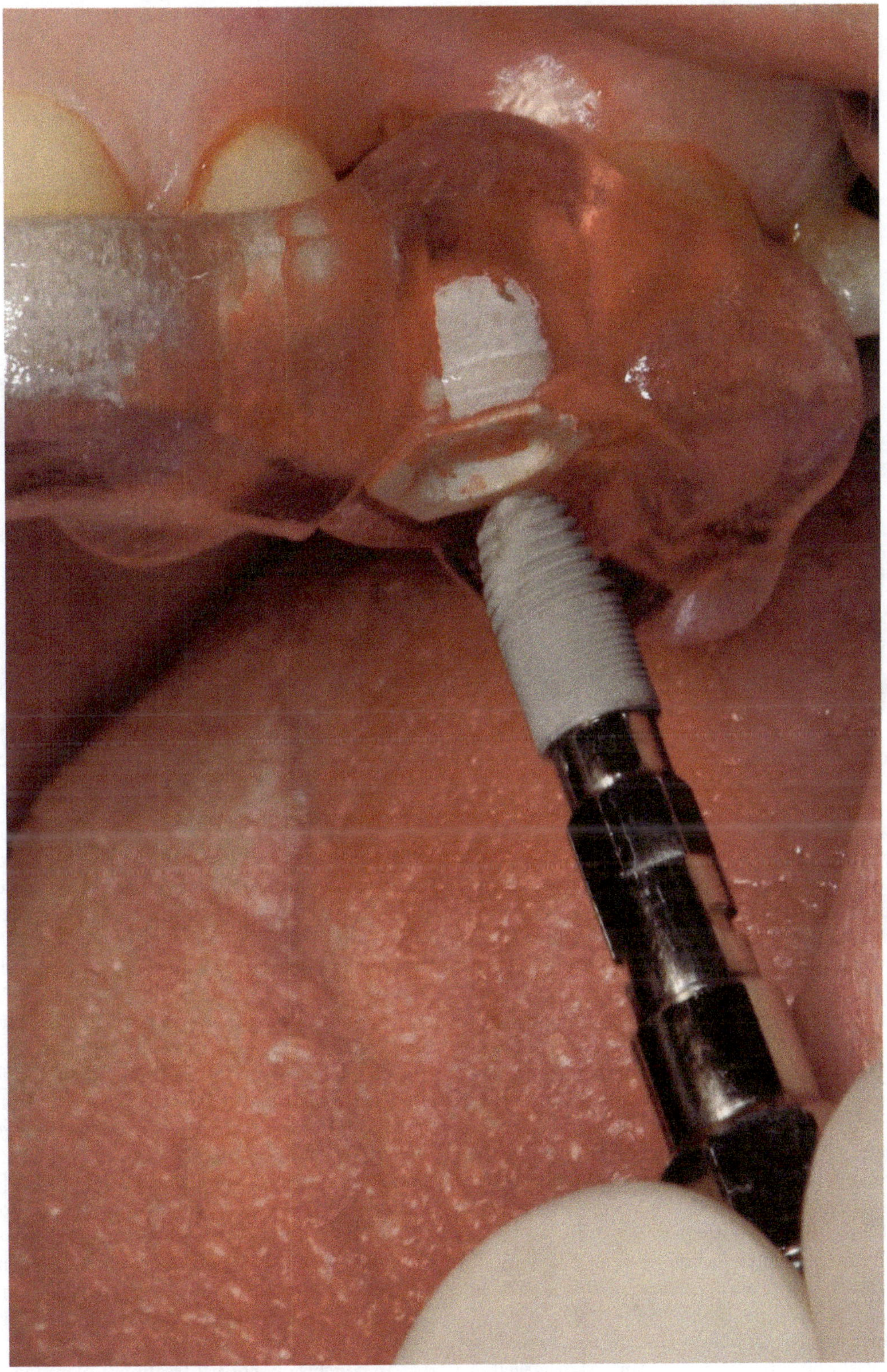

(e)

FIGURE 5: Continued.

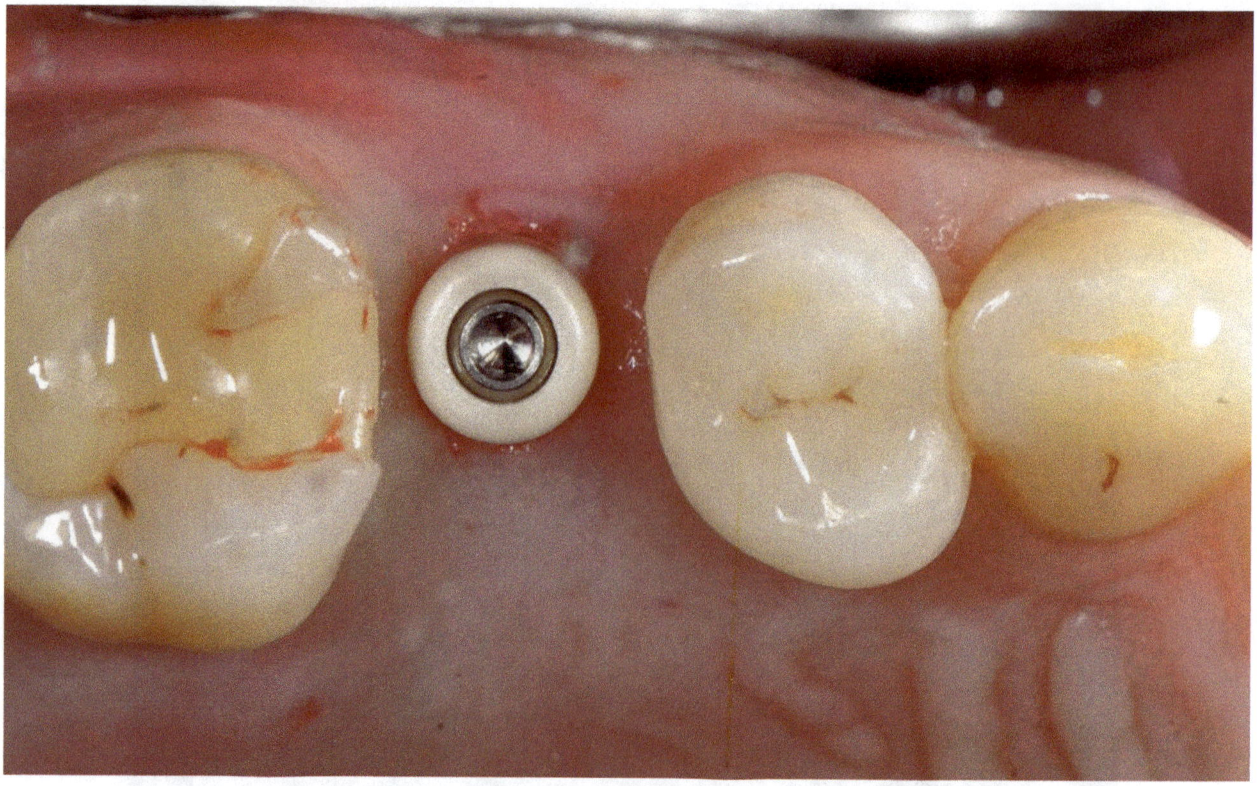

(f)

Figure 5: (a–c) Osteotomy by manual bone compactors (B&B Dental guided surgery kit, B&B Dental, San Benedetto, BO, Italy). (d) Filling of the implant site with inorganic bovine bone-derived mineral. (e) Dental implant positioning. (f) Positioning of the prosthetic abutment.

moment, a number of modifications to Summers' technique have been introduced [9–43].

Exploiting the teachings from techniques proposed in literature, the "Duravit Crestal Sinus Lift" systematics of the B&B Dental Implant Company presents some modifications which permit, with minimal surgical invasion, the obtainment of good results in cases of maxillary bone atrophy with residual bone of at least 4 mm in height. Moreover, the use of a manual technique permits a notable increase in the sensibility of the surgeon during the operation; avoiding the use of a hammer for bone compaction also makes the surgery less traumatic for the patient.

The simplicity of the use of this method also allows the less expert surgeon to speed up the learning curve and to safely position an implant of standard dimensions in areas with important atrophy in an outpatient setting.

The application of digital technologies in the various branches of dentistry represents another topic that is gaining increasing interest in literature. In the field of oral implantology, digital technologies find various possible uses, including optimizing the planning of the therapeutic program as well as developing a computer-guided surgical procedure [44].

The introduction of technologies such as intraoral optical scanners and CBCT in dental practice has made possible to develop diagnostic and planning protocols through the digital processing of anatomical data by means of virtual models, which represent a precise representation of anatomy of the patient [44]. Among the several possible applications, we have the possibility of planning the proper dental implant position and obtain surgical templates through the digital matching of the anatomical data obtained from the optical scans of the intraoral surface with those obtained from the CBCT [45]. According to the evidence in literature, indications for guided implant surgery could be the need for minimally traumatic or flapless surgery, optimal implant positioning, and immediate loading [46].

To date, several authors have studied these procedures using different systems and measuring the deviation between the planned position for the implant and the actual one after its insertion. In particular, the parameters most frequently used to measure the degree of precision of given systematics are the deviation of the implant position in its most coronal and apical portions, as well as its angulation [18, 47–49]. In the present report, a dental implant was positioned contextually to transcrestal sinus elevation, resulting in 1.88 mm of deviation on the position of the apex, 0.96 mm of deviation at the head of the implant, and an angle deviation of 4.73°. However, these data are in line with those documented in literature [18, 47–49].

In conclusion, correct treatment planning is fundamental for prosthetic-guided oral implantology and modern technologies can help to position dental implants in the most suitable location. Furthermore, the development of increasingly less invasive surgical procedures represents a topic of crucial importance in modern medicine as it allows, among other things, reducing discomfort for patients and treatment times.

The systematics presented by the authors in this case report allows the simultaneous insertion of dental implants

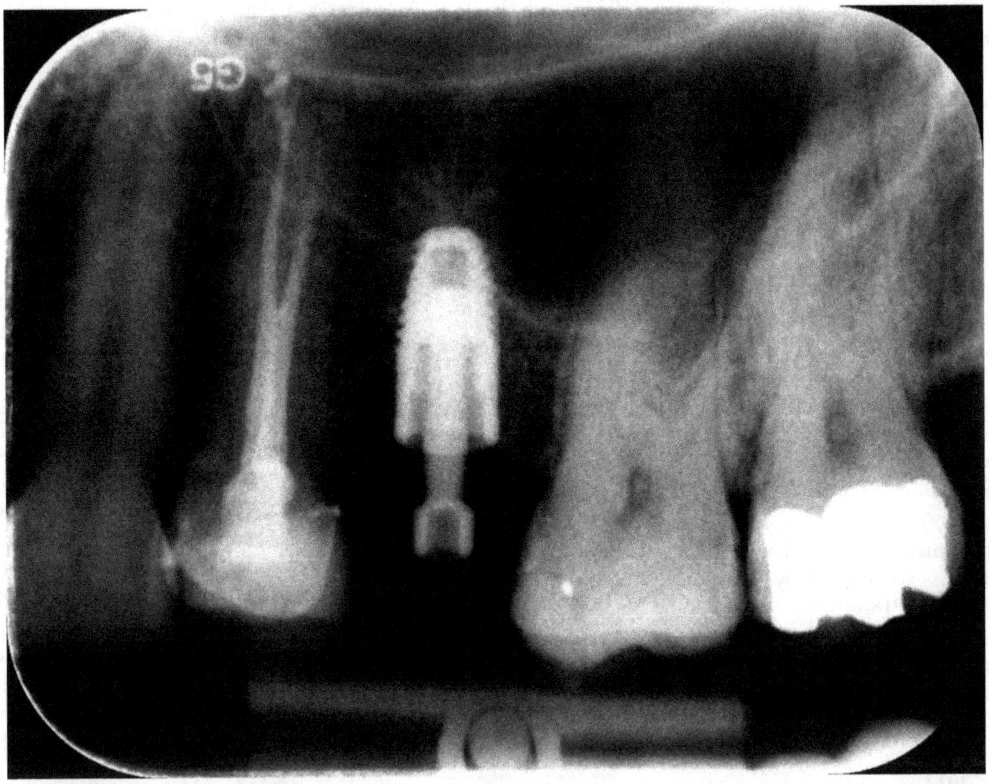

(a)

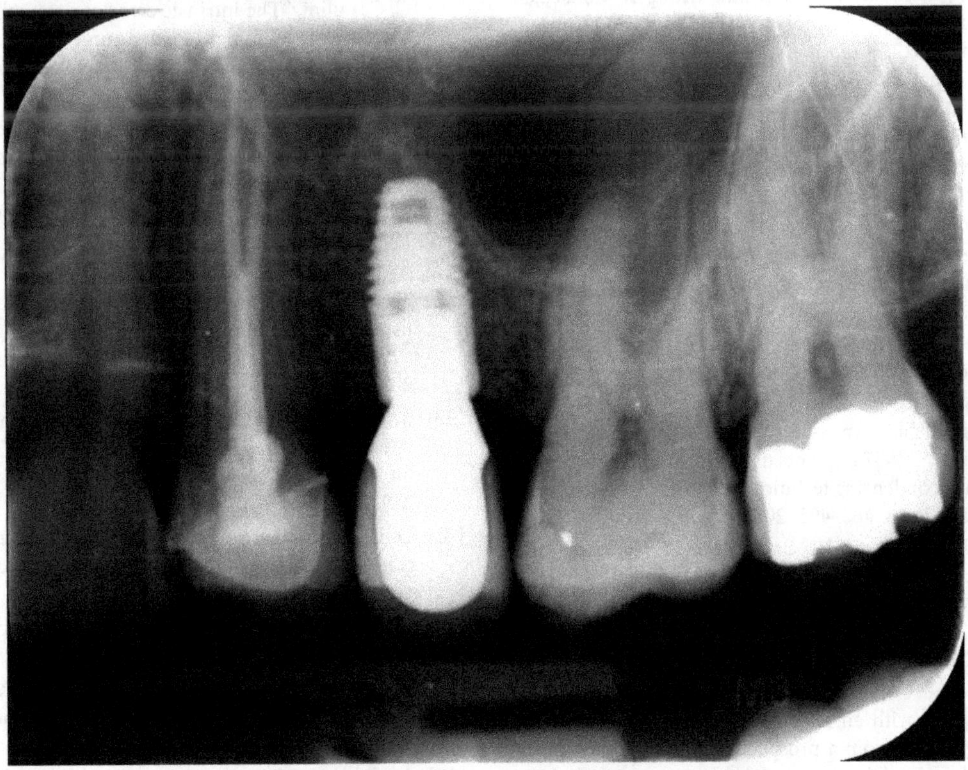

(b)

FIGURE 6: (a) Postoperatory endoral radiography. (b) Endoral radiography taken after 9 months from the surgery.

with simultaneous elevation of the maxillary sinus floor with a transcrestal approach, without performing access flaps or invasive maneuvers such as hammering of osteotomes. The minimally invasive surgical procedure is digitally planned and guided through a custom-made surgical template.

References

[1] A. Sharan and D. Madjar, "Maxillary sinus pneumatization following extractions: a radiographic study," *The International Journal of Oral & Maxillofacial Implants*, vol. 23, pp. 48–56, 2008.

[2] M. G. Araújo and J. Lindhe, "Dimensional ridge alterations following tooth extraction. An experimental study in the dog," *Journal of Clinical Periodontology*, vol. 32, no. 2, pp. 212–218, 2005.

[3] M. C. Cavalcanti, T. E. Guirado, V. M. Sapata et al., "Maxillary sinus floor pneumatization and alveolar ridge resorption after tooth loss: a cross-sectional study," *Brazilian Oral Research*, vol. 32, article e64, 2018.

[4] M. Del Fabro and T. Testori, *Maxillary Sinus Surgery and Alternatives in Treatment: Anatomy of the Maxillary Sinus*, Quintessence, Berlin, 2009.

[5] O. Hoffmann and G. G. Zafiropoulos, "Tooth-implant connection: a review," *The Journal of Oral Implantology*, vol. 38, no. 2, pp. 194–200, 2012.

[6] K. Gotfredsen, A. Wiskott, and Working Group 4, "Consensus report - reconstructions on implants. The Third EAO Consensus Conference 2012," *Clinical Oral Implants Research*, vol. 23, Supplement 6, pp. 238–241, 2012.

[7] R. Nedir, N. Nurdin, P. Khoury et al., "Osteotome sinus floor elevation with and without grafting material in the severely atrophic maxilla. A 1-year prospective randomized controlled study," *Clinical Oral Implants Research*, vol. 24, no. 11, pp. 1257–1264, 2012.

[8] R. B. Summers, "A new concept in maxillary implant surgery: the ostotome technique," *Compendium*, vol. 15, no. 152, pp. 154–156, 1994.

[9] R. B. Summers, "The ostotome technique. Part 3. Less invasive methods of elevating the sinus floor," *Compendium*, vol. 15, pp. 698–700, 1994.

[10] L. Chen and J. Cha, "An 8-year retrospective study: 1, 100 patients receiving 1, 557 implants using the minimally invasive hydraulic sinus condensing technique," *Journal of Periodontology*, vol. 76, no. 3, pp. 482–491, 2005.

[11] H. Better, D. Slavescu, H. Barbu, D. L. Cochran, and G. Chaushu, "Minimally invasive sinus lift implant device: a multicenter safety and efficacy trial preliminary results," *Clinical Implant Dentistry and Related Research*, vol. 16, no. 4, pp. 520–526, 2014.

[12] M. Tallarico, D. L. Cochran, E. Xhanari et al., "Crestal sinus lift using an implant with an internal L-shaped channel: 1-year after loading results from a prospective cohort study," *European Journal of Oral Implantology*, vol. 10, no. 3, pp. 325–336, 2017.

[13] E. Mijiritsky, H. Barbu, A. Lorean, I. Shohat, M. Danza, and L. Levin, "Use of implant-derived minimally invasive sinus floor elevation: a multicenter clinical observational study with 12- to 65-month follow-up," *The Journal of Oral Implantology*, vol. 42, no. 4, pp. 343–348, 2016.

[14] F. Attanasio, A. Antonelli, Y. Brancaccio et al., "Primary stability of three different osteotomy techniques in medullary bone: an in vitro study," *Dentistry Journal*, vol. 8, no. 1, p. 21, 2020.

[15] A. Pacifici, D. Carbone, G. Soda, A. Polimeni, and L. Pacifici, "Guided bone regeneration procedure with platelet rich fibrin (PRF) membranes in the resolution of a severe maxillary bone defect: report of a case," *Senses and Sciences*, vol. 2, no. 1, pp. 64–70, 2015.

[16] T. Testori, S. S. Wallace, M. del Fabbro et al., "Repair of large sinus membrane perforations using stabilized collagen barrier membranes: surgical techniques with histologic and radiographic evidence of success," *The International Journal of Periodontics & Restorative Dentistry*, vol. 28, no. 1, pp. 9–17, 2008.

[17] M. Cassetta, M. Giansanti, A. Di Mambro, S. Calasso, and E. Barbato, "Accuracy of two stereolithographic surgical templates: a retrospective study," *Clinical Implant Dentistry and Related Research*, vol. 15, no. 3, pp. 448–459, 2013.

[18] A. Tahmaseb, V. Wu, D. Wismeijer, W. Coucke, and C. Evans, "The accuracy of static computer-aided implant surgery: a systematic review and meta-analysis," *Clinical Oral Implants Research*, vol. 29, Supplement 16, pp. 416–435, 2018.

[19] M. Cassetta, A. Di Mambro, M. Giansanti, L. V. Stefanelli, and E. Barbato, "Is it possible to improve the accuracy of implants inserted with a stereolithographic surgical guide by reducing the tolerance between mechanical components?," *International Journal of Oral and Maxillofacial Surgery*, vol. 42, no. 7, pp. 887–890, 2013.

[20] M. Cassetta, A. Di Mambro, M. Giansanti, L. V. Stefanelli, and C. Cavallini, "The intrinsic error of a stereolithographic surgical template in implant guided surgery," *International Journal of Oral and Maxillofacial Surgery*, vol. 42, no. 2, pp. 264–275, 2013.

[21] T. Albrektsson, G. Zarb, P. Worthington, and A. R. Eriksson, "The long-term efficacy of currently used dental implants: a review and proposed criteria of success," *The International Journal of Oral & Maxillofacial Implants*, vol. 1, pp. 11–25, 1986.

[22] A. Leonhardt, K. Gröndahl, C. Bergström, and U. Lekholm, "Long-term follow-up of osseointegrated titanium implants using clinical, radiographic and microbiological parameters," *Clinical Oral Implants Research*, vol. 13, no. 2, pp. 127–132, 2002.

[23] M. Chiapasco, P. Casentini, and M. Zaniboni, "Bone augmentation procedures in implant dentistry," *THE International Journal of Oral & Maxillofacial Implants*, vol. 24, pp. 237–259, 2009.

[24] O. H. Tatum, *Lecture presented to the Alabama Implant Congress*, Clinical Implant Dentistry and Related Research, 1976.

[25] H. Tatum Jr., "Maxillary and sinus implant reconstructions," *Dental Clinics of North America*, vol. 30, no. 2, pp. 207–229, 1986.

[26] P. J. Boyne and R. A. James, "Grafting of the maxillary sinus floor with autogenous marrow and bone," *Journal of Oral Surgery*, vol. 38, no. 8, pp. 613–616, 1980.

[27] A. Jokstad, *Osseointegration and Dental Implants*, 2009, Wiley–Blackwell.

[28] J. Jensen and S. Sindet-Pedersen, "Autogenous mandibular bone grafts and osseointegrated implants for reconstruction of the severely atrophied maxilla: a preliminary report," *Journal of Oral and Maxillofacial Surgery*, vol. 49, no. 12, pp. 1277–1287, 1991.

[29] J. E. Blomqvist, P. Alberius, and S. Isaksson, "Retrospective analysis of one-stage maxillary sinus augmentation with endosseous implants," *International Journal of Oral & Maxillofacial Implants*, vol. 11, no. 4, pp. 512–521, 1996.

[30] J. E. Blomqvist, P. Alberius, and S. Isaksson, "Two-stage maxillary sinus reconstruction with endosseous implants: a prospective study," *The International Journal of Oral & Maxillofacial Implants*, vol. 13, no. 6, pp. 758–766, 1998.

[31] B. R. Johansson, K. Wannfors, J. Ekenbäck, J. I. Smedberg, and J. Hirsch, "Implants and sinus-inlay bone grafts in a 1-stage procedure on severely atrophied maxillae: surgical aspects of a 3-year follow-up study," *The International Journal of Oral & Maxillofacial Implants*, vol. 14, no. 6, pp. 811–818, 1999.

[32] J. N. Kent and M. S. Block, "Simultaneous maxillary sinus floor bone grafting and placement of hydroxylapatite-coated implants," *Journal of Oral and Maxillofacial Surgery*, vol. 47, no. 3, pp. 238–242, 1989.

[33] D. G. Smiler, P. W. Johnson, J. L. Lozada et al., "Sinus lift grafts and endosseous implants. Treatment of the atrophic posterior maxilla," *Dental Clinics of North America*, vol. 36, no. 1, pp. 151–186, 1992.

[34] D. P. Tarnow, S. S. Wallace, S. J. Froum, M. D. Rohrer, and S. C. Cho, "Histologic and clinical comparison of bilateral sinus floor elevations with and without barrier membrane placement in 12 patients: part 3 of an ongoing prospective study," *The International Journal of Periodontics & Restorative Dentistry*, vol. 20, no. 2, pp. 117–125, 2000.

[35] S. S. Wallace, S. J. Froum, S. Cho et al., "Sinus augmentation utilizing anorganic bovine bone (Bio-Oss) with absorbable and nonabsorbable membranes placed over the lateral window: histomorphometric and clinical analyses," *The International Journal of Periodontics & Restorative Dentistry*, vol. 25, no. 6, pp. 551–559, 2005.

[36] T. Starch-Jensen, D. Deluiz, K. Duch, and E. M. B. Tinoco, "Maxillary sinus floor augmentation with or without barrier membrane coverage of the lateral window: a systematic review and meta-analysis," *Journal of Oral & Maxillofacial Research*, vol. 10, no. 4, 2019.

[37] G. M. Raghoebar, P. Onclin, G. C. Boven, A. Vissink, and H. J. Meijer, "Long-term effectiveness of maxillary sinus floor augmentation: a systematic review and meta-analysis," *Journal of Clinical Periodontology*, vol. 46, Supplement 21, pp. 307–318, 2019.

[38] S. S. Wallace and S. J. Froum, "Effect of maxillary sinus augmentation on the survival of endosseous dental implants. A systematic review," *Annals of Periodontology*, vol. 8, no. 1, pp. 328–343, 2003.

[39] M. Davarpanah, H. Martínez, J. F. Técucianu, G. Hage, and R. Lazzara, "The modified osteotome technique," *The International Journal of Periodontics & Restorative Dentistry*, vol. 21, no. 6, pp. 599–607, 2001.

[40] M. Toffler, "Site development in the posterior maxilla using osteocompression and apical alveolar displacement," *The Compendium of Continuing Education in Dentistry*, vol. 22, pp. 775–790, 2001.

[41] E. Kfir, V. Kfir, E. Mijiritsky, R. Rafaeloff, and E. Kaluski, "Minimally invasive antral membrane balloon elevation followed by maxillary bone augmentation and implant fixation," *The Journal of Oral Implantology*, vol. 32, no. 1, pp. 26–33, 2006.

[42] E. Kfir, V. Kfir, E. Eliav, and E. Kaluski, "Minimally invasive antral membrane balloon elevation: report of 36 procedures," *Journal of Periodontology*, vol. 78, no. 10, pp. 2032–2035, 2007.

[43] Z. Mazor, E. Kfir, A. Lorean, E. Mijiritsky, and R. A. Horowitz, "Flapless approach to maxillary sinus augmentation using minimally invasive antral membrane balloon elevation," *Implant Dentistry*, vol. 20, no. 6, pp. 434–438, 2011.

[44] L. Pacifici and A. Pacifici, "Digital flow in medicine and dentistry: what's new?," *Journal of Biological Regulators and Homeostatic Agents*, vol. 32, no. 4, pp. 1027–1031, 2018.

[45] H. Noh, W. Nabha, J.-H. Cho, and H.-S. Hwang, "Registration accuracy in the integration of laser-scanned dental images into maxillofacial cone-beam computed tomography images," *American Journal of Orthodontics and Dentofacial Orthopedics*, vol. 140, no. 4, pp. 585–591, 2011.

[46] M. Colombo, C. Mangano, E. Mijiritsky, M. Krebs, U. Hauschild, and T. Fortin, "Clinical applications and effectiveness of guided implant surgery: a critical review based on randomized controlled trials," *BMC Oral Health*, vol. 17, no. 1, p. 150, 2017.

[47] D. Schneider, P. Marquardt, M. Zwahlen, and R. E. Jung, "A systematic review on the accuracy and the clinical outcome of computer-guided template-based implant dentistry," *Clinical Oral Implants Research*, vol. 20, Supplement 4, pp. 73–86, 2009.

[48] N. Van Assche, M. Vercruyssen, W. Coucke, W. Teughels, R. Jacobs, and M. Quirynen, "Accuracy of computer-aided implant placement," *Clinical Oral Implants Research*, vol. 23, pp. 112–123, 2012.

[49] T. Joda, U. Brägger, and G. Gallucci, "Systematic literature review of digital three-dimensional superimposition techniques to create virtual dental patients," *The International Journal of Oral & Maxillofacial Implants*, vol. 30, no. 2, pp. 330–337, 2015.

A Double Case: Socket Shield and Pontic Shield Techniques on Aesthetic Zone

Carlos Polis-Yanes,[1] **Carla Cadenas-Sebastián**,[1] **Claudia Oliver-Puigdomenech**,[1] **Raul Ayuso-Montero**,[2] **Antoni Marí-Roig**,[3,4] **and José López-López**[5]

[1]*School of Dentistry, University of Barcelona, University Campus of Bellvitge, Barcelona, Spain*
[2]*School of Dentistry, University of Barcelona, Oral Health and Masticatory System Group (Bellvitge Biomedical Research Institute) IDIBELL, University of Barcelona, University Campus of Bellvitge, L'Hospitalet de Llobregat, Barcelona, Spain*
[3]*Department of Maxillofacial Surgery, University Hospital of Bellvitge, Catalonia, Spain*
[4]*Oral Health and Masticatory System Group (Bellvitge Biomedical Research Institute) IDIBELL, University of Barcelona, L'Hospitalet de Llobregat, Barcelona, Spain*
[5]*Department of Odontostomatology, Faculty of Medicine and Health Sciences (Dentistry), Odontological Hospital University of Barcelona-University of Barcelona/Oral Health and Masticatory System Group (Bellvitge Biomedical Research Institute) IDIBELL, University of Barcelona, L'Hospitalet de Llobregat, Barcelona, Spain*

Correspondence should be addressed to José López-López; 18575jll@gmail.com

Academic Editor: Rui Amaral Mendes

When a tooth is extracted, a bone remodeling of the alveolar process occurs irretrievably. Various techniques have emerged over time to maintain the thickness of the bone crest in fixed prosthetics on teeth and implants. The socket shield and pontic shield techniques are aimed at minimizing buccal bone remodeling, especially in the aesthetic area. We present a case of an aesthetic sector rehabilitated with partial fixed denture using the socket shield and pontic shield techniques.

1. Introduction

When a tooth is extracted, the healing of the socket inevitably involves reshaping of the periodontal alveolar process with horizontal and vertical bone loss. Postextraction immediate implant placement has been proven to be a reliable and safe process, with an osseointegration success rate similar to that of conventional implants, but it does not prevent bone remodeling after extraction [1]. It has also been suggested that various regenerative treatments, such as soft or hard tissue grafts, help to compensate this alveolar process reduction [1, 2].

Among bone grafts that have been studied for immediate implantology, we can find allogenic, xenogenic, and alloplastic grafts. All of them are successful, and they have minimal differences in reabsorption [1].

The socket shield technique (SST) was published for the first time in 2010 as a feasible technique to avoid buccal bone reshaping after tooth extraction, in combination with immediate implant placement. A thin buccal and interproximal layer or fragment of the tooth needs to be maintained in order to avoid buccal bone resorption [3].

2. Objectives

The purpose of this article is to present a clinical case of a patient who underwent immediate implant placement with the SS technique in the superior aesthetic area.

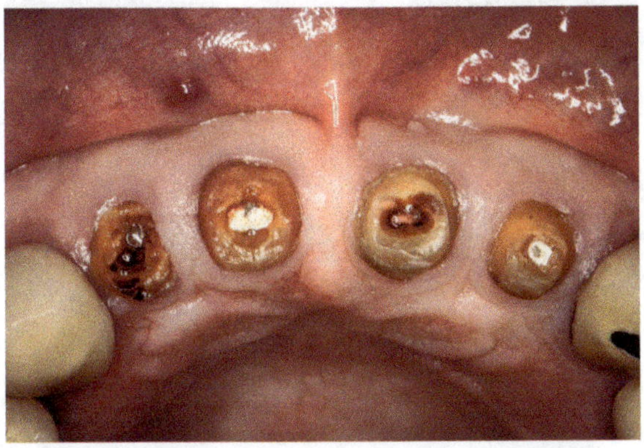

Figure 1: Image of the roots before the treatment.

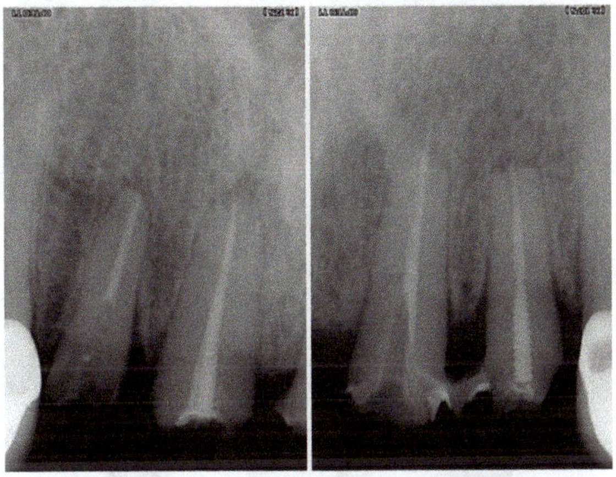

Figure 2: Periapical X-rays of the 4 incisive roots.

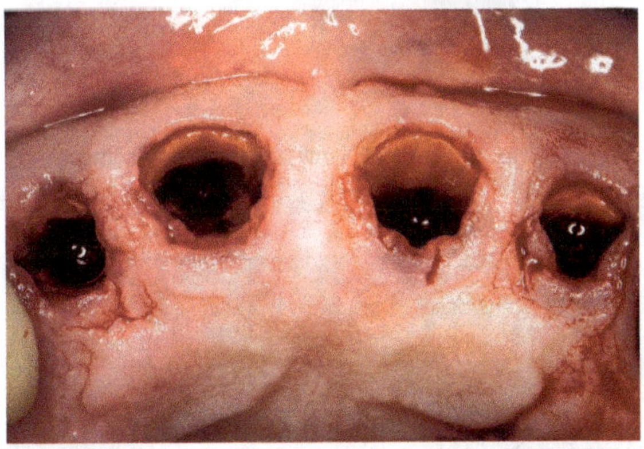

Figure 3: Intraoperative image of the root shield's preparation after extraction.

3. Case Report

A 50-year-old man was referred to us having a decemented bridge from 1.2 to 2.2, with inadequate ferrule and metal posts in each root (1.1 and 2.2), both fractured (Figures 1 and 2). Given this miserable condition of the roots and their poor prognosis, rehabilitation of the area with fixed prostheses supported by two implants was proposed.

The socket shield technique was performed on central incisors and pontic shield on lateral incisors (Figure 3) in

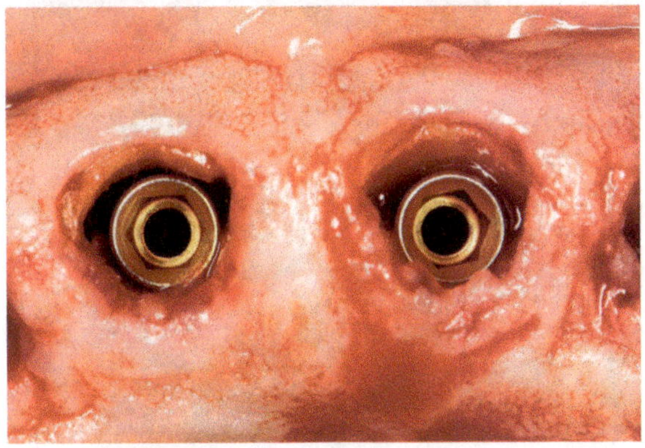

Figure 4: Intraoperative image of the implants placed, not being in contact with the buccal surface of the roots.

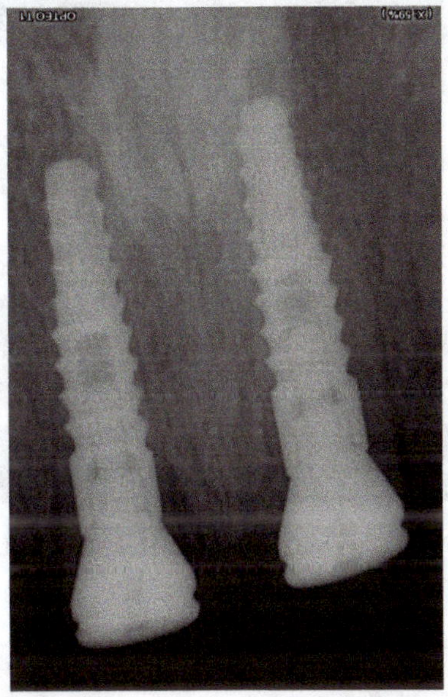

Figure 5: Postoperative periapical X-ray, taken immediately after implant placement.

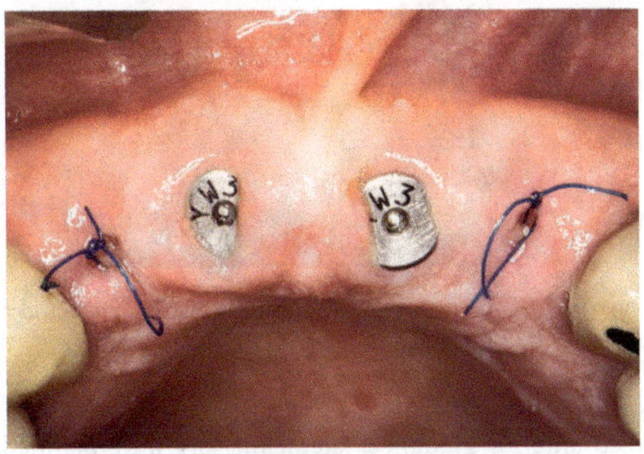

Figure 6: One-week follow-up.

order to minimize resorption and reshaping of the bone crest in implants and pontics. Haemostatic collagen sponges were placed both in 1.2 and in 2.2, and immediate implant placement was performed in 1.1 and 2.1 (Figures 4 and 5). In order

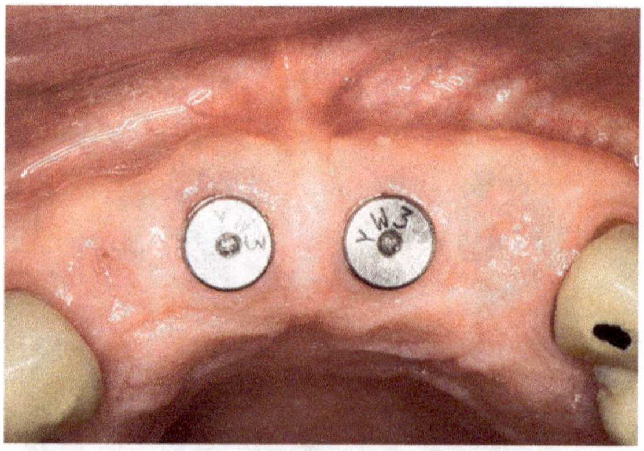

FIGURE 7: Three-month follow-up, after implant placement.

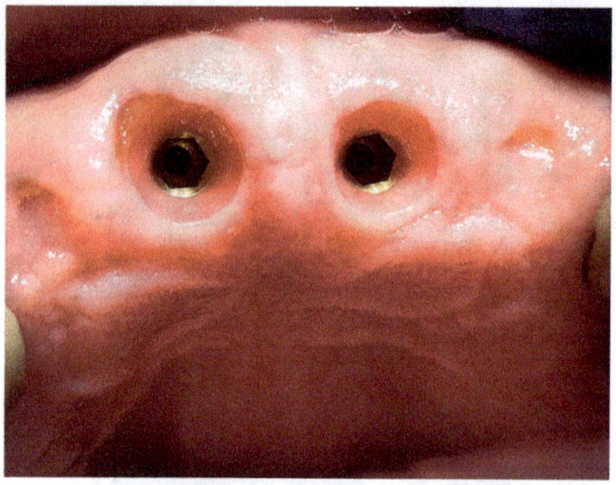

FIGURE 8: Shield exposure on 1.1 implant.

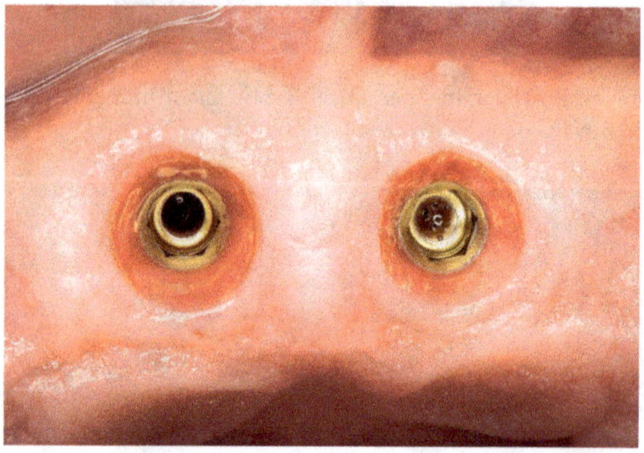

FIGURE 9: One-month follow-up, after high-speed handpiece reshaping of the shield exposure on 2.1.

to keep anterior guidance, lateral incisors were planned in cantilever, contactless during disclusion movements.

Two Biohorizons Tapered Internal 3.8 × 12 mm implants with 3.5 mm diameter internal hexagonal connection (Biohorizons®, Spain) with an insertion torque of 25 N/cm were placed, as well as the healing abutments, because the patient did not request provisional teeth. After one week, healing was proper (Figure 6).

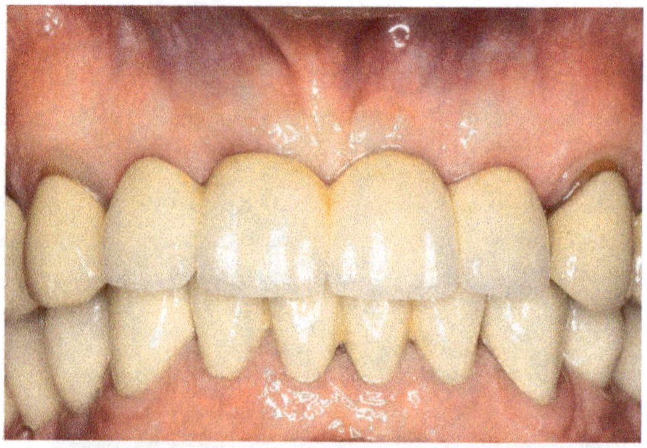

FIGURE 10: Final bridge delivery.

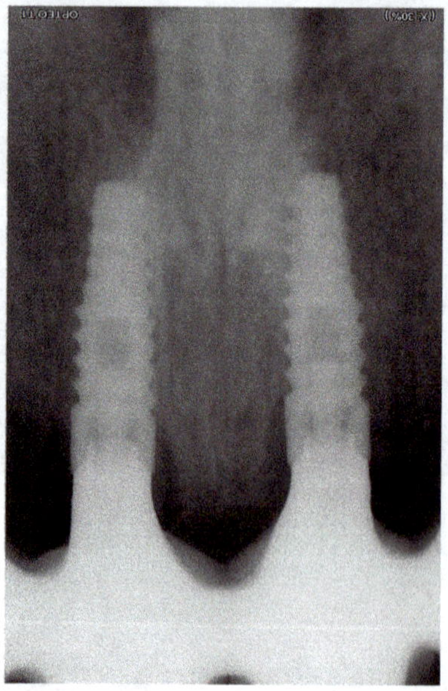

FIGURE 11: Control X-ray after bridge placing.

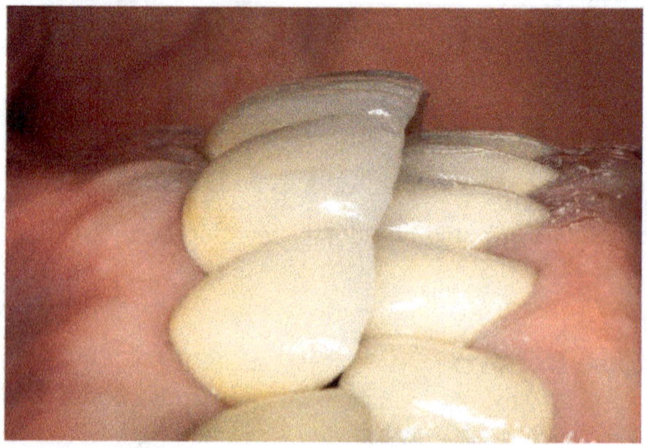

FIGURE 12: Clinical lateral vision. A good maintenance of the buccal thickness is seen.

Three months after, the osseointegration of the implants was corrected (Figure 7), but teeth 1.1 had a superficial exposure of the shield (Figure 8), which was reshaped with the

Table 1: Partial extraction therapies (PET) and their indications, adapted from Siormpas et al. [7].

PET	Clinical situation(s) indicated
Root submergence	(i) Unrestorable tooth crown or tooth indicated for extraction absence of apical pathology (ii) Healthy amputated pulp or endodontic therapy completed intention to preserve the alveolar ridge (ii) Planned removable full or partial prosthesis (iv) Planned pontic site beneath fixed prosthesis (v) Cantilever pontic site as an alternative to two adjacent implants (vi) Actively growing young patient planned for implant treatment later (vii) Ridge preservation in conjunction with other PET
Socket shield	(i) Unrestorable tooth crown or tooth indicated for extraction tooth root with or without apical pathology (ii) Intention to preserve the alveolar ridge, specifically to prevent buccopalatal collapse (iii) Immediate implant placement (iv) Ridge preservation in conjunction with other PET
Pontic shield	(i) Unrestorable tooth crown or tooth indicated for extraction tooth root with or without apical pathology (ii) Intention to preserve the alveolar ridge (iii) Planned pontic site(s) beneath fixed prosthesis (iv) Cantilever pontic site as an alternative to two adjacent implants (v) Ridge preservation in conjunction with other PET
Proximal socket shield	(i) Unrestorable tooth crown or tooth indicated for extraction tooth root with or without apical pathology (ii) Intention to preserve interdental papillae (iii) Planned immediate implant placement sites of two or more adjacent implants (iv) Papillae preservation in conjunction with other PET

high-speed handpiece using a diamond bur, without needing anesthesia. After one more month, the clinical appearance was corrected (Figure 9) and a partial fixed denture was screwed at 30 N/cm to the implant (Figures 10 and 11). Good maintenance of buccal volume and natural appearance is seen (Figure 12).

These partial extraction techniques have allowed us to maintain the volume of the buccal crest without the need to fill the gap with bone grafts and give the gingiva a natural appearance.

The authors want to emphasize that the value of this study is limited, since it is a case report of a single patient.

4. Discussion

Already in 2009, Davarpana and Szmukler-Moncler [4] presented a limited series of 5 cases with a follow-up between 12 and 42 months, in which the implants were drilled and placed through the roots of ankylosed teeth, leaving the fragments that remained stable in the socket. They found no complications derived from tooth remains in contact with the implant, and the cases were successful throughout the follow-up. They present the technique as an alternative to tooth extraction when it can cause morbidity.

Several studies have been published regarding the socket shield technique since its first reference by Hürzeler et al. [3]. Thus, Kan and Rungcharassaeng [5] and later Cherel and Etienne [6] used the SST in order to preserve the interdental papilla in between implants, in cases where adjacent teeth need to be restored.

Siormpas et al. [7] conducted a study on 46 patients with single implants, performing the "root-membrane" technique, similar to the TSS, and leaving the vestibular fragment at least 1 millimeter above the bone level and in contact with the implant surface. They obtained 100% success in a follow-up between 24 and 60 months and correct maintenance of the buccal bone volume. They concluded that it is a predictable technique for the placement of implants in aesthetic areas in healthy adults.

Gluckman et al. [8] described the pontic shield technique in which they performed a treatment similar to SST but, in these cases, filling the socket with xenogeneic graft in the pontics. Among the presented series, 13 cases were successful and one case required reshaping and advancement flap due to shield exposure. They conclude their study, describing the technique as a feasible option in bone preservation in pontics and assuming the need for more studies in this regard.

Afterwards, the same authors (in 2016 [9] and 2017 [10]) carried out two consecutive studies. The first study defined partial extraction techniques in three groups: (i) root submergence when the entire root volume is kept under the gum to preserve the volume, being very important the fact that the teeth do not have apical pathology; (ii) socket shield as a preparation of the root's buccal surface and 1 mm above the bony crest in anterior teeth and with simultaneous placement of immediate implants in the palatal surface of the socket, having eliminated any possible apical pathology before; (iii) pontic shield, which means preparing the socket shield exactly the same as SST but recommends filling the socket with osteoconductive material. They also advise soft tissue sealing and a three-month follow-up before pressing with ovoid pontics. Table 1 shows the indications for the different partial extraction techniques based on this study and review. The study finishes by concluding that partial extraction techniques should be considered by clinicians as a conservative strategy to maintain bone crest in oral rehabilitation [9].

Table 2: Instruments and materials required for PET [8].

Socket shield
(1) Long shank root resection bur
(2) Extralarge round diamond head bur (to reduce the inner aspect of shield into concavity)
(3) End-cutting diamond head bur (to reduce coronal aspect of shield) 4. Gingival protector
(4) Irrigated surgical motor
(5) Contra-angled surgical fast handpiece
(6) Microperiotomes
(7) Microforceps
Pontic shield
As for socket-shield, plus:
(1) Socket grafting instruments: plugger, particulate graft spoon, crucible
(2) SM 69 blade (or other suitable microblade, mandatory for split thickness dissection of facial and palatal pouches to tuck CTG into) 3. 6/0 nylon sutures
Root submergence
(1) Irrigated surgical motor
(2) Contra-angled surgical fast handpiece
(3) Extralarge round diamond head bur (for reducing coronal aspect root into concavity)
(4) SM 69 blade (or other suitable microblade, mandatory for split thickness dissection of facial and palatal pouches to tuck CTG into)
(5) 6/0 nylon sutures

In his second work, he focuses on the technical aspects and the management of complications. The necessary materials for partial extraction techniques described in this article are presented in Table 2. They conclude by defining partial extraction techniques as a very promising set for the future management of bone ridges after the removal of nonpreservable teeth [10].

In 2017, Gharpure & Bhatavadekar wrote in a systematic review reporting limited scientific support regarding TSS, with evidence of less osseointegration, some biological complications and short follow-up cases. They suggest the need of more studies to obtain scientific support [11]. More recently, Han et al. [12] presented a modified TSS with a series of 40 implants maintaining the buccal shield at bone crest level and with an approximate thickness of 1.5 mm, without biological complications and with a 100% success rate. They conclude that modified TSS appears to be a successful procedure combined with immediate implants because the root surface does not interfere with osseointegration and is beneficial for the aesthetics and maintenance of bone.

Bramanti et al. [13] reported a sample of forty patients who received an immediate single implant in the esthetic zone with SST versus immediate implants with the conventional technique and filling the gap with bone graft. No clinical complications were recorded at 3, 6, and 36 months from implant placement. A lower rate of crestal bone resorption was recorded in the TSS group in all checks over time.

Based on the published studies and the case we present, we can confirm that complications arise more easily when the tooth fragment remains above the bone crest. The filling of the socket does not seem necessary when performing this technique since the blood clot achieves a regeneration of the socket and the shield prevents buccal reshaping.

5. Conclusion

The conclusion that we can draw from this case report and the subsequent review of the literature is that partial extraction techniques, such as the socket shield and the pontic shield, are procedures that should be considered in oral rehabilitation in selected cases.

This kind of intervention is dependent on the surgical technique of the operator, and its reproducibility must be assessed.

References

[1] J. Majzoub, A. Ravida, T. Starch-Jensen, M. Tattan, and F. Suárez-López del Amo, "The Influence of Different Grafting Materials on Alveolar Ridge Preservation: a Systematic Review," *Journal of Oral and Maxillofacial Research*, vol. 10, no. 3, article e6, 2019.

[2] M. G. Araújo, C. O. Silva, A. B. Souza, and F. Sukekava, "Socket healing with and without immediate implant placement," *Periodontology 2000*, vol. 79, no. 1, pp. 168–177, 2019.

[3] M. B. Hürzeler, O. Zuhr, P. Schupbach, S. F. Rebele, N. Emmanouilidis, and S. Fickl, "The socket-shield technique: a proof-of-principle report," *Journal of Clinical Periodontology*, vol. 37, no. 9, pp. 855–862, 2010.

[4] M. Davarpanah and S. Szmukler-Moncler, "Unconventional implant treatment: I. Implant placement in contact with ankylosed root fragments. A series of five case reports," *Clinical Oral Implants Research*, vol. 20, no. 8, pp. 851–856, 2009.

[5] J. Y. K. Kan and K. Rungcharassaeng, "Proximal socket shield for interimplant papilla preservation in the esthetic zone," *The International Journal of Periodontics & Restorative Dentistry*, vol. 33, no. 1, pp. e24–e31, 2013.

[6] F. Cherel and D. Etienne, "Papilla preservation between two implants: a modified socket-shield technique to maintain the scalloped anatomy? A case report," *Quintessence International*, vol. 45, no. 1, pp. 23–30, 2014.

[7] K. D. Siormpas, M. E. Mitsias, E. Kontsiotou-Siormpa, D. Garber, and G. A. Kotsakis, "Immediate implant placement in the esthetic zone utilizing the "root-membrane" technique: clinical results up to 5 years postloading," *The International Journal of Oral & Maxillofacial Implants*, vol. 29, no. 6, pp. 1397–1405, 2014.

[8] H. Gluckman, J. Du Toit, and M. Salama, "The pontic-shield: partial extraction therapy for ridge preservation and pontic site development," *The International Journal of Periodontics & Restorative Dentistry*, vol. 36, no. 3, pp. 417–423, 2016.

[9] H. Gluckman, M. Salama, and J. Du Toit, "Partial extraction therapies (PET) part 1: maintaining alveolar ridge contour at pontic and immediate implant sites," *The International Journal of Periodontics & Restorative Dentistry*, vol. 36, no. 5, pp. 681–687, 2016.

[10] H. Gluckman, M. Salama, and J. Du Toit, "Partial extraction therapies (PET) part 2: procedures and technical aspects," *The International Journal of Periodontics & Restorative Dentistry*, vol. 37, no. 3, pp. 377–385, 2017.

[11] A. S. Gharpure and N. B. Bhatavadekar, "Current evidence on the socket-shield technique: a systematic review," *The Journal of Oral Implantology*, vol. 43, no. 5, pp. 395–403, 2017.

[12] C.-H. Han, K.-B. Park, and F. G. Mangano, "The modified socket shield technique," *Journal of Craniofacial Surgery*, vol. 29, no. 8, pp. 2247–2254, 2018.

[13] E. Bramanti, A. Norcia, M. Cicciù et al., "Postextraction dental implant in the aesthetic zone, socket shield technique versus conventional protocol," *The Journal of Craniofacial Surgery*, vol. 29, no. 4, pp. 1037–1041, 2018.

New Implant Design with Midcrestal and Apical Wing Thread for Increased Implant Stability in Single Postextraction Maxillary Implant

Antonio Scarano[1,2,3] **Bartolomeo Assenza,**[1] **Francesco Inchingolo,**[4] **Filiberto Mastrangelo**[5] **and Felice Lorusso**[1]

[1]*Department of Medical, Oral and Biotechnological Sciences and CeSi-MeT, University of Chieti-Pescara, Via dei Vestini, 31, 66100 Chieti, Italy*
[2]*Zirconia Implant Research Group (Z.I.R.G), International Academy of Ceramic Implantology, USA*
[3]*Department of Oral Implantology, Dental Research Division, College Ingà, UNINGÁ, Cachoeiro de Itapemirim 29312, Brazil*
[4]*Department of Interdisciplinary Medicine, University of Bari "Aldo Moro", 70121 Bari, Italy*
[5]*Department of Clinical and Experimental Medicine, University of Foggia, Foggia, Italy*

Correspondence should be addressed to Antonio Scarano; ascarano@unich.it

Academic Editor: Giuseppe Alessandro Scardina

Background. The immediate placement of a dental implant could represent an option treatment for the rehabilitation of a postextractive missing tooth socket to replace compromised or untreatable teeth, with the advantage of single-session surgery. In this way, the anatomy of the alveolar bone defect, the preservation of the buccal cortical bone, and the primary stability of the fixture represent the critical factors that consent a precise implant placement. *Objective.* This case report describes a novel fixture design for postextractive alveolar socket immediate implant. *Methods.* Two patients (25 and 31 years old) were treated for postextractive dental implant placement to replace both central upper incisor teeth with four implants. The residual bone implant gap was not filled with graft or bone substitute. The restoration was provided following a standard loading protocol by a cement-sealed prosthetic abutment. *Results.* Clinically, all implants positioned showed an excellent insertion torque. No postoperative complications were reported. At 6 months of healing, the buccal cortical bone and the implant stability were present and well maintained. *Conclusion.* The evidence of this study allows us to underline the possible advantages of this new fixture design for postextractive implant technique.

1. Introduction

Nowadays, dental implants are recognized as a reliable treatment option for replacing missing teeth for periodontal defects, endodontic problems, trauma, fracture, and bone tissue atrophy is often present, which is more marked in a horizontal direction [1, 2].

The presence of vertical and horizontal lack of bone tissue represents an indispensable condition in order to reach stable implant-prosthetic rehabilitation over time [3–5]. Primary implant stability is a key factor that influences the success rate of these implants and determines the timing of prosthetic loading [6]. Many factors influence implant stability such as quality and quantity [7], shape, size, length, and the variety of surfaces [8, 9]. Primary implant stability is also important in case of immediate implant placement into fresh extraction sockets [10].

In this clinical situation, there is a bone defect and primary implant stability is very difficult to achieve. The surgical method allows reaching aspired aesthetical results, but a certain failure percentage has been reported [11, 12] due to different causes such as the presence of bacteria, absence of good primary stability, and lack of adequate bone support. Nowadays, the most used surgical protocol constitutes

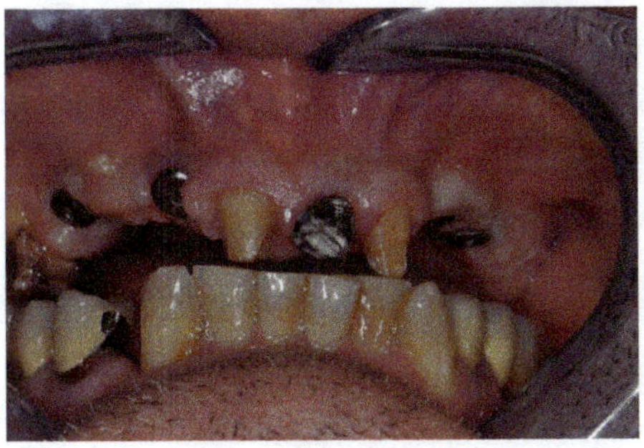

FIGURE 1: The teeth before extraction.

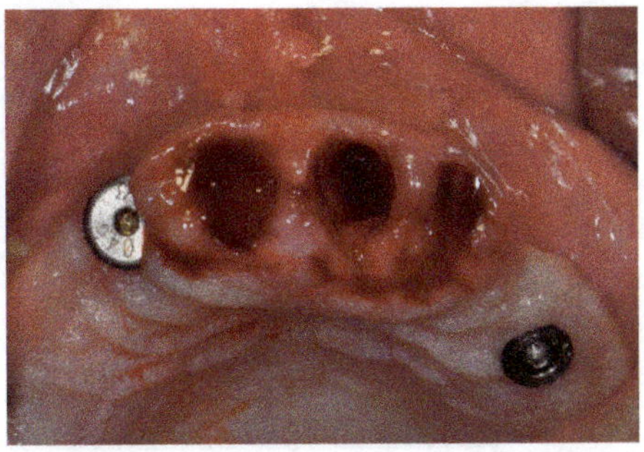

FIGURE 2: Extraction of the compromised element without flap elevation.

removing the causal element and waiting 2 months or more in order to reach socket healing. In a case of inadequate bone tissue where regenerative surgery is used to rehabilitate function and aesthetics [12, 13], it is necessary to wait an additional healing period.

In case of immediate postextractive implants for increasing the implant stability, a new implant geometry was introduced, aimed specifically at enabling better initial and long-term stability. This implant has a specially designed expanded diameter and a midcrestal and apical "wing" thread, which provides added bone contact for a higher insertion torque for primary stability.

The aim of this case report was to evaluate this novel implant design in two patients with immediate postextractive implant in an aesthetic area.

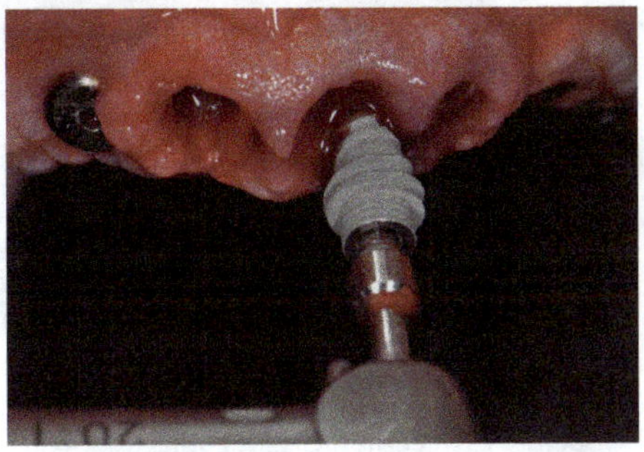

FIGURE 3: Placement of the implant with expanded diameter thread in the midcrestal and apical area.

2. Case Report

A total of two patients, a 25-year-old male and a 31-year-old female, who required extraction of both central upper incisor teeth because of caries were selected. Neither patient presented chronicle or acute diseases that could influence osseointegration. The patients were nonsmokers with a good and correct domiciliary oral hygiene. A three-dimensional radiographic tomography scan (CBCT) (Vatech Ipax 3D PCH-6500, Fort Lee, NJ, USA) was performed before and after 6 months of implant placement. Two grams of amoxicillin was prescribed to both patients 2 hours before surgery. Chlorhexidine digluconate mouthwashes (Curaden Healthcare S.p.A., Saronno, Italy) were also recommended for at least 7 days after every meal or beverage, avoiding rinsing by water.

The extraction of the teeth was executed without flap in order to allow postextractive implant placement (Figures 1 and 2). To prepare the implant site, a 2 mm diameter bur was first used that was 15° palatally inclined and worked along the socket remaining after extraction; this inclination allows the palatal direction preserving greater quantity of vestibular bone tissue. It must be emphasized that the implant sites did not respect socket length completely, since they had to move apically in a palatal direction. Compared to the implant, the site has to have a smaller section (0.5 mm) in order to guarantee greater quantity of vestibular bone tissue and assure valid primary stability. The final bur length has to be equal to the inserting fixture, which was 12 mm in these two cases. The implant site was prepared with dedicated surgical cutters, as indicated by the manufacturer with a sequential cutter passage: pilot cutter 2 mm and 3.1 mm, 3.9 mm then 4.25 mm terminal cutter. To verify the height of the implant site preparation, a 2 mm diameter and 12 mm length measurer was inserted. The insertion of a 4.5 mm diameter and 12 mm length X-Space implant (Bone System® Implant System, Milano, Italy) completed the surgery (Figure 3). This dental implant has a rounded apex and two sharp and highly engaging threads, located close to each other to facilitate implant insertion.

The implants were placed with a mean insertion torque of 35.5 ± 4 Ncm measured with a manual torque wrench by the dentist and recorded for statistical analysis (GraphPad 6.0, Prism, San Diego, USA). No bone substitute was used for filling the implant gap. The implants were loaded with standard protocol, and the reverse torque was evaluated at 6 months after healing in the second phase surgery [14, 15].

3. Results

The four implant implants showed good radiologic osseointegration (Figure 4). The application of a 60 Ncm torque by a manual torque after 6 months of implant placement was not sufficient for detaching them from the bone. This confirms the good integration of the implants. A three-dimensional radiographic tomography scan (CBCT) (Vatech Ipax 3D PCH-6500, Fort Lee, NJ, USA) was performed before the procedure. The CBCT image after 6 months of implant placement showing the preserved buccal plate and the gap was filled by a new bone (Figure 4).

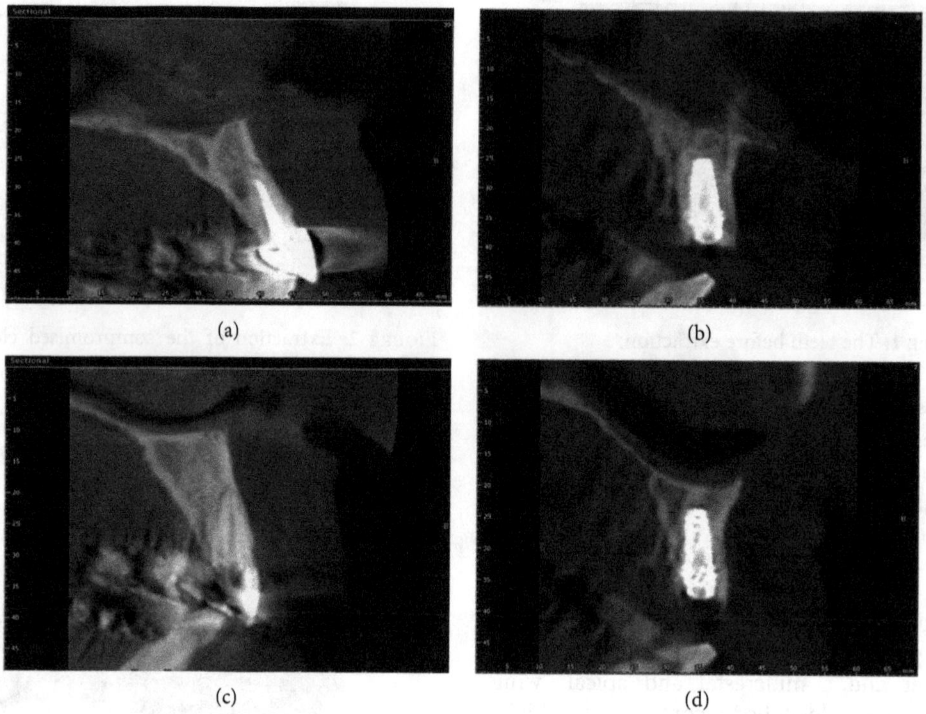

Figure 4: (a) Before extraction the CBCT image showing a thin buccal plate. (b) After 6 months of implant placement, the buccal plate was preserved and the gap was filled by new a bone. (c) Second clinical case. Before extraction, there is a thin buccal plate. (d) After 6 months of implant placement. Also in this case, the buccal plate was preserved.

4. Discussion

The application of this new implant design in immediate postextractive socket guarantees a valid primary stability that is indispensable for following implant osseointegration. The use of the studied implant with an expanded diameter and midcrestal and apical "wing" thread, inserted by dynamometer ratchet pressure, determines preservation of the postextractive site and increases implant stability. Immediate implant placement into fresh extraction sockets is extensively used in clinical practice and is considered a predictable and acceptable procedure [16, 17]. In this report, the procedure for immediate implant placement with an expanded diameter thread in the midcrestal and apical area was conducted as planned and a favourable result was obtained, as shown by the initial postoperation images. Ever since the immediate implant placement procedure was developed, the maintenance of the buccal bony wall and implant stability has always been a major concern for implantologists.

5. Conclusion

After 6 months of clinical observation, this report demonstrates that the stability of immediately placed implants can be ensured by an expanded diameter thread in the midcrestal and apical area. However, due to the limitations associated with the use of only two case reports and four implants, further research is required to confirm it.

References

[1] C. E. Jansen and A. Weisgold, "Presurgical treatment planning for the anterior single-tooth implant restoration," *Compendium of Continuing Education in Dentistry*, vol. 16, no. 8, 1995.

[2] P. S. Wöhrle, "Single-tooth replacement in the aesthetic zone with immediate provisionalization: fourteen consecutive case reports," *Practical Periodontics and Aesthetic Dentistry*, vol. 10, no. 9, pp. 1107–1114, 1998.

[3] A. Scarano, A. Piattelli, G. Murmura, G. Iezzi, B. Assenza, and C. Mancino, "Delayed expansion of the atrophic mandible by ultrasonic surgery: a clinical and histologic case series," *The International Journal of Oral & Maxillofacial Implants*, vol. 30, no. 1, pp. 144–149, 2015.

[4] A. Scarano, G. Murmura, G. Vantaggiato et al., "Delayed expansion of atrophic mandible (deam): a case report," *Oral & Implantology*, vol. 10, no. 2, pp. 190–196, 2017.

[5] A. Scarano, F. Carinci, B. Assenza, M. Piattelli, G. Murmura, and A. Piattelli, "Vertical ridge augmentation of atrophic posterior mandible using an inlay technique with a xenograft without miniscrews and miniplates: case series," *Clinical Oral Implants Research*, vol. 22, no. 10, pp. 1125–1130, 2011.

[6] L. Sennerby and N. Meredith, "Implant stability measurements using resonance frequency analysis: biological and biomechanical aspects and clinical implications," *Periodontology 2000*, vol. 47, no. 1, pp. 51–66, 2008.

[7] F. Javed and G. E. Romanos, "The role of primary stability for successful immediate loading of dental implants. A literature review," *Journal of Dentistry*, vol. 38, no. 8, pp. 612 620, 2010.

[8] P. Cappare, G. Sannino, M. Minoli, P. Montemezzi, and F. Ferrini, "Conventional versus digital impressions for full

arch screw-retained maxillary rehabilitations: a randomized clinical trial," *International Journal of Environmental Research and Public Health*, vol. 16, no. 5, p. 829, 2019.

[9] P. Capparé, R. Vinci, D. A. di Stefano et al., "Correlation between initial BIC and the insertion torque/depth integral recorded with an instantaneous torque-measuring implant motor: an in vivo study," *Clinical Implant Dentistry and Related Research*, vol. 17, Supplement 2, pp. e613–e620, 2015.

[10] A. Scarano, "Traditional postextractive implant site preparation compared with pre-extractive interradicular implant bed preparation in the mandibular molar region, using an ultrasonic device: a randomized pilot study," *The International Journal of Oral & Maxillofacial Implants*, vol. 32, no. 3, pp. 655–660, 2017.

[11] A. Piattelli, A. Scarano, and M. Piattelli, "Microscopical aspects of failure in osseointegrated dental implants: a report of five cases," *Biomaterials*, vol. 17, no. 12, pp. 1235–1241, 1996.

[12] L. Huys, "Replacement therapy and the immediate post-extraction dental implant," *Implant Dentistry*, vol. 10, no. 2, pp. 93–102, 2001.

[13] D. P. Tarnow and R. N. Eskow, "Considerations for single-unit esthetic implant restorations," *Compendium of Continuing Education in Dentistry*, vol. 16, no. 8, 1995.

[14] N. Mall, B. Dhanasekar, and I. N. Aparna, "Validation of implant stability: a measure of implant permanence," *Indian Journal of Dental Research*, vol. 22, no. 3, pp. 462–467, 2011.

[15] S. G. Simeone, M. Rios, and J. Simonpietri, ""Reverse torque of 30 Ncm applied to dental implants as test for osseointegration"-a human observational study," *International Journal of Implant Dentistry*, vol. 2, no. 1, p. 26, 2016.

[16] L. Tettamanti, C. Andrisani, M. A. Bassi, R. Vinci, J. Silvestre-Rangil, and A. Tagliabue, "Post extractive implant: evaluation of the critical aspects," *Oral & Implantology*, vol. 10, no. 2, pp. 119–128, 2017.

[17] A. Barone, P. Toti, A. Quaranta, G. Derchi, and U. Covani, "The clinical outcomes of immediate versus delayed restoration procedures on immediate implants: a comparative cohort study for single-tooth replacement," *Clinical Implant Dentistry and Related Research*, vol. 17, no. 6, pp. 1114–1126, 2015.

Decompression and Enucleation of a Mandibular Radicular Cyst, Followed by Bone Regeneration and Implant-Supported Dental Restoration

M. AboulHosn,[1] Z. Noujeim,[1] N. Nader,[1] and A. Berberi[2]

[1]*Department of Oral & Maxillofacial Surgery, Faculty of Dental Medicine, Lebanese University, Beirut, Lebanon*
[2]*Professor and Head Department of Oral & Maxillofacial Surgery, Faculty of Dental Medicine, Lebanese University, Beirut, Lebanon*

Correspondence should be addressed to A. Berberi; anberberi@gmail.com

Academic Editor: Daniel Torrés-Lagares

Odontogenic cysts are usually treated by enucleation (cystectomy). Limited cysts (less than 5 cm) are usually managed by primary excision (total cystectomy), whereas larger ones (exceeding 5 cm) are often decompressed or marsupialized. Because it consists only of opening a much smaller surgical window, decompression is regarded as a more conservative method of treatment: this method associates the creation of an opening (window) into the cystic cavity with the suturing of a decompressing device (plastic tube or stent) at the periphery of the cyst. Apart from releasing intraluminal pressure in the pathological cavity, this procedure helps the lesion to progressively decrease in volume "with a gradual increase in bone apposition" and preserves pulp vitality and periodontal integrity of the adjacent teeth. We are reporting a case of a mandibular radicular cyst that was treated by decompression, followed by enucleation, bone reconstruction, and restoration with two osseointegrated dental implants. The cystic cavity progressively decreased in volume and increased in bone density.

1. Introduction

Marsupialization of odontogenic cystic lesions was described by Partsch in 1892; it is a technique where a large window is made in cystic wall and then sutured to the oral mucosa [1]. Decompression, proposed by Thoma [2], can be performed by using devices such as tube or stent [3], it's based on creation a window between the cyst and the oral cavity by fixing the device [4]. The decompression procedure may be easier to perform and more conservative than marsupialization [3, 4].

Bone defects can occur inevitably after mandibular cyst enucleation. A bone graft can be planned to promote bone regeneration of this bony defect [5, 6]. The remaining cystic cavity can be filled with different grafting materials to accelerate bone healing and anatomical regeneration and provide adequate support to the teeth and alveolar bone [2, 7, 8].

The aim of the present study is to present a clinical case report of a radicular cyst in a female patient that was treated by decompression, followed by cyst's enucleation, bone reconstruction of the cyst cavity, and dental implant placement and restoration.

2. Case Report

A 45-year-old female patient consulted our office with a chief complaint of left facial swelling and numbness of her chin, left lower lip, and a part of her left buccal mucosa and mandibular posterior vestibule. The patient had a history of endodontic treatment of her mandibular second left premolar (tooth 35) that was not accomplished by her restorative dentist; she also revealed that the swelling increased and reached her mid lower face, extending to the left anterior triangle of her neck, as well. She was treated by her restorative dentist

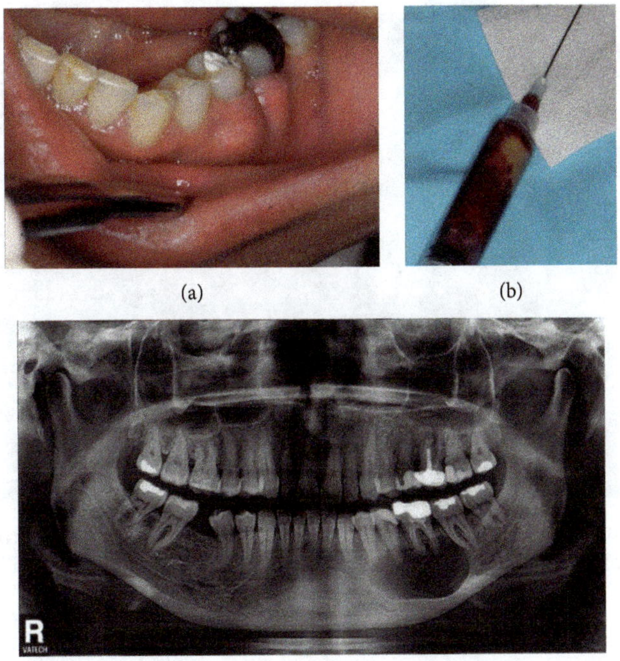

(a) (b) (c)

Figure 1: (a) Clinical aspect of left mandibular vestibule (premolar and molar regions). (b) Aspiration syringe yielding blood and pus from the radiolucent image. (c) OPG of the patient displaying the radiolucent image in left mandible (34 to 37).

with intramuscular injections of Rocephin® (ceftriaxone) during 4 weeks without remission.

Patient originally consulted for left facial swelling and paresthesia of left lower lip and chin. The left posterior mandibular vestibule, and particularly apical regions of 34 to 37, was spontaneously painful.

Intraoral examination displayed two swellings (in the left mandibular vestibule in relation to teeth 35 and 36) that were tender to palpation. On clinical examination, teeth 35 and 36 showed extreme mobility and were painful on horizontal and vertical percussion. Tooth 35 was open to access pulpal cavity, and thermal pulp test was negative on teeth 34 and 36 and positive on tooth 37.

An orthopantomogram (OPG) was taken in order to determine a possible bony pathology underneath the swollen left mandibular vestibule: OPG displayed a well-limited radiolucent image, extending from tooth 34 to tooth 37 and occupying most of the mandibular basal bone, in this sector. Periapical radiolucent lesion measured around 3-4 cm in length with around 2 cm width. It appeared unilocular, with well-defined, nonsclerotic borders, extending from mesial aspect of 34 to mesial aspect of mesial root of tooth 37, and almost reaching lower border of the mandible. Aspiration of the lesion was performed under local analgesia and it released pus and blood and a presumptive diagnosis of infected radicular cyst was made (Figures 1(a)–1(c)).

Axial and coronal cuts of a cone beam computed tomography (CBCT) showed a radiolucency, ball shaped, measuring approximately 30.7 mm × 19.7 mm with discontinuity of the buccal wall, and the mandibular canal is repressed toward the basic bone of the mandible (Figures 2(a)–2(c)).

Treatment plan was decided and discussed with the patient, and the agreement was to undertake root canal treatment of tooth 34 and extract teeth 35 and 36 and to perform decompression of the radiolucent lesion through their alveolar cavities, after extractions of these teeth.

Block analgesia of the left inferior alveolar nerve was implemented with block 2% articaine with 1 : 100,000 adrenaline (3M ESPE, Seefeld, Germany); teeth 35 and 36 were extracted using elevators and forceps.

An incision through alveolar processes of 35 and 36 was made with no. 15 blade and the lesion's lining was fenestrated with a scalpel's blade: two transparent plastic tubes, sectioned from the tubing of a standard saline bag, were inserted in each alveolar cavity, and two interrupted sutures, from each side of the tubes, were placed to stabilize them (Figures 3(a) and 3(b)).

The patient was instructed to self-irrigate the lesion with a plastic disposable syringe with needle, with two antiseptic solutions, normal saline solution (0.9% sodium chloride in water) during the day (once every 3 hours and after each meal) and 0.12% chlorhexidine gluconate in the morning and in the evening before bedtime.

The patient was recalled every week for irrigation of the lesion and check-up. What is special in this irrigation modality is that the antiseptic solution (saline and/or chlorhexidine gluconate) was injected through one tube and drained from the other one, instantaneously. At biweekly intervals, the length of the tube was monitored and cut in order to keep it far from occlusion (Figure 4).

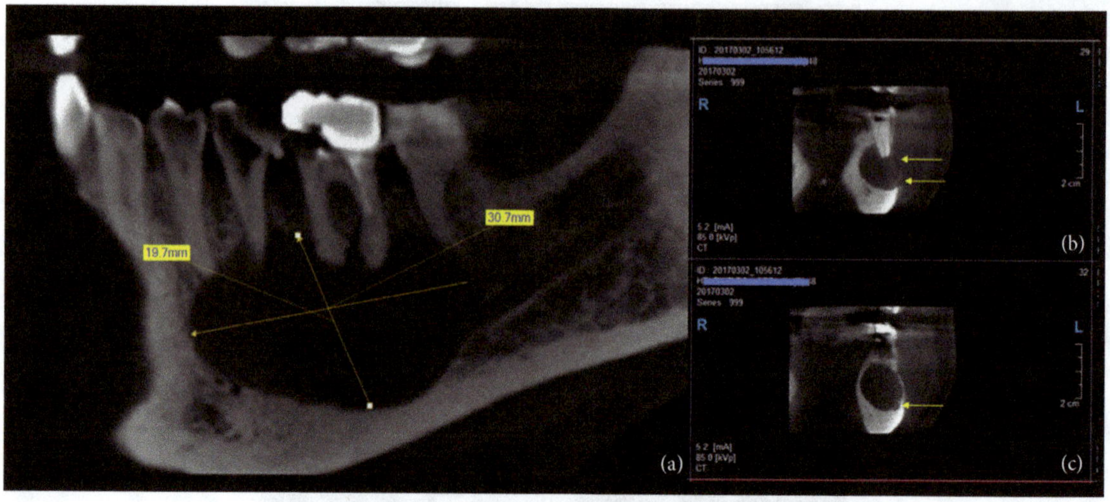

FIGURE 2: CBCT reconstruction of the left mandible. (a) The sagittal reconstruction with the approximative measurement of the bone destruction (30.7 mm × 19.7 mm). (b) Para-axial cut showing the discontinuity of the buccal cortical bone. (c) Para-axial cut showing the position of the mandibular canal.

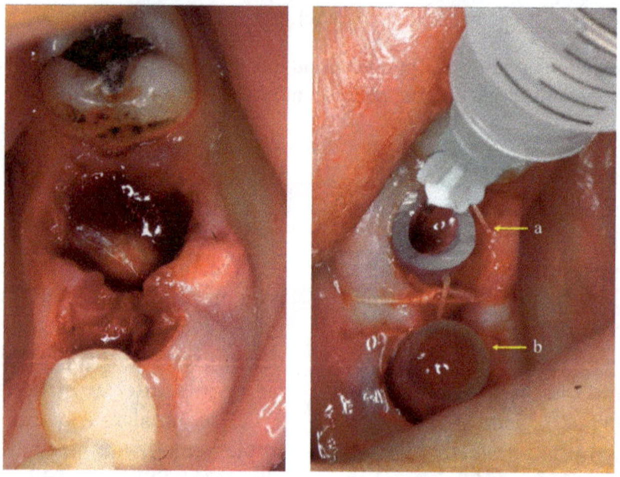

FIGURE 3: (a) Clinical aspect of alveolar cavities of 35 and 36, immediately after their extraction. (b) Plastic tubes secured in alveolar cavities of teeth 35 and 36 with sutures. A disposable syringe (with needle) injecting a normal saline solution (sodium chloride in water) in distal tube in order to regularly irrigate the lesions. After injection of antiseptic solution in distal tube (A), irrigating liquid is evacuated from mesial tube (B).

The lesion's enucleation was planned to be implemented 6 months after decompression that would reduce its size. Indeed, 6 months after the first lesion's irrigation, a panoramic radiograph was taken in order to evaluate the bone apposition: bone formation took place within the lesion as observed on CBCT performed after 7 months, with an almost complete formation of buccal cortical and bone apposition buccally (±4 mm) and lingually (±2.4 mm) as shown on the para-axial cut and lesion volume reduction as shown on the sagittal reconstruction (±25.1 mm × 15.2 mm), all along the lesion (Figures 5(a)–5(c)).

At first week of the 7th postoperative month, the decompression tubes were removed. With a blade #15, a crestal incision followed by 2 relaxing incisions was performed before raising a full-thickness flap. After separating the lesion's membrane from the flap, enucleation was accomplished with a Lucas curette and the entire pathological specimen was collected and immersed in a fixative solution (20% formol) for histopathological examination.

During operation, it was noticed that the buccal bone wall took the same shape of drainage tubes after reformation. After the lesion's enucleation, the bony cavity was filled with Puros® cortico-cancellous particulate allograft (Zimmer Biomet Dental, Carlsbad, California, USA) due to its osteoconductive properties. The flap was relocated with 5/0 nylon interrupted sutures, and tube opening locations were covered with collagen (CollaTape®) over bone graft (Figures 6(a)–6(d)).

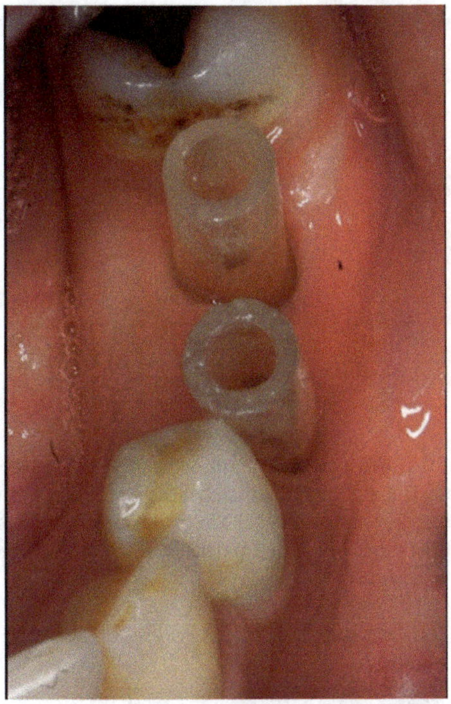

FIGURE 4: Gingival healing around decompressing devices (tubes), 3 weeks after their placement and suturing.

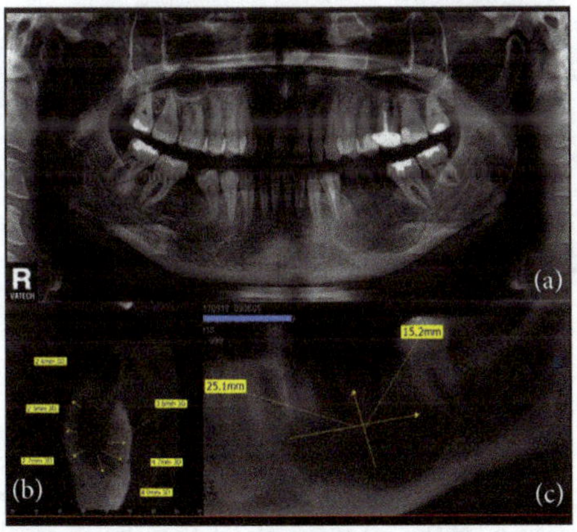

FIGURE 5: (a) Panoramic radiograph 7 months after decompression, showing a reduction of the volume of the lesion. (b) CBCT of the same time period time, the para-axial cut shows a bone healing toward the center of the lesions with approximately ±4 mm buccally and ±2.4 mm lingually. (c) Sagittal reconstruction of the CBCT shows a volume reduction of the lesion approximately.

The patient consulted us again one week after the cyst enucleation with less than 20% of left lower lip/chin numbness remaining, and two weeks later, she almost recovered her normal sensation, with a mild left lower lip "heaviness" remaining (Figures 7(a) and 7(b)).

Pathological report concluded that the lesion was a radicular cyst (Figure 8).

Six months following bone grafting, CBCT shows a complete bone regeneration of the whole area (Figure 9) and two SwissPlus Zimmer® implants were placed in locations of teeth 35 and 36 and were restored with cemented prostheses 3 months after their surgical placement (Figures 10(a)–10(e)).

3. Discussion

Radicular cyst is the most frequent odontogenic cyst observed in tooth-bearing areas: it is usually associated with carious, nonvital, discolored, or fractured tooth. Dental caries are known to provocate dental pulp inflammation that leads, ultimately, to pulp necrosis; infection will then spread to periradicular space, causing periodontitis that usually precedes either periradicular acute abscess, chronic granuloma, or radicular cyst. This cyst usually follows persistent chronic infection, and it is believed to form by proliferation of the epithelial cell rests of Malassez in inflamed periradicular tissues [9].

Several treatment options are nowadays available for a radicular cyst such as nonsurgical root canal therapy (endodontic treatment), extraction of the offending tooth if unrestorable, decompression, marsupialization, and enucleation with primary closure, when the lesion is large [6]. The treatment of choice depends on the size and localization of the lesion, integrity of the cystic epithelial lining, proximity of the cyst to adjacent vital teeth and anatomical structures (such as inferior alveolar canal, mental foramen, infraorbital foramen, maxillary sinus, nasal cavity, and infratemporal space), and behavior of the cyst (clinical aggressively and radiological invasiveness) [10].

Decompression procedure is "an alternative plan of treatment and a more conservative approach; this procedure allows for continuous drainage, which removes those conditions that favor cyst expansion" [8]. In the present case report, an aspiration of a serosanguinous purulent fluid confirmed the provisional, presumptive diagnosis of a "cystic" lesion (presumptive radicular cyst), knowing that cystic content may be straw colored, cloudy, or serosanguinous. Failure to withdraw any kind of intracystic fluid or repeated aspirations of blood warrant a reevaluation of the provisional diagnosis and absence of any aspirate liquid may suggest a solid cellular lesion of neoplastic origin or a fibrous one [11].

Decompression devices (tubes) aim to maintain drainage of jaw pathological lesions and facilitate their repeated irrigations [4]: in our case, fabrication of these tubes consisted of a section of the tubing from a standard saline solution bag. We decided to use this kind of tubing because it is not collapsible, readily available, and sufficient in diameter to prevent clogging; they can be adjusted and fashioned for patient comfort as well and their insertion and removal are easy and appropriate.

Decompression tubes were immersed in 0.12% chlorhexidine gluconate for 15 minutes and then sterilized before placement in the pathological cavity. They were inserted using a slight rotary motion and gently pushed downwards into the depth of the lesion until resistance was met at the lesion's lower level. Initial drainage occurred immediately after their insertion.

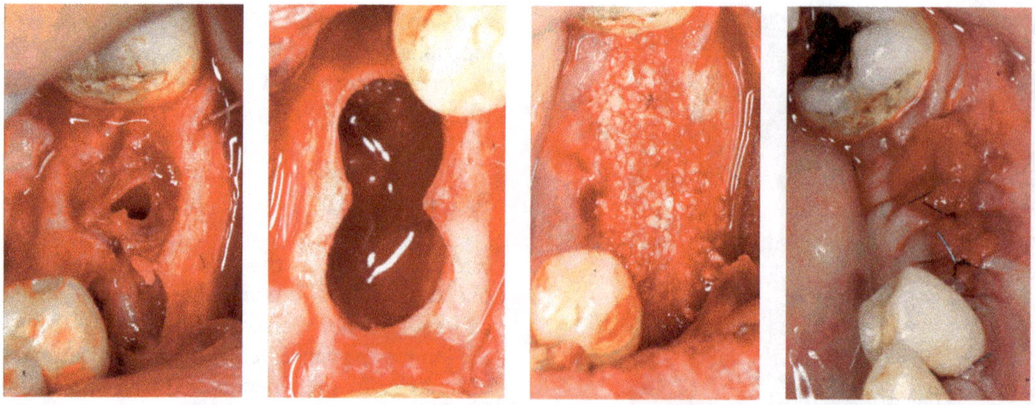

(a) (b) (c) (d)

FIGURE 6: (a) Six months after the beginning of decompression, a mucoperiosteal flap was performed and decompression tubes removed, leading to the roof of the radiolucent lesion. (b) Upper aspect of the bony pathological cavity, immediately after the lesion's enucleation. Notice that the bone was formed all around external surfaces of both decompression devices (tubes). (c) The pathological cavity filled with Puros® cortico-cancellous particulate allograft, a mixture of 70% cortical and 30% cancellous bone particulate. (d) Puros® biomaterial covered with collagen cones (CollaPlug®) and mucosal wound sutured with 5/0 nylon sutures.

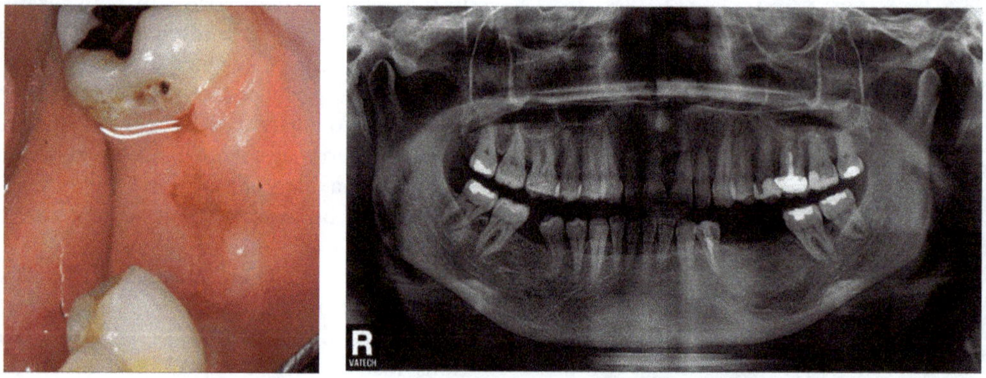

(a) (b)

FIGURE 7: (a) Clinical mucosal healing after one week. (b) Radiological aspect of the graft and surrounding bone.

It is widely known that decompression and marsupialization are conservative treatment modalities that involve an opening to reduce intracystic pressure and induce bony formation [2, 3, 12]: both procedures provide good surgical access to lesions with low postoperative morbidity and low incidence of peroperative complications [13, 14], help in maintaining pulp vitality of intracystic teeth, shrink the lesions' volume, and reduce their recurrence rates [15, 16].

In our case, decompression led to reduce the volume of the cyst from 30.7 mm × 19.7 mm to 25.1 mm × 15.2 mm approximately. The CBCT shows a complete bone formation of the cortical buccal plate and bone apposition from the buccal bone and lingual bone in a central direction measured as ±4 mm and ±2.4 respectively.

The effects of decompression based on age are controversial: it was reported that younger patients had higher reduction rates [12], but it was also known that decompression and incidence of recurrence are not correlated with age [17].

Another advantage of these two methods, particularly decompression, is the positive effect they have on the histological nature of the cyst's epithelial lining. In a study on 14 decompressed odontogenic keratocysts (OKCs) with 65% of mean shrinkage of the radiolucency, August and coworkers reported a dedifferentiation and loss of cytokeratin-10 production in 64% of decompression and irrigation patients after a 9-month average treatment time: changes in cystic epithelium appeared to be a gradual process and their results suggested that a treatment time of at least 9 months may be required to induce epithelial dedifferentiation [18].

Schlieve and coworkers [19] studied the possible histological diagnostic changes after decompression of odontogenic cysts and cyst-like lesions: the purpose of their study was to report the histopathological findings after postdecompression definitive treatment, thereby answering the clinical question "does decompression change the histologic diagnosis?" Twenty-five cysts and cyst-like lesions in 25 patients were decompressed before being enucleated and curetted.

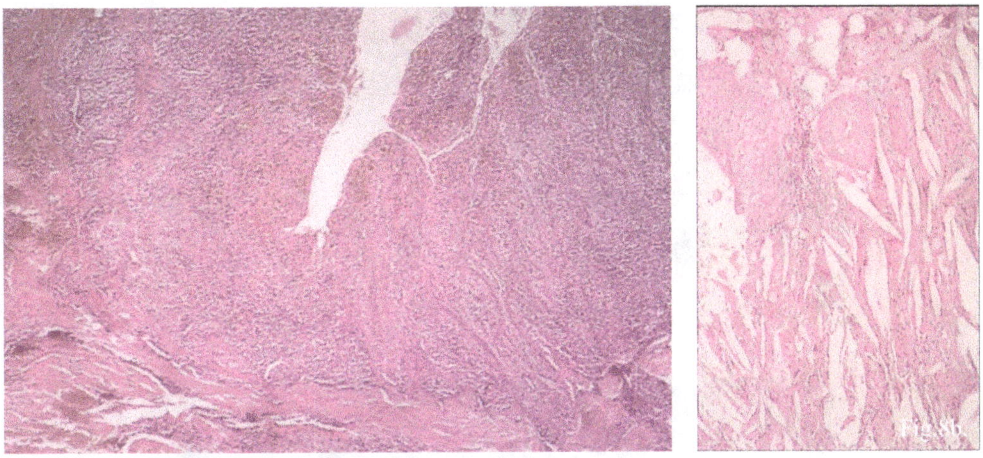

(a) (b)

FIGURE 8: Histopathology of the cyst. (a) Stratified squamous nonkeratinized epithelium with rete ridges and inflamed connective tissue wall (H&E × 20). (b) Cystic lumen is filled with liquid containing cholesterol crystals (H&E × 40). Mucoperiosteal flap showing the buccolingual thickness of mandibular ridge before implant placement.

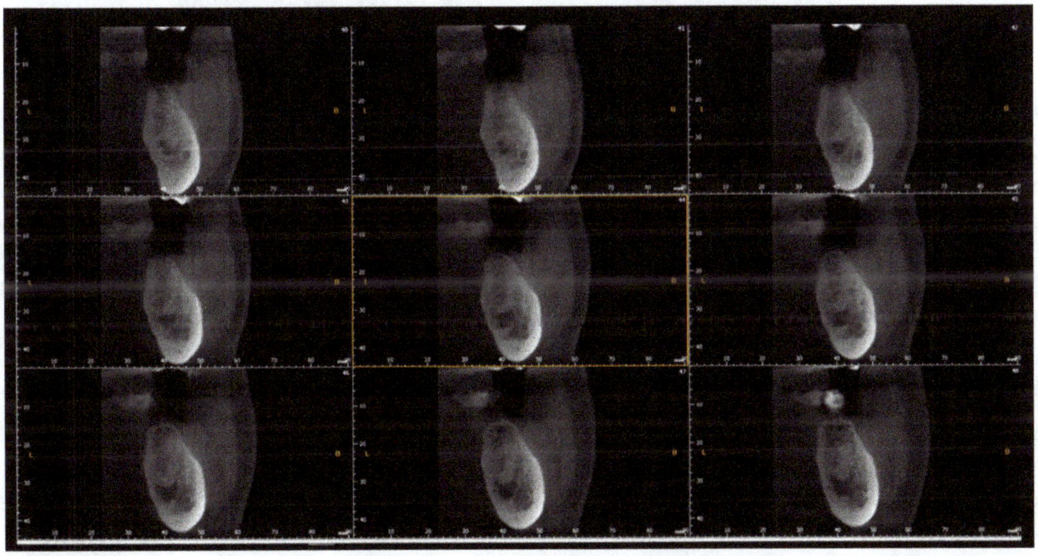

FIGURE 9: Para-axial cuts of a control CBCT before implant placement showing a complete bone regeneration of the cyst area.

Postdecompression histological examination at the time of definitive surgical treatment was found consistent with the preoperative biopsy diagnosis in 91% of keratocystic odontogenic tumors, 67% of glandular odontogenic cysts, 75% of dentigerous cysts, and 100% of cystic ameloblastomas. Authors concluded that all decompressed lesions should be definitely treated based on the initial diagnosis, with all patients placed on an appropriate follow-up protocol dependent on the original diagnosis [19]. However, other authors found no statistical evidence that decompression influences expression of proliferation markers in the lining, indicating that the potential for recurrence may not be restricted to cellular level [20, 21].

The most important requisites for bone deposition in a bone cavity includes the presence of blood clot, a source of osteoblasts, a contact with living tissue, and prevention of soft tissue invasion [22]. There have been controversies regarding bony regeneration in cystic cavities with or without bone grafts [23]. Some authors reported treating cyst cavities without using any graft materials and found new bone apposition after a period of one year [24, 25]. Others have reported using resorbable and nonresorbable grafts for bone defects secondary to the removal of cysts with good outcomes [26–28].

In our case, after the cyst's enucleation, we grafted the cavity with allograft, an osteoconductive material [29], knowing that osteoconductive materials are thought to stabilize blood clot and advance bone regeneration providing a scaffold, thus enhancing the migration of osteoprogenitor cells [8]. Without filling the cavity, we believe that there would

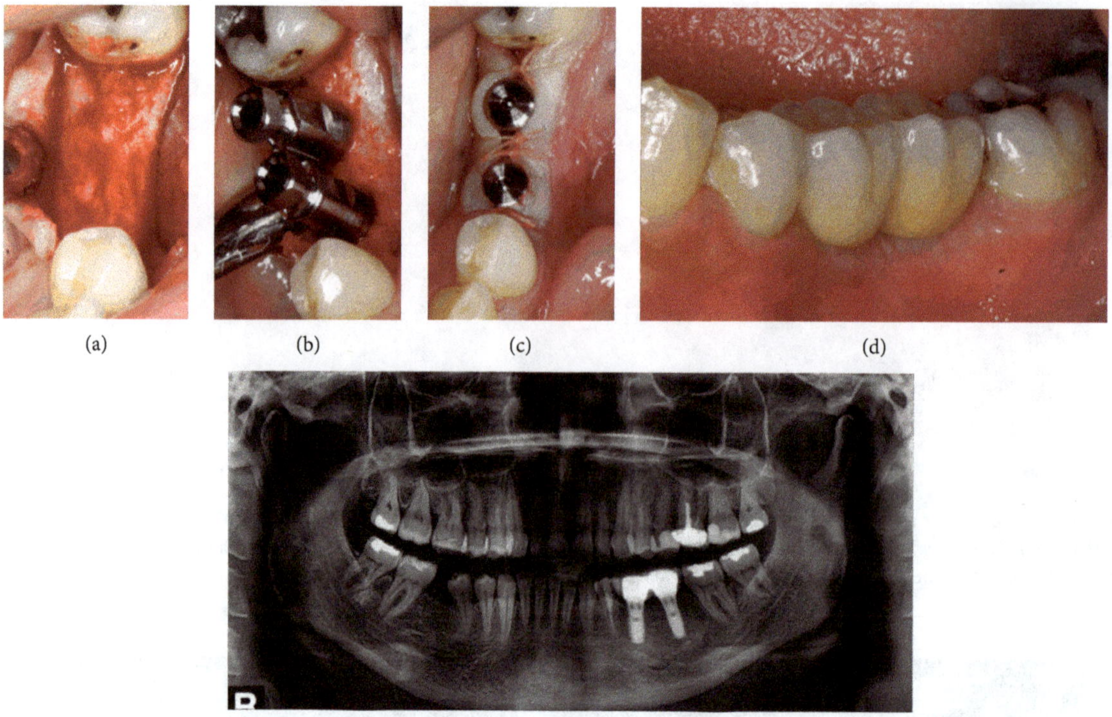

(a) (b) (c) (d) (e)

FIGURE 10: (a) Clinical view of the bone healing before implant placement. (b) Two Swiss Plus Zimmer® implants placed in postalveolar locations of teeth 35 and 36. (c) Clinical aspects of cover screws and sutures, immediately after implants placement. (d) Clinical aspect of restored implants (35 and 36). (e) Panoramic radiograph showing the final situation of the bone and the restored implants.

have been tissue collapse in the cavity. The bone regeneration was observed after 6 months and allowed to place dental implants with a good primary stability.

4. Conclusion

Radicular cyst is commonly found in the jaws. This case report illustrates the successful management of a mandibular radicular cyst by decompression, enucleation, grafting, and site rehabilitation.

References

[1] C. Partsch, "Uber kiefercyzten," *Dtsch Mschr Zahnheilkd*, vol. 10, pp. 271–304, 1892.

[2] K. H. Thoma, *Oral Surgery*, Mosby, St. Louis, MO, USA, 3rd edition, 1958.

[3] L. Tolstunov, "Marsupialization catheter," *Journal of Oral and Maxillofacial Surgery*, vol. 66, no. 5, pp. 1077–1079, 2008.

[4] E. J. Neaverth and H. A. Burg, "Decompression of large periapical cystic lesions," *Journal of Endodontics*, vol. 8, no. 4, pp. 175–182, 1982.

[5] M. A. Rawashdeh and H. Telfah, "Secondary alveolar bone grafting: the dilemma of donor site selection and morbidity," *British Journal of Oral and Maxillofacial Surgery*, vol. 46, no. 8, pp. 665–670, 2008.

[6] T. Ettl, M. Gosau, R. Sader, and T. E. Reichert, "Jaw cysts – filling or no filling after enucleation? A review," *Journal of Cranio-Maxillofacial Surgery*, vol. 40, no. 6, pp. 485–493, 2012.

[7] W. Pradel, U. Eckelt, and G. Lauer, "Bone regeneration after enucleation of mandibular cyst: comparing autogenous grafts from tissue-engineered bone and iliac bone," *Oral Surgery, Oral Medicine, Oral Pathology, Oral Radiology, and Endodontics*, vol. 101, no. 3, pp. 285–290, 2006.

[8] P. Stoor, S. Apajalahti, and R. Kontio, "Regeneration of cystic bone cavities and bone defects with bioactive glass S53P4 in the upper and lower jaws," *The Journal of Craniofacial Surgery*, vol. 28, no. 5, pp. 1197–1205, 2017, -1205, 2017.

[9] M. Shear, *Cysts of the Oral Regions*, Wright. Radicular and residual cysts, Boston, 3rd edition, 1992.

[10] R. P. Domingos, S. Goncalves Eduardo, and E. S. Neto, "Surgical approaches of extensive periapical cyst. Considerations about surgical technique," *Salusvita Bauru*, vol. 23, pp. 317–328, 2004.

[11] R. Bellizzi and R. Loushine, *Decompression in "A clinical atlas of endodontic surgery"*, Quintessence books, quintessence publishing co, Inc., Chicago, London, Berlin, 1991.

[12] Y. Kubota, I. Imajo, R. Itonaga, and Y. Takenoshita, "Effects of the patient's age and the size of the primary lesion on the speed of shrinkage after marsupialisation of keratocystic odontogenic tumours, dentigerous cysts, and radicular cysts," *British Journal of Oral and Maxillofacial Surgery*, vol. 51, no. 4, pp. 358–362, 2013.

[13] G. Enislidis, N. Fock, I. Sulzbacher, and R. Ewers, "Conservative treatment of large cystic lesions of the mandible: a prospective study of the effect of decompression," *The British Journal of Oral & Maxillofacial Surgery*, vol. 42, no. 6, pp. 546–550, 2004.

[14] L. Oliveros-Lopez, A. Fernandez-Olavarria, D. Torres-Lagares et al., "Reduction rate by decompression as a treatment of

odontogenic cysts," *Medicina Oral Patología Oral y Cirugia Bucal*, vol. 22, no. 5, pp. e643–e650, 2017.

[15] F. Asutay, Y. Atalay, O. Turamanlar, E. Horata, and M. C. Burdurlu, "Three-dimensional volumetric assessment of the effect of decompression on large mandibular odontogenic cystic lesions," *Journal of Oral and Maxillofacial Surgery*, vol. 74, no. 6, pp. 1159–1166, 2016.

[16] S.-T. Lee, S.-G. Kim, S.-Y. Moon, J. S. Oh, J. S. You, and J. S. Kim, "The effect of decompression as treatment of the cysts in the jaws: retrospective analysis," *Journal of the Korean Association of Oral and Maxillofacial Surgeons*, vol. 43, no. 2, pp. 83–87, 2017.

[17] A. Kolokythas, R. P. Fernandes, A. Pazoki, and R. A. Ord, "Odontogenic keratocyst: to decompress or not to decompress? A comparative study of decompression and enucleation versus resection/peripheral ostectomy," *Journal of Oral and Maxillofacial Surgery*, vol. 65, no. 4, pp. 640–644, 2007.

[18] M. August, W. C. Faquin, M. J. Troulis, and L. B. Kaban, "Dedifferentiation of odontogenic keratocyst epithelium after cyst decompression," *Journal of Oral and Maxillofacial Surgery*, vol. 61, no. 6, pp. 678–683, 2003.

[19] T. Schlieve, M. Miloro, and A. Kolokythas, "Does decompression of odontogenic cysts and cystlike lesions change the histologic diagnosis?," *Journal of Oral and Maxillofacial Surgery*, vol. 72, no. 6, pp. 1094–1105, 2014.

[20] S. Awni and B. Conn, "Decompression of keratocystic odontogenic tumors leading to increased fibrosis, but without any change in epithelial proliferation," *Oral Surgery, Oral Medicine, Oral Pathology, Oral Radiology*, vol. 123, no. 6, pp. 634–644, 2017.

[21] J. T. Rodrigues, H. Dos Santos Antunes, L. Armada, and F. R. Pires, "Influence of surgical decompression on the expression of inflammatory and tissue repair biomarkers in periapical cysts," *Oral Surgery, Oral Medicine, Oral Pathology and Oral Radiology*, vol. 124, no. 6, pp. 561–567, 2017.

[22] F. Stavropoulos, J. C. Nale, and J. D. Ruskin, "Guided bone regeneration," *Oral and Maxillofacial Surgery Clinics of North America*, vol. 14, no. 1, pp. 15–27, 2002.

[23] M. H. Seo, M. Y. Eo, Y. J. Cho, S. M. Kim, and S. K. Lee, "Autogenous partial bone chip grafting on the exposed inferior alveolar nerve after cystic enucleation," *Journal of Craniofacial Surgery*, vol. 29, no. 2, pp. 1–490, 2018.

[24] J. A. Meltzer, "Lateral periodontal cyst: report of a case with 1-year reentry," *International Journal of Periodontics & Restorative Dentistry*, vol. 19, no. 3, pp. 299–303, 1999.

[25] E. Angelopoulou and A. P. Angelopoulos, "Lateral periodontal cyst. Review of the literature and report of a case," *Journal of Periodontology*, vol. 61, no. 2, pp. 126–131, 1990.

[26] M. Pearrocha-Diago, J. M. Sanchis-Bielsa, J. Bonet-Marco, and J. M. Minguez-Sanz, "Surgical treatment and follow-up of solitary bone cyst of the mandible: a report of seven cases," *British Journal of Oral and Maxillofacial Surgery*, vol. 39, no. 3, pp. 221–223, 2001.

[27] S. Pappalardo, M. Coronella, M. L. Lanza et al., "Multidetector CT Dentascan evaluation of bone regeneration obtained with deproteinised bovine graft in residual cavity after mandibular cyst enucleation," *La Radiologia Medica*, vol. 118, no. 4, pp. 523–533, 2013.

[28] S. Sivolella, C. Perin, M. Capecchi, V. Buongiorno, and M. Valente, "Guided bone regeneration in the treatment of a lateral periodontal cyst: 2-year clinical and radiologic follow-up," *The International Journal of Periodontics & Restorative Dentistry*, vol. 38, no. 5, pp. 747–754, 2018.

[29] S. S. Noumbissi, J. L. Lozada, P. J. Boyne et al., "Clinical, histologic, and histomorphometric evaluation of mineralized solvent- dehydrated bone allograft (Puros) in human maxillary sinus grafts," *The Journal of Oral Implantology*, vol. 31, no. 4, pp. 171–179, 2005.

30

A Novel Approach for Rehabilitation of a Subtotal Maxillectomy Patient with Immediately Loaded Basal Implant-Supported Prosthesis: 4 Years Follow-Up

Motaz Osman,[1] **Abdelnasir G. Ahmad**,[2] **and Fadia Awadalkreem**[3]

[1]*Department of Implantology, Khartoum Teaching Dental Hospital, Federal Ministry of Heath, Khartoum, Sudan*
[2]*Department of Oral and Maxillofacial Surgery, Faculty of Dentistry, International University of Africa, Khartoum, Sudan*
[3]*Department of Oral Rehabilitation, Prosthodontic Division, Faculty of Dentistry, University of Khartoum, Sudan*

Correspondence should be addressed to Motaz Osman; motazdent@yahoo.com

Academic Editor: John H. Campbell

The prosthetic rehabilitation of maxillary defect can be achieved successfully by using an implant-supported prosthesis. The use of remote bony areas such as the zygomatic bone in cases of large defects provides an innovative substitute for free vascularized osteocutaneous flaps and the solution to flap failures. This report describes the rehabilitation of a 22-year-old female with a subtotal maxillectomy using an immediately loaded basal implant-supported prosthesis. Four basal cortical screw implants (BCS®) are inserted; 1 on the contralateral nasal floor, 2 implants in the pterygoid plates, and the last in the zygomatic bone using cone beam computed tomography scans. The prosthesis was constructed and cemented in 3 days. The surgical and prosthetic procedures were performed without any obstacles. After 4 years in function, the patient was highly satisfied with the treatment as it improved her mastication, speech, aesthetic and returned her self-esteem. To our knowledge, this is the first clinical report detailing the use of basal implant-retained obturator in a subtotal maxillectomy patient.

1. Introduction

The maxilla is a fundamental structure in the face that plays a critical role in esthetics, speech, swallowing, and mastication [1]. It separates the oral, antral, and orbital cavities and provides support to many vital structures such as the lower eyelids, cheeks, lips, and nose [1]. Any maxillary defect regardless of its size affects speech, swallowing, and mastication; may result in cosmetic disfigurement; and compromised the patient's quality of life [1, 2]. Reconstruction of maxillary defects is one of the most challenging works the maxillofacial surgeons and prosthodontists are facing [1, 2].

The aims of maxillary defect reconstruction should include closure of the defect, separation of the oral cavity from the sinus and nasal cavities [2–4], maintenance of orbital content support, preservation of eyelid functions, cleared nasal airways, replacement of masticatory units, improving esthetics, and restoring normal or near to normal patient life [2–5]. Subtotal maxillectomy is a term used to define "any maxillary resection involving the removal of at least two walls, including the floor of the antrum (the hard palate) with the exception of the posterior wall" [6]. Reconstruction of subtotal maxillectomy can be achieved either through surgical reconstruction, prosthetic reconstruction (obturator), or a combination of both techniques [2–4].

Many surgical techniques such as local/regional flaps [2, 3], soft tissue, and/or bone free flaps have been reported although their use alone in massive defect reconstruction was limited [3].

Consequently, large maxillary defects can be repaired using obturators or a combination of both techniques [1, 3].

The main advantages of an obturator are shorter treatment time, reduced cost, and easy visualization of the maxillectomy cavity [2, 3]. However, obturator therapy has many disadvantages, including lack of retention in cases of large defects, reduction in supportive dentition, discomfort associated with prosthesis wear, the potential of hypernasal speech, and regurgitation of foods and liquids into the nasal cavity in cases of an inadequate seal [2, 3]. In addition, other drawbacks include the inconvenience of prosthesis removal and cleaning to maintain defect hygiene and the periodic need for prosthesis adjustments following healing and bone remodeling [2].

Many methods of maxillofacial prosthesis retention and support have been reported, such as engagement of the remaining teeth, bony anatomic undercuts, and lateral scar band [2–4].

Unfortunately, in A very large defect and/or when primary closure of soft tissue defects is achieved immediately after resection, the gingivobuccal sulcus is reduced, and the undercuts required for prosthesis retention are deficient or even eliminated [3]. In such cases, implants can improve obturator retention, support, and stability and therefore improve the patient's quality of life [7–13].

Following maxillectomy, a limited amount of maxillary bone remains; therefore, implant placement utilizes the use of more distant sites [7–12] such as the zygomatic bone [8, 10, 11] and pterygoid bone [12]. In 1989, Bidra et al. and Tulasne [12, 13] introduced the Tubero-pterygoid implants, which are inserted through the maxillary tuberosity in an oblique direction proceeding deeply to the pterygoid plate. On the other hand, zygomatic implants were firstly described by Branemark [14] in 1989. Several authors [3, 8, 10, 11, 15, 16] have reported the use of zygomatic implants to eliminate the need for bone grafting, reduce the risk of implant failure, and shorten treatment time.

Basal Cortical Screw (BCS ®) implants are basal implants with specific characteristics [17–19].

They are designed in an extended length, up to 55 mm, to be inserted from the crestal direction and anchored securely (osseofixated) into the remaining remote basal bone such as the pterygoid plate of the sphenoid and zygomatic bones providing a 2nd or even 3rd cortex engagement [17, 18]. The insertion of conventional implants into the pterygoid and zygomatic bones has been previously described [10–16]. However, evidence concerning the use of basal implants in these areas is limited.

This clinical report describes a successful case of maxillary defect reconstruction via fixed implant-supported prosthesis using basal implants inserted into the nasal floor, zygomatic, and pterygoid plate bones.

2. Case Presentation

A 22-year-old female patient presented at the Khartoum Teaching Dental Hospital with a swelling on the right side of her face. She was diagnosed with odontogenic myxoma. Subtotal maxillectomy was performed, and the intraoral defect was closed using soft tissue approximation (Figures 1(a) and 1(b)). One year later, the patient returned with esthetic complaints and reported masticatory inefficiency; she requested a fixed prosthesis. The patient was very depressed. During the previous 6 months, she visited a dentist who inserted one implant in the area of the maxillary tuberosity to construct an implant-supported prosthesis, but unfortunately, the prosthesis was not retained. This treatment failure had led to further deterioration of her emotional status.

A multidisciplinary team was formed, including an expert oral maxillofacial surgeon and a removable and fixed prosthodontists to avoid any technical complication. Preoperative radiographs (digital panorama and cone beam CT) was performed in order to evaluate the treatment options and identify optimal bone areas for implant anchorage (Figure 1(c)). The formulated treatment plan included the construction of immediately loaded fixed basal implant-supported obturator. The treatment plan was fully discussed with the patient, and informed consent was obtained.

Four BCS® implants (Dr. Ihde Dental, Switzerland) were inserted using local anesthesia (2% lidocaine with epinephrine 1 : 100,000) and flapless technique. Implant anchored are as follows: one implant in the contralateral nasal floor, two pterygoid implants, and one implant in the zygomatic bone with 3.5 mm width and 29, 32, 35, and 35 mm length, respectively. (Figure 2(a)).

More than 60 N cm insertion torque was obtained [20]. The anterior implant (inserted in the contralateral nasal floor) was bent using a special bending tool provided by the implant's company for more favorable prosthetic orientation [19, 21] (Figure 2(b)).

Postoperative panoramic and cone beam computed tomography views were performed to verify the implant's positions (Figures 3(a)–3(f)).

Impression coping was attached to the implants' head (Figure 4). An impression was taken using monophase vinyl polysiloxane (VPS, Ivoclar Vivadent AG). Amoxicillin and clavulanate potassium 1 mg (Megamox, HIKMA), diclofenac potassium 50 mg (Rapidus, Tabuk), and xylometazoline adult nasal drops (Otrivin, GlaxoSmithKline) were prescribed.

One day later, a metal framework try-in was performed, followed by silicone jaw relation (Figures 5(a) and 5(b)).

Both acrylic teeth and veneer material were added, and a wax try-in was done to verify the patient esthetic and occlusion (Figure 6).

The labial and palatal flanges were shortened (not extended to the full depth of the sulcus, i.e., hygienic design) for hygienic purposes. On the third day, the final prosthesis was inserted and cemented using Fuji cement (GC Fuji I Luting Cement, Japan) (Figures 7(a) and 7(b)).

The patient was scheduled for follow-up after 1 week, and 3, 6, 9, 12, and 18 months and 6 months, therefore. At each follow-up, the patient was examined both clinically and radiographically. She had no complaints, and her speech, mastication, and esthetics had improved significantly. She was highly satisfied with the result and had become married. After 4 years of function, the patient presented with an optimum peri-implant health, a stable prosthesis without complaints, and a high satisfaction level. The panoramic view showed an increase in bone-implant contact and no evidence of peri-implant radiolucency (Figure 8). The patient gave the investigators a signed consent for the publication of this case.

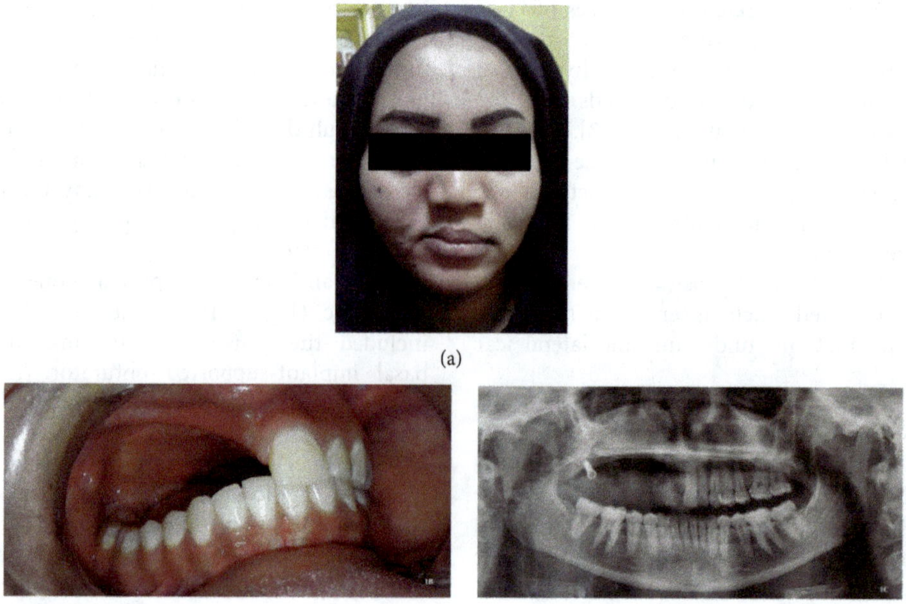

(a)

(b) (c)

FIGURE 1: (a) Patient's frontal view at the time of presentation showing depressed check. (b) Patient's intraoral view showing right partial maxillectomy after soft tissue healing. (c) A preoperative panoramic view showing previously placed implant at the right tuberosity area.

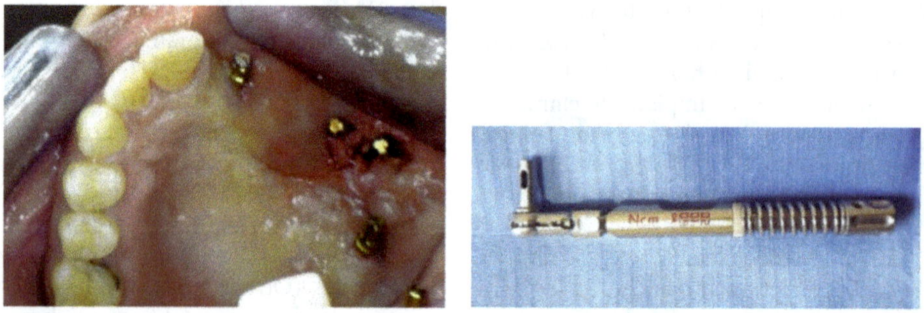

(a) (b)

FIGURE 2: (a) Patient's intraoral view showing implant's distribution (image using mirror). (b) Tool used for implant bending.

3. Discussion

The primary objective of maxillary resection rehabilitation is the restoration of the patient's previous appearance and function [2–5]. Procedure success depends on both the dentist's judgment and skill, and the postoperative anatomical, physiological, and psychological condition of the patient.

The function of obturator prostheses is directly influenced by the location and size of the maxillectomy defect and the quality and quantity of the remaining teeth, soft, and bone tissues [2–4].

Even though numerous advances in surgical reconstruction have been documented, it is not always possible because of the general health condition of the patient, defect size, probability of tumor recurrence, and patient preference. In such situations, prosthetic rehabilitation is considered the treatment of choice [8].

In the present case, the nature of the tumor and the patient preference limited the immediate surgical reconstruction approach; only soft approximation was encountered [22]. Although this approximation reduced the size of the defect and closed the oroantral communication, it adversely affects the final prosthesis's retention, stability, and support. Bidra et al. [12] reported that sometimes both the bulky and flaccid nature of the remaining tissue preclude conventional prosthesis support; therefore, other means of support should be used, such as implant therapy.

Many authors [7–16] reported the successful use of the pterygoid and zygomatic implants for cases of severely resorbed maxilla and maxillary defects reconstruction. Both implants offered the utilization of the thick cortical bone for implant anchorage and increased the possibility of bicortical or even tricortical anchorage, it eliminates donor-site morbidity and/or graft material infection [17].

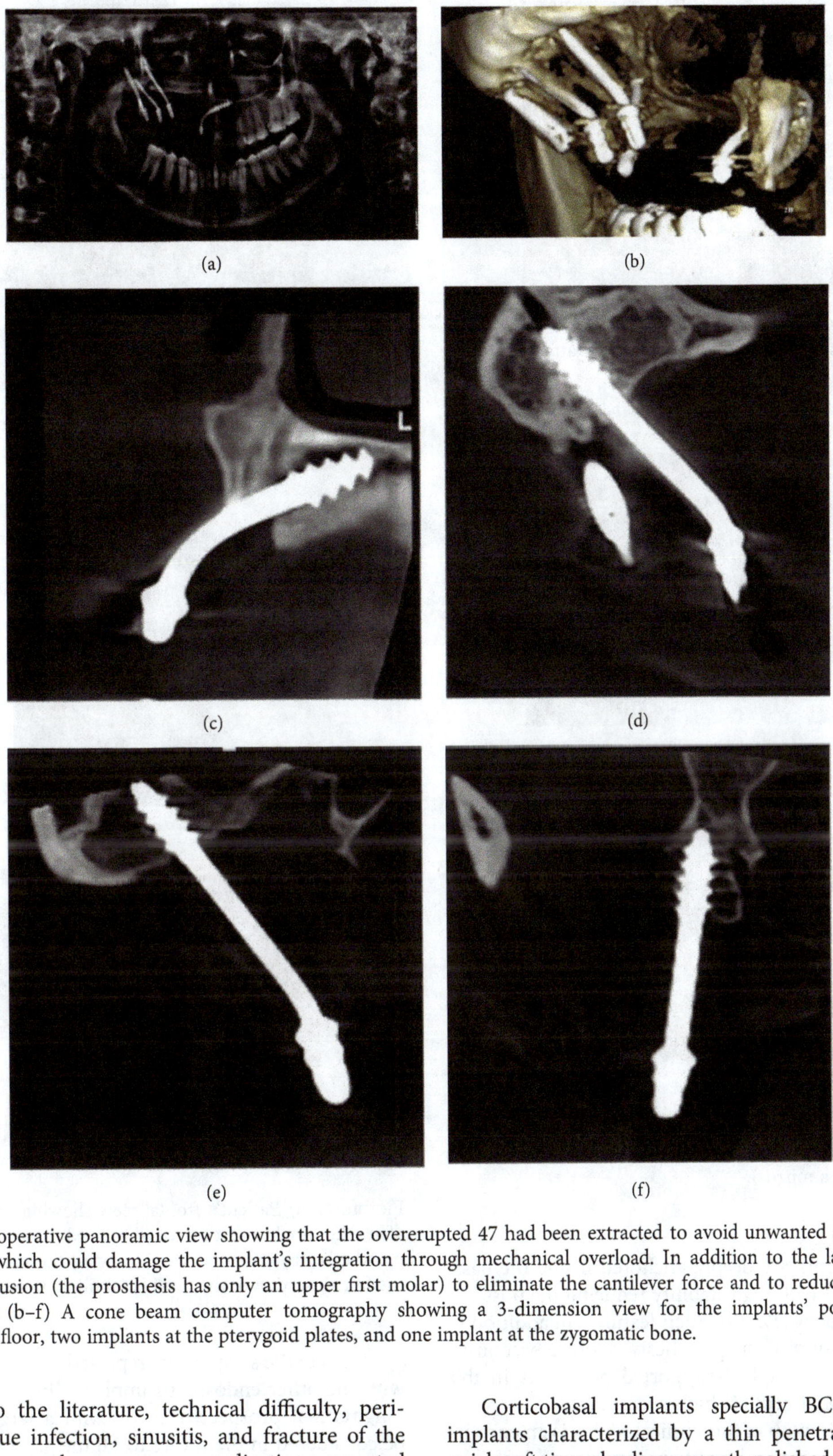

FIGURE 3: (a) Postoperative panoramic view showing that the overerupted 47 had been extracted to avoid unwanted and noncontrollable further eruption, which could damage the implant's integration through mechanical overload. In addition to the lake of the opposing artificial teeth occlusion (the prosthesis has only an upper first molar) to eliminate the cantilever force and to reduce and ensure better force distribution. (b–f) A cone beam computer tomography showing a 3-dimension view for the implants' positions; one in the contralateral nasal floor, two implants at the pterygoid plates, and one implant at the zygomatic bone.

According to the literature, technical difficulty, peri-implant soft tissue infection, sinusitis, and fracture of the prosthetic veneer are the common complications reported with zygomatic implants [8]. These complications may have been related to the characteristics of the implant surface, the implant-abutment connection, the surgical procedure, occlusal overload, and implant's micromovement during functioning [8].

Corticobasal implants specially BCs® are one-piece implants characterized by a thin penetrating tip ensuring quick soft tissue healing, smooth polished surface improving the peri-implant soft tissue health [17, 18], isoelastic prosperity offering implant bending without compromising its survival [19, 21], and implants splinting with a supporting metal framework for better force distribution and to counteract the implant length cantilever [17, 19]; the horizontal

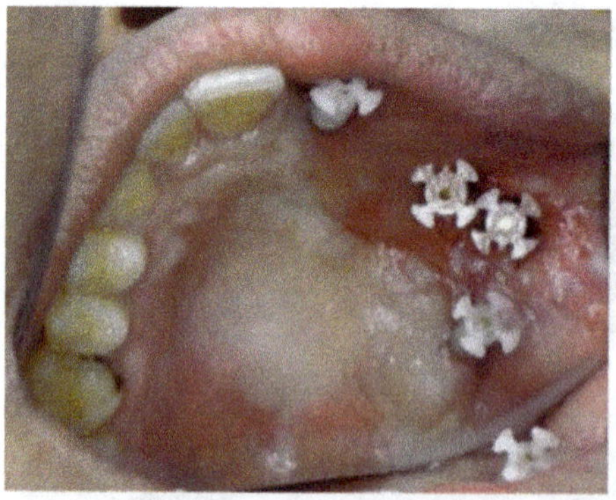

Figure 4: Image showing impression copping attached to the abutments head (image using mirror).

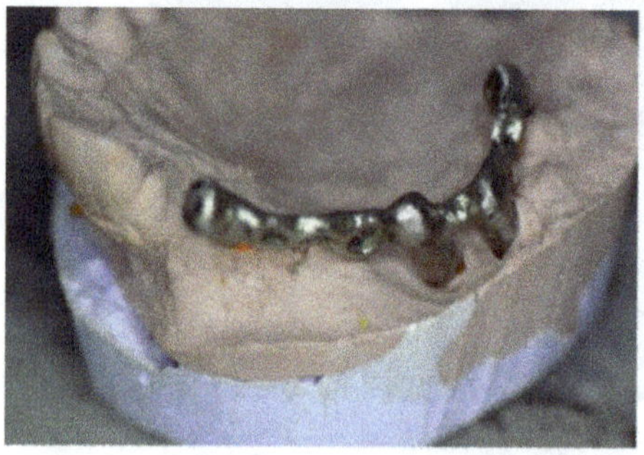

(a)

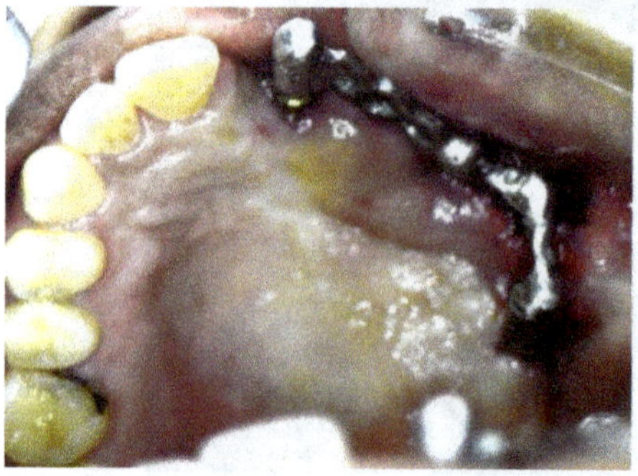

(b)

Figure 5: (a) Image showing the metal framework in the cast. (b) Image showing the metal framework try-in inside the patient's mouth (image using a mirror).

plates of the implants are deeply anchored inside the basal bone (osseofixated) with high stability reducing the possibility of micromovement [17–19]. Such features, in addition to the hygienic extension of the prosthesis, denture base justified the use of these implant-supported prosthesis in this present case with a susceptible high success rate.

The 4 years follow-up of this clinical report is an encouraging result as according to the systemic review conducted by Goiato et al. [8]; they studied 1541 zygomatic implants among which 33 implants failed; they reported that failure generally occurred during the first-year interval. In our knowledge, this is the first study reporting the use of basal implant in a patient with maxillectomy.

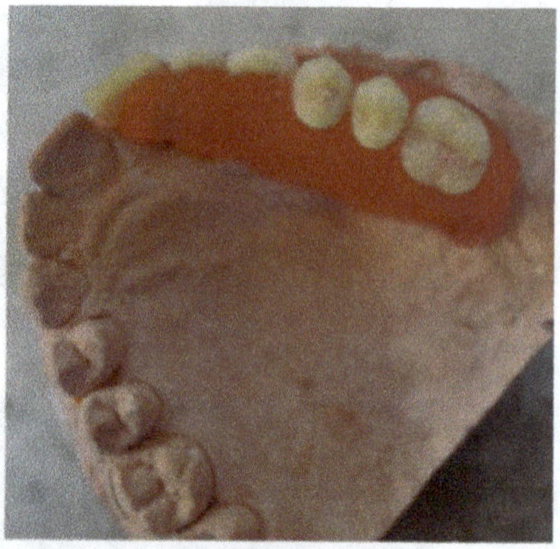

Figure 6: Image showing the wax try-in in the cast.

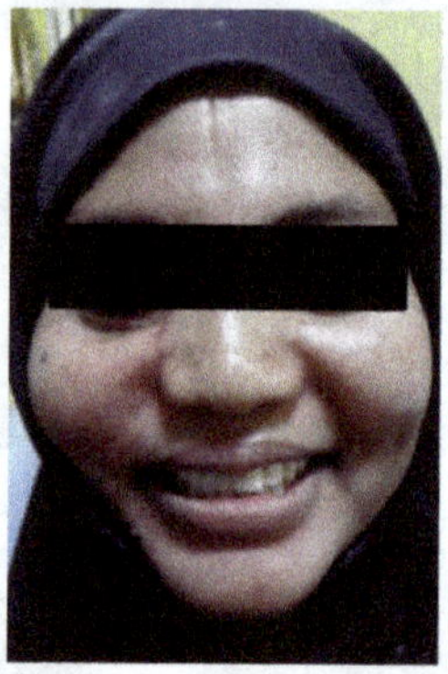

(a)

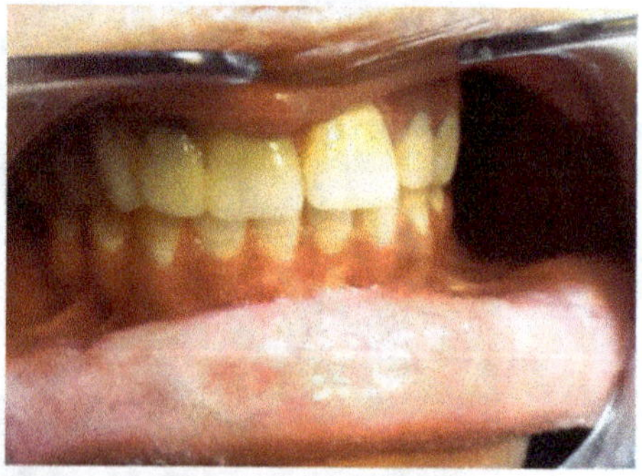

(b)

Figure 7: (a) Patient's frontal view showing the clinical outcome after the final insertion of the fixed basal implant-supported prosthesis. (b) Intraoral view showing the clinical outcome after the final insertion of the fixed basal implant-supported prosthesis.

Despite the success rate reported in this case being in line with the other endosseous implant's literature [8, 15, 16], a longitudinal prospective study with a large sample should be considered in the future to fill the gap of knowledge.

4. Conclusion

This clinical case highlighted the feasibility of basal implant-supported prosthesis as a successful treatment modality for

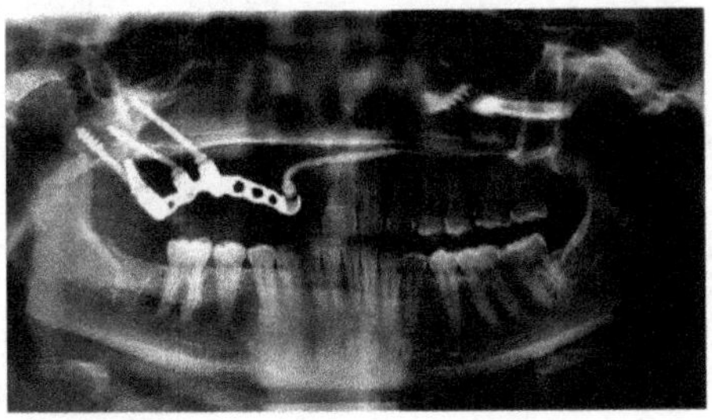

FIGURE 8: The panoramic view of the patients after 4 years of function showing an increased bone-implant contact without peri-implant radiolucency.

patients with subtotal maxillectomy after soft tissue closure. It restored the patient's masticatory function, esthetics, and phonetics and improved her self-esteem and quality of life.

Consent

Written informed consent was obtained from the patient for publication of this case report and supplementary images.

Authors' Contributions

All the authors contribute in the treatment of the patient and in writing and in the finalization of the manuscript.

References

[1] S. Iyer and K. Thankappan, "Maxillary reconstruction: current concepts and controversies," *Indian Journal of Plastic Surgery*, vol. 47, no. 1, pp. 8–19, 2014.

[2] P. Andrades, O. Militsakh, M. M. Hanasono, J. Rieger, and E. L. Rosenthal, "Current strategies in reconstruction of maxillectomy defects," *Archives of Otolaryngology–Head & Neck Surgery*, vol. 137, no. 8, pp. 806–812, 2011.

[3] C. Chen, W. Ren, L. Gao et al., "Function of obturator prosthesis after maxillectomy and prosthetic obturator rehabilitation," *Brazilian Journal of Otorhinolaryngology*, vol. 82, no. 2, pp. 177–183, 2016.

[4] D. J. Okay, E. Genden, D. Buchbinder, and M. Urken, "Prosthodontic guidelines for surgical reconstruction of the maxilla: a classification system of defects," *The Journal of Prosthetic Dentistry*, vol. 86, no. 4, pp. 352–363, 2001.

[5] R. Chigurupati, N. Aloor, R. Salas, and B. L. Schmidt, "Quality of life after maxillectomy and prosthetic obturator rehabilitation," *Journal of Oral and Maxillofacial Surgery*, vol. 71, no. 8, pp. 1471–1478, 2013.

[6] R. H. Spiro, E. W. Strong, and J. P. Shah, "Maxillectomy and its classification," *Head & Neck*, vol. 19, no. 4, pp. 309–314, 1997.

[7] S. M. Parel, P.-I. Brånemark, L.-O. Ohrnell, and B. Svensson, "Remote implant anchorage for the rehabilitation of maxillary defects," *Journal of Prosthetic Dentistry*, vol. 86, no. 4, pp. 377–381, 2001.

[8] M. C. Goiato, E. P. Pellizzer, A. Moreno et al., "Implants in the zygomatic bone for maxillary prosthetic rehabilitation: a systematic review," *International Journal of Oral and Maxillofacial Surgery*, vol. 43, no. 6, pp. 748–757, 2014.

[9] T. Sumida, H. Nakano, H. Hamakawa, and Y. Mori, "Dental implants in oral rehabilitation of a maxillary cancer reconstruction: a case report," *Journal of Oral Implantology*, vol. 41, no. 6, pp. 737–739, 2015.

[10] A. AntonioD', P. Pasquale, F. Ferrari, L. Trevisiol, and N. P. Francesco, "Zygoma implant-supported prosthetic rehabilitation of a patient after subtotal bilateral maxillectomy," *Journal of Craniofacial Surgery*, vol. 24, no. 2, pp. e159–e162, 2013.

[11] R. A. Zwahlen, K. W. Grätz, C. K. Oechslin, and S. P. Studer, "Survival rate of zygomatic implants in atrophic or partially resected maxillae prior to functional loading: a retrospective clinical report," *International Journal of Oral & Maxillofacial Implants*, vol. 21, no. 3, pp. 413–420, 2006.

[12] A. S. Bidra, G. W. May, G. E. Tharp, and M. S. Chambers, "Pterygoid implants for maxillofacial rehabilitation of a patient with a bilateral maxillectomy defect," *Journal of Oral Implantology*, vol. 39, no. 1, pp. 91–97, 2013.

[13] J. F. Tulasne, "Implant treatment of missing posterior dentition," in *Pterygoid Implants for Maxillofacial Rehabilitation of a Patient with a Bilateral Maxillectomy Defect*, A. S. Bidra, G. W. May, G. E. Tharp, G. E. Tharp, and M. S. Chambers, Eds., vol. 39, pp. 91–97, Journal of Oral Implantology, 2013.

[14] P. I. Branemark, *Surgery and fixture installation: zygomaticus fixture clinical procedures*, vol. 1, Nobel Biocare, Go teborg, Sweden, 1998.

[15] J. F. Valerón and P. F. Valerón, "Long-term results in placement of screw-type implants in the pterygomaxillary-pyramidal region," *International Journal of Oral and Maxillofacial Implants*, vol. 22, no. 2, pp. 195–200, 2007.

[16] S. F. Balshi, G. J. Wolfinger, and T. J. Balshi, "Analysis of 164 titanium oxide-surface implants in completely edentulous arches for fixed prosthesis anchorage using the pterygomaxillary region," *International Journal of Oral and Maxillofacial Implants*, vol. 20, no. 6, pp. 946–952, 2005.

[17] S. Ihde and A. Ihde, *Immediate Loading: Guideline to Successful Implantology*, International Implant Foundation, Munich, 2010.

[18] M. Singh, R. Batra, D. Das, S. Verma, and M. Goel, "A novel approach for restoration of hemisected mandibular first molar with immediately loaded single piece BCS implant: a case report," *Journal of Oral Biology and Craniofacial Research*, vol. 7, no. 2, pp. 141–146, 2017.

[19] A. Lazarov, "Immediate functional loading: results for the concept of the strategic implant®," *Annals of Maxillofacial Surgery*, vol. 9, no. 1, pp. 78–88, 2019.

[20] G. J. P. L. de Oliveira, M. S. Brackmann, L. C. Trojan, P. D. Ribeiro Júnior, and L. E. M. Padovan, "Oral rehabilitation with zygomatic implants in a patient with cleft palate," *Case Reports in Dentistry*, vol. 2019, Article ID 6591256, 5 pages, 2019.

[21] T. Goldmann, S. Ihde, J. Kuzelka, and L. Himmlova, "Bendable vs. angulated dental implants: consideration of elastic and plastic material properties based on experimental implant material data and FEA," *Biomedical Papers*, vol. 152, no. 2, pp. 309–316, 2008.

[22] C. Shivashankara, M. Nidoni, S. Patil, and K. T. Shashikala, "Odontogenic myxoma: a review with report of an uncommon case with recurrence in the mandible of a teenage male," *The Saudi Dental Journal*, vol. 29, no. 3, pp. 93–101, 2017.

Permissions

All chapters in this book were first published by Hindawi Publishing Corporation; hereby published with permission under the Creative Commons Attribution License or equivalent. Every chapter published in this book has been scrutinized by our experts. Their significance has been extensively debated. The topics covered herein carry significant findings which will fuel the growth of the discipline. They may even be implemented as practical applications or may be referred to as a beginning point for another development.

The contributors of this book come from diverse backgrounds, making this book a truly international effort. This book will bring forth new frontiers with its revolutionizing research information and detailed analysis of the nascent developments around the world.

We would like to thank all the contributing authors for lending their expertise to make the book truly unique. They have played a crucial role in the development of this book. Without their invaluable contributions this book wouldn't have been possible. They have made vital efforts to compile up to date information on the varied aspects of this subject to make this book a valuable addition to the collection of many professionals and students.

This book was conceptualized with the vision of imparting up-to-date information and advanced data in this field. To ensure the same, a matchless editorial board was set up. Every individual on the board went through rigorous rounds of assessment to prove their worth. After which they invested a large part of their time researching and compiling the most relevant data for our readers.

The editorial board has been involved in producing this book since its inception. They have spent rigorous hours researching and exploring the diverse topics which have resulted in the successful publishing of this book. They have passed on their knowledge of decades through this book. To expedite this challenging task, the publisher supported the team at every step. A small team of assistant editors was also appointed to further simplify the editing procedure and attain best results for the readers.

Apart from the editorial board, the designing team has also invested a significant amount of their time in understanding the subject and creating the most relevant covers. They scrutinized every image to scout for the most suitable representation of the subject and create an appropriate cover for the book.

The publishing team has been an ardent support to the editorial, designing and production team. Their endless efforts to recruit the best for this project, has resulted in the accomplishment of this book. They are a veteran in the field of academics and their pool of knowledge is as vast as their experience in printing. Their expertise and guidance has proved useful at every step. Their uncompromising quality standards have made this book an exceptional effort. Their encouragement from time to time has been an inspiration for everyone.

The publisher and the editorial board hope that this book will prove to be a valuable piece of knowledge for researchers, students, practitioners and scholars across the globe.

List of Contributors

Gustavo Vargas da Silva Salomão
Department of Oral Rehabilitation, School of Dentistry, Ibirapuera University (Unib), Av. Interlagos, 1329, Chácara Flora, São Paulo, SP 04661-100, Brazil

Eliseo Pablo Chun, Renato dos Santos Panegaci and Fernando Toledo Santos
Department of Prosthodontics, School of Dentistry, Ibirapuera University (Unib), Av. Interlagos, 1329, Chácara Flora, São Paulo, SP 04661-100, Brazil

Mounika Ayinala and Gautam Shetty
Department of Prosthodontics, Rajarajeswari Dental College and Hospital, Bengaluru, Karnataka, India

Fawaz Alzoubi
Department of General Dental Practice, Faculty of Dentistry, Kuwait University, Jabriya, Kuwait

Hsiu-Wan Meng
Department of Periodontics and Dental Hygiene, The University of Texas Health Science Center School of Dentistry, Houston TX, USA

Esther Yun Chien
Private Practice, Columbus OH, USA

Hua-Hong Chien
Division of Periodontology, College of Dentistry, The Ohio State University, Columbus OH, USA

Sharaf Eldeen M. Abbas and Mohamed A. ELKhashab
Department of Prosthodontics, Faculty of Dentistry, Cairo University, Cairo, Egypt

Carlos Polis-Yanes, Carla Cadenas-Sebastián, Patricia Gual-Vaqués and Claudia Oliver-Puigdomenech
School of Dentistry, University of Barcelona, University Campus of Bellvitge, Barcelona, Spain

Raúl Ayuso-Montero
School of Dentistry, University of Barcelona, University Campus of Bellvitge, Barcelona, Spain
Oral Health and Masticatory System Group (Bellvitge Biomedical Research Institute) IDIBELL, University of Barcelona, L'Hospitalet de Llobregat, Barcelona, Spain

Antoni Marí-Roig
Oral Health and Masticatory System Group (Bellvitge Biomedical Research Institute) IDIBELL, University of Barcelona, L'Hospitalet de Llobregat, Barcelona, Spain
Department of Maxillofacial Surgery, University Hospital of Bellvitge, Catalonia, Spain

José López-López
Oral Health and Masticatory System Group (Bellvitge Biomedical Research Institute) IDIBELL, University of Barcelona, L'Hospitalet de Llobregat, Barcelona, Spain
Department of Odontostomatology, Faculty of Medicine and Health Sciences (Dentistry), Odontological Hospital University of Barcelona, University of Barcelona, Spain

Ni Putu Mira Sumarta and Andra Rizqiawan
Department of Oral and Maxillofacial Surgery, Faculty of Dental Medicine, Universitas Airlangga, Surabaya, Indonesia

David Buntoro Kamadjaja
Department of Oral and Maxillofacial Surgery, Faculty of Dental Medicine, Universitas Airlangga, Surabaya, Indonesia
Stem Cell Research and Development Center, Universitas Airlangga, Surabaya, Indonesia

Joseph Bassil and Stephanie Mrad
Department of Oral Surgery, Faculty of Dental Medicine, Saint Joseph University of Beirut, Lebanon

Alain Abi Sleiman
Attending Oral Surgeon, Lebanese Army Dental Department, Beirut, Lebanon

Ziad Noujeim
Department of Oral and Maxillofacial Surgery, Faculty of Dental Medicine, Lebanese University, Beirut, Lebanon

Igor Smojver and Ivan Katalinić
St. Catherine Specialty Hospital, Zagreb, Croatia

Marko Vuletić and Dragana Gabrić
Department of Oral Surgery, School of Dental Medicine, University of Zagreb, Croatia

Luka Stojić
Private Dental Clinic, Zagreb, Croatia

Dražena Gerbl
Clinic of Anesthesiology, University Hospital Clinic Zagreb, Croatia

Ivica Pelivan
Department of Prosthodontics, School of Dental Medicine, University of Zagreb, Zagreb, Croatia

Gregor-Georg Zafiropoulos
University of Sharjah, College of Dental Medicine, Sharjah, UAE

Tae Ho Yoon and Moosa Abuzayda
Hamdan Bin Mohammed College of Dental Medicine, Mohammed Bin Rashid University, Dubai, UAE

Guilherme José Pimentel Lopes de Oliveira
Department of Periodontology/Implantology, Dental School, Federal University of Uberlândia-UFU, Uberlândia 38405-266, Brazil

Mariana Schaffer Brackmann
Department of Diagnosis and Surgery, Univ. Est. Paul.-UNESP, Araraquara 14801-903, Brazil

Luis Eduardo Marques Padovan
Instituto Latino Americano de Ensino e Pesquisa Odontológico-ILAPEO, Curitiba 80710-150, Brazil

Paulo Domingos Ribeiro Júnior
Univ. Sagrado Coração, Bauru 17011-160, Brazil

Ferdinando Attanasio and Amerigo Giudice
Department of Health Sciences, Magna Graecia, University of Catanzaro, Catanzaro, Italy

Andrea Pacifici, Antonella Polimeni, Luciano Pacifici and Daniele Carbone
Department of Oral and Maxillo-Facial Science, Sapienza University of Rome, Rome 00100, Italy

Bruno Freitas Mello, Márcio de Carvalho Formiga and Jamil Awad Shibli
Department of Periodontology and Oral Implantology, Dental Research Division, University of Guarulhos, Sao Paulo, Brazil

Luiz Fernando de Souza da Silva and Gustavo dos Santos Coura
Department of Implantology, Unisociesc, Florianópolis, Brazil

Gerardo La Monaca, Nicola Pranno, Giorgio Pompa, Susanna Annibali and Iole Vozza
Department of Oral and Maxillo-Facial Sciences, Sapienza University of Rome, Rome, Italy

Maria Paola Cristalli
Department of Biotechnologies and Medical Surgical Sciences, Sapienza University of Rome, Rome, Italy

Lincoln Lara Cardoso, Giovanni Gasperini, Leandro Carvalho Cardoso and Guilherme Romano Scartezini
Department of Oral and Maxillofacial Surgery, Aparecida de Goiânia Hospital, Goiânia, Goiás, Brazil

Annika Ingrid Maria Soderberg Campos and Heloisa Fonseca Marão
Department of Implantology, University of Santo Amaro, São Paulo, São Paulo, Brazil

Eliana de Souza Bastos Mazuqueli Pereira and Rachel Gomes Eleutério
School of Dentistry, University of Marília (UNIMAR), Marília 17525-902, Brazil

Fernando Accetturi
Private Dental Clinic, Fernando Accetturi Implants and Aesthetic Dentistry, Marília 17525-170, Brazil

Daniela Vieira Buchaim
School of Dentistry, University of Marília (UNIMAR), Marília 17525-902, Brazil
Medical School, University Center of Adamantina (UniFAI), Adamantina 17800-000, Brazil

Rogério Leone Buchaim
School of Dentistry, University of Marília (UNIMAR), Marília 17525-902, Brazil
Bauru School of Dentistry, University of São Paulo (FOB/USP), Bauru 17012-901, Brazil

Juliana Trindade Clemente-Napimoga
School of Dentistry, São Leopoldo Mandic (SLMANDIC), Campinas 13045-755, Brazil

Minou Hélène Nilius, Charlotte Mueller and Anna Krahe
Niliusklinik, Londoner Bogen 6, D-44269 Dortmund, Germany

Bernhard Weiland, Dominik Haim and Guenter Lauer
Department of Oral and Maxillofacial Surgery, University Hospital "Carl Gustav Carus", Technische Universität Dresden, Fetscherstr 74, D-01307 Dresden, Germany

Manfred Nilius
Niliusklinik, Londoner Bogen 6, D-44269 Dortmund, Germany
Department of Oral and Maxillofacial Surgery, University Hospital "Carl Gustav Carus", Technische Universität Dresden, Fetscherstr 74, D-01307 Dresden, Germany

Algirdas Puisys and Viktorija Auzbikaviciute
Vilnius Implantology Center, Vilnius, Lithuania
Vilnius Research Group, Vilnius, Lithuania

Renata Simkunaite-Rizgeliene
Vilnius University, Vilnius, Lithuania

Dainius Razukevicius
Lithuanian University of Health Science, Kaunas, Lithuania

Rokas Linkevicius
Vilnius Research Group, Vilnius, Lithuania
Lithuanian University of Health Science, Kaunas, Lithuania

Tomas Linkevicius
Vilnius Research Group, Vilnius, Lithuania
Vilnius University, Vilnius, Lithuania

Francesco Campione, Ludovica Campione and Mario Francesco Campione
Dottor Francesco Campione Clinic, via de Caro 104 Catania, Italy

Michele Melillo and Claudia Arena
Department of Experimental and Clinical Medicine-University of Foggia, Italy

Francesc Abella
Department of Endodontics, Universitat Internacional de Catalunya, Sant Cugat del Vallès, Barcelona, Spain

Luca Boschini
Ambulatorio Polispecialistico Dottor Boschini Srl, Rimini, Italy

Andrew Sotirios Melenikiotis
Implantology at Ilapeo College, Curitiba, Brazil

Camila Pereira Vianna
Pathology, Curitiba, Brazil

Waleska Caldas
Orthodontics, Curitiba, Brazil

Larissa Carvalho Trojan
Instituto Latino Americano de Ensino e Pesquisa Odontológico-ILAPEO, Curitiba 80710-150, Brazil
Biomechanics, Curitiba, Brazil

Rubens Moreno de Freitas
Ilapeo College, Curitiba, Brazil

Caroliene M. Meijndert
Department of Oral and Maxillofacial Surgery, University of Groningen, University Medical Center Groningen, Groningen, Netherlands

Gerry M. Raghoebar and Arjan Vissink
Department of Implant Dentistry, Dental School, University of Groningen, University Medical Center Groningen, Groningen, Netherlands

Henny J. A. Meijer
Department of Oral and Maxillofacial Surgery, University of Groningen, University Medical Center Groningen, Groningen, Netherlands
Department of Implant Dentistry, Dental School, University of Groningen, University Medical Center Groningen, Groningen, Netherlands

Salah Sakka, Ali Al Rafedah, Nasser Alqhtani and Adel Alenazi
Department of Oral and Maxillofacial Surgery and Diagnostic Sciences, Prince Sattam Bin Abdulaziz University, Al-Kharj, KSA, Saudi Arabia

Sušić Mato and Vuletić Marko
School of Dental Medicine, Department of Oral Surgery, Zagreb, Croatia

Smojver Igor and Katalinić Ivan
St. Catherine Specialty Hospital, Zagreb, Croatia

Stojić Luka
Private Dental Office, Zagreb, Croatia

Gerbl Draženа
Department of Anaesthesiology & Critical Care, University Hospital Centre Zagreb, Zagreb, Croatia

Anna Paula da Rosa Possebon and Ana Paula Pinto Martins
Graduate Program in Dentistry, School of Dentistry, Federal University of Pelotas, RS, Brazil

Alessandra Julie Schuster, Amália Machado Bielemann, Luciana de Rezende Pinto and Fernanda Faot
Department of Restorative Dentistry, School of Dentistry, Federal University of Pelotas, RS, Brazil

Samille Biasi Miranda
School of Dentistry, Federal University of Pelotas, RS, Brazil

Otacílio Luiz Chagas-Júnior
Department of Oral and Maxillofacial Surgery and Maxillofacial Prosthodontics, School of Dentistry, Federal University of Pelotas, RS, Brazil

Sergio Bortolini
CHIMOMO, Università di Modena e Reggio Emilia, Largo del Pozzo 71, 41125 Modena, Italy

Raul Ayuso-Montero
School of Dentistry, University of Barcelona, Oral Health and Masticatory System Group (Bellvitge Biomedical Research Institute) IDIBELL, University of Barcelona, University Campus of Bellvitge, L'Hospitalet de Llobregat, Barcelona, Spain

Bartolomeo Assenza and Felice Lorusso
Department of Medical, Oral and Biotechnological Sciences and CeSi-MeT, University of Chieti-Pescara, Via dei Vestini, 31, 66100 Chieti, Italy
Zirconia Implant Research Group (Z.I.R.G), International Academy of Ceramic Implantology, USA
Department of Oral Implantology, Dental Research Division, College Ingà, UNINGÁ, Cachoeiro de Itapemirim 29312, Brazil

Francesco Inchingolo
Department of Interdisciplinary Medicine, University of Bari "Aldo Moro", 70121 Bari, Italy

Filiberto Mastrangelo
Department of Clinical and Experimental Medicine, University of Foggia, Foggia, Italy

Antonio Scarano
Department of Medical, Oral and Biotechnological Sciences and CeSi-MeT, University of Chieti-Pescara, Via dei Vestini, 31, 66100 Chieti, Italy
Zirconia Implant Research Group (Z.I.R.G), International Academy of Ceramic Implantology, USA
Department of Oral Implantology, Dental Research Division, College Ingà, UNINGÁ, Cachoeiro de Itapemirim 29312, Brazil

M. AboulHosn, Z. Noujeim and N. Nader
Department of Oral & Maxillofacial Surgery, Faculty of Dental Medicine, Lebanese University, Beirut, Lebanon

A. Berberi
Professor and Head Department of Oral & Maxillofacial Surgery, Faculty of Dental Medicine, Lebanese University, Beirut, Lebanon

Motaz Osman
Department of Implantology, Khartoum Teaching Dental Hospital, Federal Ministry of Heath, Khartoum, Sudan

Abdelnasir G. Ahmad
Department of Oral and Maxillofacial Surgery, Faculty of Dentistry, International University of Africa, Khartoum, Sudan

Fadia Awadalkreem
Department of Oral Rehabilitation, Prosthodontic Division, Faculty of Dentistry, University of Khartoum, Sudan

Index

Printed in the USA
CPSIA information can be obtained
at www.ICGtesting.com
LVHW082107141123
763883LV00008B/585

9 798887 406053